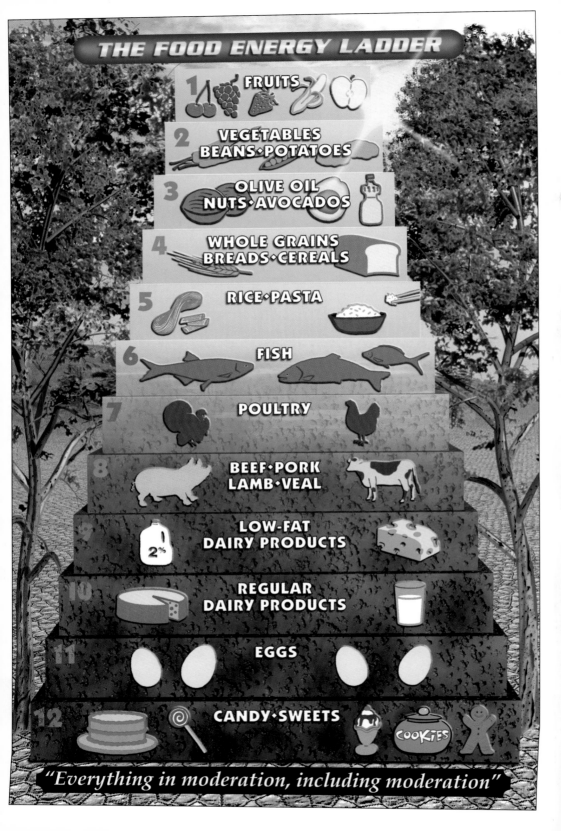

BALANCE YOUR BODY

BALANCE YOUR LIFE

BALANCE YOUR BODY

BALANCE YOUR LIFE

Total Health Rejuvenation

EDWARD A. TAUB, M.D.

KENSINGTON BOOKS
http://www.kensingtonbooks.com

The contents of this book are a reflection of the author's philosophy, beliefs, and clinical experience. The ideas, suggestions, and procedures contained in the book are not intended to be a substitute for consultation with your own physician.

KENSINGTON BOOKS are published by

Kensington Publishing Corp.
850 Third Avenue
New York, NY 10022

A co-publishing venture with
Health Ventures Partners
1200 Wilson Drive
West Chester, PA 19380

Library of Congress Card Catalog Number: 98-067106
ISBN 1-57566-503-4

First Revised Printing: November, 1999
10 9 8 7 6 5 4 3 2 1

Printed in the United States of America

Text design by Stanley S. Drate/Folio Graphics Co. Inc.

To David and Debbie Oliphant

L'Chaim, To Life!

ACKNOWLEDGMENTS

◆

David Oliphant, my friend and partner, first envisioned this book and then wove the vision into reality by encouraging me to believe that I could discover a new theory of nature. He nurtured and strengthened my work with an enormous personal effort that challenged me to new heights.

Debbie Oliphant, my friend and partner, contributed hard work, loving skills, unwavering patience, and artistic ingenuity to this book. Along the way, her courage and personal healing power provided inspiration to everyone in this project.

I'm grateful to Claire Oliphant and Alieta Kalman Fresenius for giving David and Debbie such keen intelligence and imagination.

Lora E. Taub, Ph.D., my daughter and editor, helped me to shape and inspire this book from conception to completion. Her devotion, skills, and sage guidance continue to define my career as an author; every page of this book lives up to her high ideals. Mostly, I hope that my work reflects her best hopes for me. *Namaste.*

Anneli Taub, my wife and cookbook writer, cares for me every day with friendship, unending patience, and wholesome food. How she manages to make green bean soup taste better than boeuf bourguignon is a tribute to my mother-in-law, too.

At Kensington Books, I owe a great debt of gratitude to Walter Zacharius, Steve Zacharius, Lynn Brown, Paul Dinas, Laura Shatzkin, Diane Wright, and Richard Ember, for their grasp, understanding, and belief in my work. My heartfelt thanks also go to Senior Editor Allan Graubard, who critically evaluated each of my ideas and applied his keen intelligence to bring this book to fruition.

I am deeply grateful to all friends and colleagues at QVC for making a Wellness Medical Doctor's dreams come true. Douglas Briggs, Darlene Daggett, Robert Ayd, Judy Grishaver, Jeanine Gendrachi, Jackie Mack, Kim Sheller, Scott Sentell, Kevin Else, Marty Rusnak, Lena Hoover, John Link, Robb Cadigan, Babette Burns, and Betty Broder helped me refocus my career into one continuing house call to over 65-million homes.

I want to express my sincere appreciation to Gale Bensussen, Scott Rexinger, Peter Cosgrove, Craig Angell and the rest of the team at Leiner Health Products.

Kathryn Koether contributed a long labor of love by typing the manuscript, providing sound grammatical advice, and keeping us all on deadline. Denise Lerner rose to an urgent task with energy and grace. Publicist Anita Halton, assisted me with dignity and skill. Michelle Di Vincenzo, a former student of the Culinary Institute of America, gave sensitive help with preparing, testing, and tasting recipes.

Justine Amadeo helped me to organize my thoughts and provided me with invaluable insight and editorial assistance for this revision. Artist Mark Hannon depicted the Food Energy Ladder beautifully. Marcus Laux N.D. was very kind to allow me to use his strength training drawings by artist Barbara Mindell. Clint Thompson, C.P.T. inspired the strength training aspect of this revision by keeping me motivated and helping my body feel better at 60 than at 50.

I am grateful to Doug Batezel, Bob Myers, Fred Stern and Julie Schneider of the Bergen Brunswig Company for their support.

I am especially thankful for my friends at Media Productions International, Inc. The trust and skills of Bob Marty, Bill Marty, Jim Scalem, JoAnn Young and Sven Nebelung are responsible for making this revision for the PBS Special into a reality.

Lanny Taub, M.D., served me with brotherly kindness and advice. Marc Taub, M.D., provided me with much food for thought, and the joy of my first grandchild, Lucas. My parents, Daniel and Roslyn, continuously demonstrated that, after all, love is really all there is.

CONTENTS

◆

Part Three

TRUTH IS ON THE MARCH AND NOTHING WILL STOP IT

Part Four

ENERGY NUTRITION AND THE CYCLE OF LIFE

Part Five

BUILDING A NEW PATH OF LEAST RESISTANCE 139

Part Six

FOOD IS ENERGY:
A New Mindset and Plan for Permanent Weight Loss and Balanced Energy Throughout the Cycle of Life . . . The Blueprint 171

Part Ten

NUTRITIONAL SUPPLEMENTS . . . BEYOND DEFICIENCY

Part Eleven

PREVENTIVE THEOLOGY

◆

FOREWORD

By Harvey Diamond

◆

My colleague and friend, Dr. Edward Taub, is a man fulfilling his life's purpose. He teaches patients how to assume responsibility for their personal health destiny, and shows physicians how to be gentler and more noble. Ever since he first glimpsed the paradigm of wellness, not illness, he has been spreading the word that health is primarily determined by personal responsibility, self-value, and reverence for life. At the same time, he has diagnosed the illness that is undermining Western medicine: *It is based almost entirely on repairing the human body rather than stimulating the will to be well.*

Fifteen years ago, Dr. Taub's powerful foreword for my book, *Fit For Life,* conferred upon it the scientific credibility that helped it become a success. I was grateful for his generous words designating the book a "giant step forward in extending life's span and life's quality." Amazingly, ever since writing that foreword, Dr. Taub has devotedly conveyed its nutritional principles to thousands of patients around the world. Now, on the basis of his extensive clinical experience, he has created *the next step forward in extending life's span and life's quality.*

Readers should cherish this work and take it seriously; Dr. Taub has written a practical guide to the link between nutrition and wellness. His message is essential: Food is nourishment for body, mind, and spirit.

Here is a book from a physician who sees the presence of God in all life, and defines wellness as the graceful dance of energy in balance. I can think of no words that more accurately describe Dr. Taub's contribution to wellness than those in which Albert Einstein described himself and his work: *"The ideals which have lighted me on my way and time and time again given me new courage to face life cheerfully, have been truth, goodness, and beauty."*

These ideals grace the principles that Dr. Taub shares with you in this book, the first modern scientific update of *Fit For Life*. When I was first asked to write this foreword, I unhesitatingly and enthusiastically agreed to do so. As we make our way through this life, on occasion we are fortunate enough to cross paths with others whose integrity and desire to improve the human experience is exceeded only by their love and genuine caring. Just such a man is Dr. Edward Taub, who exemplifies these high-minded ideals. I wholeheartedly support his healing and educational work, for I know his intent is for personal, community, and planetary transformation. I feel honored to have been asked to write this foreword.

—Harvey Diamond,
co-author, *Fit For Life*

INTRODUCTION

◆

What a wonderful opportunity to update my book to help you live life to the fullest! When I originally wrote this book, my intent was to help as many readers as possible by setting the record straight on some disturbing misinformation about nutrition. I created a scientifically sound plan for a healthy way to eat foods you love and still lose weight. But since this book was first published just one year ago, stress, obesity and degenerative diseases have soared to record levels in America. Now even people of other nations who are following our example are becoming as stressed, obese and ill as we are. The truth about good food and nutrition has been hidden from us until now, and we are almost helpless to fight back against the so-called experts who keep assuring us they know what's best. *This is why I have updated and revised this book. It is even more important now than ever before for you to read the pages that follow—to absorb it and live it.*

As a Wellness Medical Doctor, I have always sought to help my patients and readers stay healthy and live healthy, especially women and children—*because they are our future.* In order to do this, I have developed a psychotherapeutic treatment plan to help you *prevent* and *reverse* disease, as well as lose weight permanently through *"Total Health Rejuvenation."* This requires stimulating your own natural healing force, which is equivalent to the presence of God in every one of your trillions of cells. Medical science defines the "healing force" as "merely an array of polypeptide chemicals such as endorphins and enkephalins," so no wonder your healing force beguiles physicians who search in all the wrong places and ask the wrong questions! If you will allow me to be your Wellness Medical Doctor, I promise to help create a healthier understanding and environment in which your body, mind and soul can thrive. *Please . . . just trust me to touch your life in a positive manner.*

"Total Health Rejuvenation"—stimulating your healing force— begins deep inside you, at the level of your soul, and radiates outward. This is why my plan is based on "Integrative Medicine"— combining the best of modern science with traditional spirituality. I believe your health is mostly determined by your own personal responsibility, self-value and reverence for life. Therefore, I have now introduced the concept of "Preventive Theology." Basically, you will be asked to expand your words and beliefs into action by behaving ethically and being a loving person. "Preventive Theology" entails having faith, that if you take one step towards God, God will take a thousand steps towards you. You see, your natural healing force is like an eternal flame, perhaps neglected but still burning deeply within you. *Now you can rekindle your healing force from a tiny flicker to a brilliant flame . . . you can do it . . . you can live life to the fullest!*

I also promise you that just *reading* this book will change the way you look at food forever, and cause you to lose excess weight permanently, healthfully and naturally. In modern terminology, this phenomenon is known as *cognitive restructuring* and *conscious re-programming.* In other words, enough seeds will be planted in your mind so that one day, very soon, they will sprout. You may try to ignore what you are about to read in *Balance Your Body, Balance Your Life,* but you will always remember what you have read . . . *that's why it is so important to read on.*

The truth about good food and proper nutrition cannot be conveyed to you in mere words, because you have much too much mental baggage blocking the way and you are limited to looking at the world through rose-colored glasses placed before your eyes by the so-called nutrition experts. However, *just by reading this book,* you will begin to peel away the layers of misinformation about food that now befog your mind. Once you glimpse the truth, and then realize the full extent of the following truth, you will begin to live life to the fullest: Americans are being fed, fattened and sickened for profits; you and your loved ones, *especially women and children,* have simply become a commodity for the giant food industry, which controls our food supply as well as our minds. *Please . . . just observe the changes that will occur in you as you read on.*

I wish to bring the following news items to your attention. They were published in 1999, after the first edition of *Balance Your Body, Balance Your Life* was published.

▶ An article in the *Journal of the American Medical Association* announced that the long-term intake of *cereal fiber* decreased the risk of coronary heart disease among women by as much as 34 percent. This article provided further reason to replace refined, processed junk food with whole grain products, especially since the *already proven* benefits of fiber include preventing diverticulitis, hypertension, non-insulin dependent diabetes mellitus and cancer of the mouth, pharynx, larynx, esophagus and stomach.

▶ Yet despite the benefits of fiber—*especially cereal fiber*—an article in the *Los Angeles Times* announced that a major cereal company would probably drop its new line of healthy, grain-based, cholesterol-lowering foods by year's end because it had not achieved its "sales and distribution" goals. The products, which contained natural fibers, will be dropped because "the company stands to make a higher profit on new convenience foods and extensions of its breakfast snacks *(popular sugar-laden cereals),* rather than spend a lot of time and money trying to interest consumers in the healthier products."

▶ A 1999 article in *Pediatrics*—the professional journal of America's pediatricians—reported the stunning news that the results of a 1996 article about fruit juice in *Pediatrics* were false! The earlier article had concluded that "Excessive fruit juice intake was associated with short stature and obesity in pre-school children." However, while the results of the earlier false study were quickly sensationalized throughout the major news media, the *updated* 1999 report was virtually ignored! Unfortunately, for the last three years, America's pediatricians have not been recommending that preschool children drink much fresh fruit juice . . . *and even worse, the myth has spread to millions of parents and growing children.*

▶ Finally, the United States Department of Agriculture (USDA) announced the "Children's Food Pyramid," which actually *recommends* and features pictures of ice cream and hamburgers for kids! The National Food Processors Association, the voice of the $430 billion food processing industry, immediately sent out a press release: "We are pleased that the new 'Children's Food Pyramid' includes depictions of various processed foods. These graphics will be useful in helping children and their parents to understand that canned and frozen fruits and vegetables—as well as other processed foods—should be just as much a part of a healthful diet as fresh foods." Thankfully, the prestigious and non-profit "Center for Science In The Public Interest" headlined *its* press release this way: "The USDA's 'Children's Food Pyramid' reinforces kids' *worst* eating habits and may *increase* heart disease in the next generation. It shows once again that the USDA's mission to promote the meat and dairy industries is incompatible with its responsibility to promote good nutrition." *Wow! Wake up, Americans! Can you believe what is being recommended to our children—our future?*

Let's try a test so that you can prove to yourself what you already intuitively know. Go to your local market and buy some fresh oranges, fresh strawberries, fresh peaches and fresh tomatoes. Then buy some orange juice from concentrate, frozen strawberries, a can of peaches and a can of tomatoes. Now squeeze the oranges to make a glass of juice and place it next to a glass of juice from concentrate. Defrost the strawberries and put them next to the fresh ones. Finally, after pouring out the canned peaches and tomatoes, place them next to the freshly sliced produce. Close your eyes and do a taste test. *Which would you rather be eating or drinking?* I know this isn't exactly "rocket science," but it's time for you to stop believing all the so-called experts who insist that "freshness" doesn't matter as long as the same "scientifically measurable nutrients" are present . . . *Sure!*

It's also clearly time for the Food Energy Ladder (see Part Six) to replace the harmful and obsolete food pyramid myths. Foods that are among the top steps of the Food Energy Ladder are infused with energy and vitality transferred from the sun through photosynthesis. When you eat these foods, they transfer the sun's energy and vitality to you, igniting the healing force within you, which is the only natural and proper way to lose weight permanently. It's so very simple: *Foods at the top of the Food Energy Ladder are natural fat burners and foods at the bottom are natural fat accumulators!* Yet there are no forbidden foods and there is no sense of deprivation.

The Food Energy Ladder motto is "Everything in moderation, including moderation." *How about actually eating more and weighing less?*

For this updated and revised edition of *Balance Your Body, Balance Your Life*, I have rearranged the Food Energy Ladder based on further science and research (especially to help men and women in the second half of their natural human lifecycle (see Part Four). For instance, if you are approaching fifty years old, you will need to lessen your intake of pasta and white rice, and increase your daily intake of water. You see, *Balance Your Body, Balance Your Life* is all about learning to pinpoint where you are in your own personal human lifecycle in order to take appropriate steps for "Total Health Rejuvenation" and permanent weight loss. You will find that the Food Energy Ladder is truly a picture that is worth a thousand words . . . *and a concept that is user-friendly and easy to understand.*

Unfortunately, we have become the most overweight, hypertensive, atherosclerotic, diabetic, ulcer-ridden, cancer-, stroke- and coronary-prone people in the world. Fifty-five percent of Americans are overweight with dire consequences for health—*especially women and children.* The rate of obesity in children has doubled in the last 25 years so that we may soon be facing a major crisis in the incidence of type II Diabetes Mellitus. *In 1999, researchers at a major hospital reported a quadrupling of the disease among children and teenagers in the last few years!* Our minds have been programmed into actually expecting illness—especially diseases related to the way we eat. Media messages have led us to believe we have no choice but to accept illness and enjoy eating food that is lacking in energy and vitality. *But you do have a choice . . . and you don't have to be overweight!*

SOLUTIONS TO THE CRUEL DIET HOAX

A multibillion-dollar-a-year diet industry has grown into a cruel hoax that is threatening your health because yo-yo diets don't work *and they can harm you.* The biological makeup of men and women has not changed in thousands of years. So why are there thousands of diet books in the marketplace? Because diets don't work and we are always looking for a quick fix! The current fad diets based on

◆

eating high amounts of animal protein and avoiding fresh fruits are especially harmful. The way high protein diets work is by first causing the body to turn acidic, and then as a result, become sick. Sick bodies tend to lose weight—just as those that are afflicted with cancer. But people ought not to be tampering with their God-given metabolism in order to lose weight, especially with diets that discourage fruits—*God's food*.

The current fad diets based on eating according to your blood type are so completely ridiculous that there is little to say about them other than you might as well believe that the moon is made out of cheese! Also, reading *Balance Your Body, Balance Your Life* will be far more beneficial to you *(and a whole lot safer)* than any over-the-counter or prescription diet pills. *Please use your common sense. There is nothing new under the sun.* Food is energy that nature provides to sustain you in good health during your entire personal human lifecycle, from birth to death. So, if you are trying to lose weight, stop yo-yo dieting now! Trying to diet your excess weight off is like trying to bail water out of a rowboat without first plugging the leak. Now you have a choice—with the new Food Energy Ladder, you don't have to be overweight and you can still eat the foods you love!

All my proven clinical solutions for *"Total Health Rejuvenation"* are in this book because it's important to realize that losing excess weight is much more than just a cosmetic issue. Are you short of breath, suffering with high blood pressure, experiencing backaches or afflicted with adult-onset diabetes? *Losing weight will help you solve these problems.* Losing weight will also help you prevent, or even reverse: fibromyalgia, chronic fatigue syndrome, arthritis, varicose veins, gallbladder disease, colitis, irritable bowel syndrome, strokes, heart attacks and even cancer! By taking control of your own health destiny, you can lose weight permanently and naturally, and live longer and more lovingly. *This is not a diet book . . . it's about "Total Health Rejuvenation" . . . and I promise you that just reading this book will begin triggering your own natural healing force.*

Yes, there are no quick fixes and just a cursory reading will not cause a miracle to happen. But being overweight begins and persists in your mind, and I have written this book to instigate *change* in your mind. You will realize that food is your "energy, not your enemy." Just reading this book . . . *very carefully and very thoughtfully* . . . will cause you to lose weight permanently and naturally because it will help you to rediscover love for yourself, love for others, and love for God. This goal is crucial because being overweight means your body is ill. And in this time of incredible stress, I.L.L. has become largely equivalent to "*I* L*ack* L*ove*." Just reading this book empowers you to regain love . . . *the most powerful healer of all!*

You can lose as much as 10% of your excess body weight each year and keep it off until you approach your natural weight. Also, women will understand why they should weigh more than they imagine (weight standards are created by males with visions of beauty that are culturally driven by the widespread images of fashion models). I have also added a very simple strength training section to the book, especially to help men and women over fifty to strengthen and tone their bodies so that they can live life to the fullest.

I have expanded the scope of the book's journal writing section (Part Six), because again, more new research published in 1999 suggests that keeping a journal is far more therapeutic than even I was aware of. An article in the *Journal of the American Medical Association* showed that asthma and arthritis patients who wrote about their traumatic experiences and stress for just 15–20 minutes a day, for only three or four days, reduced their recurring symptoms of asthma and arthritis by as much as 47 percent. *Remarkably, the improvements lasted for up to four months.* An accompanying editorial praised the study and noted that if a similar outcome had been experienced with a new drug, it would be in widespread use within a short time. I surely agree, and that's why I have updated and revised the book into a psychotherapeutic and spiritual road map for just 28 days to get you going . . . *so that you can learn to live life to the fullest, forever!*

IT'S JUST FOR A DAY!

Finally, I have some more very good news that makes the book's 28-Day Plan for *Total Health Rejuvenation* and permanent weight loss even easier. Because your health is mostly determined by per-

◆

sonal responsibility, self-value and reverence for life, it's obvious that you are required to take at least one small step to prepare for the psychotherapeutic and spiritual benefits of the book. Your Personal Wellness Retreat (described in Part Five) provides you with the powerful *kick-start* necessary to trigger the internal process of *"Total Health Rejuvenation."* However, now further clinical research has allowed me to cut the time of your Personal Wellness Retreat in half. *It's just for a day!* It's a day for setting aside time for healthy food, fresh air, easy exercise, soft music, meditation, journal writing, resting and prayer. It's a day for catharsis (your Day), and for getting rid of old baggage to make room for a leaner, healthier, and more energetic you. It really sounds like a vacation, doesn't it? Please remember that you can take *"your Day"* as many times as you wish in the future—especially when life's challenges seem to be throwing you off balance and you need to get back on track. You're going to be absolutely amazed at how good you will feel when you start living life to the fullest and realize your full potential. That's just the beginning. *I know you can do it . . . please read on . . . and remember, I only have your health and well-being in my heart.*

TO-LIFE!

BALANCE YOUR BODY

◆

BALANCE YOUR LIFE

Part One

FAT IS NOT JUST A PHYSICAL PROBLEM

How to Change Your Inherited Beliefs and Emotions to Solve Your Weight Problems Forever

As Medicine has become more specialized, we have lost sight of the fact that love is the most powerful medicine of all. We forgot how a simple mother's kiss can help take away our hurt, and we also forgot how a concerned doctor's reassurance and guidance can help make us better. My patients have become healthier and lost weight permanently by following this 28 Day Plan for *"Total Health Rejuvenation."* It's based on TLC . . . *tender, loving care that keeps you well.*

Health is your most precious asset, but with all the confusing information about how to be well, and especially how to lose weight, how in the world do you know if you are even close to doing the right thing? This is why my plan for *Total Health Rejuvenation* consists of 28 daily doses of self-administered TLC! Just reading

I

this book will cause you to become a person of strength and conviction who recognizes the truth and power of your choices.

You probably know that the foods you eat affect your health, vitality, and well-being. However, it is also important to know that most of the deadly diseases that afflict Americans are influenced by food—heart disease, cancer, stroke, diabetes, chronic liver disease and atherosclerosis. Small changes in the way you eat today will help you and your family to live a healthier life in the future.

Small changes in diet, though, are not enough. What really matters are your attitudes toward food. Your thoughts, beliefs, and emotions determine which foods you choose to eat. That is why *you eat only as well as you think*. It is the reason why the path to permanent weight loss and healthy nutrition begins with what you think and how you feel about food. When it comes to beliefs about food and eating, we have been raised on a media diet of misinformation and myths. Simply put, some of our basic perceptions about food, learned as early as infancy, are unhealthy misconceptions.

Surprisingly, most of us take better care of our cars than our bodies. You surely can think of many other examples that are more applicable to you in your own life, such as your work, home, boat, garden, or even your pet. Think of one example with which you can identify and apply it to yourself as you read on. When you were born, your body, generally, was like a fine-tuned, upscale car. Just as a car requires proper care and maintenance, so does your body. If you care for your body, maintain its health, and, most of all, provide it with proper fuel, then, like a fine car, it will thrive for a long, long time. But, like an automobile, if you neglect your body, fail to maintain it, and fill it with inferior fuel, it will deteriorate into a junk heap.

Conventional Nutritional Wisdom: Separating Fact from Fiction

Now, I would like you to start giving your body the nutritional tune-up it is starving for by tuning up your attitudes and thoughts about food. Thoughts, after all, are the motor behind every action. Moreover, without a change in attitude, most people cannot make lasting changes in their diet. Your diet may change, but as long as your underlying attitudes about food remain unchanged, you will probably revert back to the eating habits from which you want to free yourself in the first place. Your thoughts are the driving force behind what you choose to eat. So, as you embark on this journey to nutritional well-being, you need to flush out the misperceptions about food that corrode and clog your mental motor. Remember: *what you eat is a response to how you think.*

Why have your thoughts about nutrition been steered in the wrong direction? Almost every month a new nutritional "theory" flashes across the television screen or splashes across the front page of newspapers. Most of these "theories" are fads, developed to market and sell some new diet product—a meal-replacement shake, a miracle herb, a cellulite-busting cream. The claims of some are so outrageous, they are almost laughable; but because we are hungry for better health and weight loss, we do pay attention to them. How can you reliably distinguish between the hype and the hope? *Balance Your Body, Balance Your Life* will teach you how by constantly reminding you of your own innate nutritional wisdom.

Why is there so much confusion? The often contradictory data on nutrition that reach us, sometimes daily, is one answer. It seems that recommendations from the halls of science are always changing: Once we were told to reduce starchy foods, now we are told to eat more starch; then we were advised that all oil is bad, only to find out later that olive oil is healthful. No wonder it's so hard for us to know exactly what we should or should not eat!

Because few of us have the time or inclination to personally track the scientific research, we rely on information filtered to us through the media. Unfortunately, most of this information just fuels the myths and misconceptions about food that dominate our culture. Most of us also acquire our nutritional information from television. But, for the most part, television is an unreliable guide to healthful eating. What can you really learn about food from TV? By today's standards, an "in-depth" television news story lasts two minutes. The average news story is closer to thirty seconds. And the result?

Diluted, oversimplified, often contradictory data that contributes more to our confusion than to our clarity.

Television is in the business of entertainment, which is supported by its advertisers. TV advertisers profit from creating new food fads. New diets and diet gurus are sensationalized on television, because sensationalism attracts audiences and boosts ratings, which in turn draws advertising dollars. The advertisers who pay billions of dollars to promote their products during the news shows, for example, are also among the leading contributors of nutritional misinformation! The food industry, fast-food chains, and diet/exercise industries generate much of the advertising revenues for the television stations.

As public awareness about nutrition and health has grown, so has our dissatisfaction with the information the media makes available to us. A recent poll revealed that people believe the most trustworthy source of nutritional information is our doctors. Yet for most people, correct nutritional advice/information has become harder and harder to come by—and it isn't free! Access to doctors is limited by HMOs and managed care. If you do get in to see your doctor and want to talk about nutrition, you may discover that he or she is among the 60 percent of physicians who are themselves overweight! In many cases, even your doctor's nutritional advice may be outdated and misleading.

Balance Your Body, Balance Your Life will help guide you out of this maze of myths that influences how you think and feel about food. Then and only then can you get back on the road to eating properly.

There is one myth in particular that you should toss from your mental baggage right away. It is the prevailing belief that, if you have been overweight for a long time, once you reach a certain age you will always be overweight. *No one is predestined to be overweight all of their life.* There is no "magic age" at which losing weight becomes improbable or impossible. And although it is commonly believed that it is easier to lose weight when you are young, recent findings suggest just the opposite. Older people trying to lose weight may actually have an advantage because they turn their past experiences with failed diets into knowledge that will help them lose weight now. In other words, people between the ages of thirty and fifty who have spent years trying to lose weight can draw from that experience in effective ways. They have greater knowledge and experience of what does *not* work, are less likely to be drawn to fads, and have great determination to succeed at last.

So, readers upwards of thirty who want to lose weight—a lot or a little—let go of the idea that you will always be overweight. *No one is born to be fat, and no one is predestined to be fat forever.* Heredity influences body shape and size, but fatness is not a biologically inherited trait. A genetic disposition toward obesity may exist, but *it is the culture of eating that you live in* that will turn a disposition into reality. The fact that you have overweight relatives does not mean that you are destined to live *your* life overweight. Even if you have dieted unsuccessfully in the past, now you can turn those experiences around—you can use them to help you.

There is a second powerful myth that discourages many people from trying to lose weight: the only way to lose weight is to eat less. Although many studies have shown that reductions in food intake will not lead to healthful, lasting weight loss, this myth refuses to die. *Eating less does not guarantee success.* You can, in fact, eat *more* of some foods and still lose weight. It is not the *amount* of food you eat, but the *kinds* of food you eat. Foods low in fat and high in fiber—like vegetables, fruits, and grains—contain fewer calories than high fat foods, so you can enjoy them in plentiful amounts without gaining weight.

As you get ready to make changes in your diet, let's get rid of the thought that *you must eat less to lose weight*. Erase the notion from your mental blackboard that deprivation is the key to dieting. Eating to *balance your body* and *balance your life* encourages you to eat less of some foods, but invites you to enjoy plenty of delicious, healthful, natural foods.

Because the lessons you have learned about food are so deeply ingrained, even going back to your childhood, they are difficult lessons to unlearn. Each one of us has in our memory a child who recalls the lessons of the four food groups. The knowledge you received as a young child was just the start of a long, misleading education about food and your relationship to food. Much of that education now hurts your health more than it helps. It is time to graduate from the school of thought you've been swimming in since childhood. It is time to change the way you think about food altogether, and forever.

Balance Your Body, Balance Your Life is not a diet. Diets, as everyone who has tried them knows, do not last. This plan doesn't begin by changing what you eat. The more important change occurs in what you know, how you think, and how you feel. *Short-term weight loss results from dietary changes, but lasting, successful weight loss results from changes in your attitudes, habits, emotions, and beliefs toward food.*

You must recognize the myths of nutrition that have contributed to the way you think about food, the majority of which took root in your mind when you were a child. As a child, you were taught to believe certain things about food; as an adult, these beliefs are reinforced on a daily basis by the food, diet, and exercise industries. These multibillion-dollar industries are so powerful and so profitable because they succeed at making people feel weak. Even though most people know from firsthand experience that diets generally do not live up to their promises, billions of dollars are spent on diet products every year. Stop giving these industries your attention and your money. They will not make you thinner, only poorer. And they may make you sick.

To change the way you think about food, you must look at the values, feelings, and thoughts about food that you were raised on, shaped by your family, your teachers, your environment, and your culture. Once you examine these long-standing misperceptions, you can redefine the value and meaning of food in your life and in the lives of your loved ones forever!

Time and time again, I've seen many patients who have struggled for years to lose weight make the final, necessary breakthrough and reach their weight loss goals. Why? Because they stopped wasting time and money on diet gimmicks. They gave up the belief that they had to suffer on starvation diets or use medicinal or surgical shortcuts. After years of unsuccessful, painful, and disappointing attempts to lose weight, they finally found the key to permanent weight loss. It wasn't in a bottle of pills, in a strict calorie-controlled diet, in meal-replacement shakes or in fanatical exercise programs. *The key was in changing their outlook on food.* Instead of feeling denied of foods that were keeping them unhealthy and overweight, they began to focus on foods that naturally promote health, energy, and weight loss.

One patient, a 45-year-old woman named Emily,* who had been on and off diets from the time she was nine, explained the change in perception that led to dramatic changes in her weight: "I used to spend all of my time worrying about the foods that I was *not allowed* to eat. Because they were fattening and forbidden, I wanted them even more, especially rich desserts. Either I was eating them all the time, or I was on a diet and *thinking* about eating them all the time. Finally, I realized that diets and denial were getting me nowhere, and what I really needed to do was get out of the dieter's mindset of deprivation." Like so many other patients with whom I have worked, when Emily redefined the meaning of food in her life, when she stopped obsessing about dead foods and just started eating live foods, she began to lose weight and has kept it off ever since.

The way you think and feel about food, and the value you give to it, is not natural. These attitudes, feelings, and meanings are as much created by the culture you grew up in as by food industries and their marketing allies. Once you understand the origins of your thoughts and emotions about food, however, you can resist the values that marketers especially attach to food. You can then create your own truly natural and healthy relationship with food.

Unfortunately, we have learned to think of food as the enemy, and to see the refrigerator as a battlefield. *But food is* not *the enemy; it is your energy!* Once you realize this, the refrigerator no longer has to be a battlefield; instead, it becomes a lively garden of health and vital energy.

Because we live in a diet-crazed culture, many of us are battling with our bodies. Diets are our weapons. But most of these weapons are just blunt knives. The only way to end the battle is to surrender to your body's nutritional needs and wisdom. Your body knows exactly what it needs for nourishment, and it knows exactly how to achieve and maintain your personal optimal weight. Your greatest resource in losing weight and keeping it off is not a weapon—it is

---

*I thank my patients who thoughtfully agreed to share their stories with my readers. To protect their privacy, the names used in this book are fictitious.

the wisdom hidden within you. Now you can learn to use that wisdom despite the roadblocks set in your path.

Since the early 1980s in particular, weight consciousness has turned into a cultural obsession fed by an over $50-billion-per-year diet and exercise industry. Our society is choked with images and messages about appearance and body weight. And with the average person encountering numerous commercial messages each day, they become very hard to resist. In fact, these images and messages create very powerful myths on their own about health, beauty, and strength. They found expectations and standards that, for the majority of us, are simply unattainable, unrealistic, and unhealthy.

Right now, as you are reading this, nearly 60 million Americans are dieting in some manner or another. At the same time, nearly another 60 million people think they need to be on a diet but are not. Diets have become a national obsession that afflicts men, women, and children. On average, males are twenty to thirty pounds heavier than their ideal weight; women are between fifteen and thirty pounds overweight; and even children carry, on average, ten to twenty percent more weight than they should. If so many of us are dieting, and spending billions of dollars to do it, ask yourself: Why are rates of obesity increasing rather than diminishing?

Along with such obesity, a shocking number of people suffer from eating disorders such as anorexia and bulimia—currently about 10 million—another indication of the ineffectiveness of the available methods of dieting. The way we think about food is hurting our health and sabotaging our efforts to lose weight and keep it off. Our nation's collective consciousness about nutrition is extremely out of balance.

How did food become the enemy? What turned the refrigerator into a place of fear rather than a Garden of Eden? Take a look at your children's attitudes or of those children close to you. Children observe and internalize their parents' eating habits—the good and the bad. From their parents, children first learn what foods to crave, to resist, to indulge in, and to avoid. Children initially learn from their parents how to *feel* and *think* about food. Children learn that some foods carry positive emotional associations while others carry just the opposite.

When I was growing up, I learned from my parents that different foods were charged with symbolic meanings. My father associated food with his success as the family provider. For him, success meant the finest beef on the table every night. My mother taught us another lesson. Even when she said she was famished, my mother never finished a meal. Only later did I realize that, for her, leaving food on her plate symbolized her restraint, her ability to resist temptation. The untouched potato and the half-eaten steak were signs that her willpower was stronger than the temptation to clean her plate.

If you don't have children, think about your experiences around the table when you were a child. What meanings did your parents attach to different kinds of food? What foods did they insist you eat? What foods were you forbidden to eat?

When I was a boy, my grandparents always encouraged my brother and I to eat second and third helpings when they were available. Do you remember this? *"Eat, eat, it's good for you."* We were never cautioned about overeating. In fact, a little bit of extra weight was considered ideal—a sign that we were well cared for. Today, the message is different.

What Children Learn About Nutrition May Be Bad for Their Health

Parents worry about their children's weight much more today than they used to. Some of this concern is justified, as the rate of overweight children has increased steadily over the past decades. Approximately one out of every four children between the ages of six and seven is overweight, which is *double* the number from just thirty years ago. This may seem surprising, but keep in mind that children's weights have followed the same patterns as their parents' weight. Statistics vary, but approximately one-half of all adults are overweight.

Parents should be proactive if their children are overweight, but worrying tends more to feed the problem than not. Often, when parents worry excessively about their children's weight, they perpetuate their children's overeating. Children learn from their parents to worry about food, to be obsessed about how much and what they eat, and this worry feeds their anxieties about food. This is where unhealthy attitudes toward food begin. What is the greatest risk for overweight children? It is that they will grow up with the mindset and emotions that will lead them to become overweight adults.

Like so many things, food often becomes a focus for children's rebellion against their parents. Unless your children are excessively overweight, *don't* worry about their weight. *Do* be a good role model and teach your children positive lessons about food. *Don't* put your children on diets or monitor how much they eat at every meal and in between. *Do* encourage physical activity. *Do* prepare healthful meals of wholesome natural foods that are low in animal fat and refined sugar, and have abundant amounts of fresh fruits available when your children want a snack. *Set the example.* This approach will not only help them shed the excess weight they carry around with them but, most importantly, it will help prevent them from becoming overweight adults. *Don't teach your children that food is the enemy. Teach them that food is a wonderful source of energy . . . food is energy!*

There is a big difference between modifying your overweight children's eating habits and putting them on a diet. Most diets are based on cutting calories. Children at any age can sense when something is being taken away from them. When food is withheld from children, they usually don't understand why. It can feel like they are being punished or deprived. Feelings of hurt then undermine the goal of the diet, because they usually lead an overweight person to seek food to heal the hurt of being punished. Remember, your children's peers may be eating the foods that you do not allow or want your children to eat.

Diets don't teach children about nutrition. Diets teach children about deprivation and craving. And every child hungers for what they feel deprived of having, whether it's a new bicycle, a trip to Disneyland, a new pair of tennis shoes, or junk food. Trying to teach children to resist the temptation of cookies, candy bars, hamburgers, pizza, and ice cream only makes those foods more appealing. What is off-limits in the fridge is, inevitably, the food your children most crave! You don't have to be a trained psychologist to understand why—it's common sense!

Growing children need proper nutrition, and diets just don't deliver. In fact, children whose parents or doctor have placed them on low-calorie or low-fat diets are known to experience many health problems: mental and physical fatigue, constipation, muscle loss, dehydration, dry skin, hair loss, and restless sleep. When kids feel this crummy, they are likely to eat poorly. For parents and children alike, the best approach is a comprehensive one, where food is perceived as part of an enjoyable, healthy, active lifestyle. Increase the amount of live, fresh foods in your diet, balance this with healthy amounts of physical activity, and set a vibrant, healthy example.

For adults and children, inactivity is often a greater culprit than eating too much. *Inactivity inspires obesity.* It has been reported that children spend more time in front of the television than they do in the classroom. And while in front of the television, they're often snacking on fat-laden or sugar-filled junk foods. Children who spend several hours watching television each day are much more likely to be overweight than those who do not. Children should take part in hobbies and interactive activities that stimulate their minds while building healthy bodies and self-esteem.

In 1996, the U.S. surgeon general reported that approximately half of the children and young adults between the ages of twelve and twenty-one do not engage in any vigorous activity. Inactivity contributes to unhealthy weight gain. The encouraging fact is that even a small increase in physical activity, coupled with proper eating habits, is the best way to healthy weight loss. Children's opportunities for physical activity are also shrinking: Nearly two-thirds of our schools have cut down on physical education classes, while after-school clubs are losing their appeal because they are too costly for schools and parents and, in some cases, even too competitive for children to enjoy them.

Computers are another issue. Today kids play more on computers than they play outdoors. And while children's computer skills and knowledge are important to develop, at the same time children are losing other skills that are just as crucial. The strength, endurance, and coordination that comes from physical activity builds children's self-confidence. Just like adults, when children feel good about themselves, they will naturally feel more motivated to take better care of themselves.

Overcoming obesity and promoting health should also be a *family affair*. Both adults and children need more physical activity than they currently get. When the whole family engages in playful physical activities—hiking, swimming, biking, or walking, to name just a few—everyone benefits. As a parent, you will also reap the benefits of physical activity for your own health—a great double benefit! You will set for your children a positive example to ensure their good health and well-being. Remember, your children will carry these lessons with them wherever they go and for the rest of their lives.

How can it be that in a culture so obsessed with dieting, one out of every four children is overweight? How can parents raise healthy, nutritionally smart children in a culture so consumed with dieting? You *can* grow healthy children in a diet-crazed culture. As I've said before, the positive examples you set are vital to your children now and as they grow up. Parents can make healthful eating and physical activities fun for their children. You can guide them on a path to nutritional awareness from the get-go. Once they are firmly on that path, they will not succumb to false promises. They will not let the diet culture's mindset about food become their own. You will build up their defenses against false premises and promises through example and education.

Involve your children in the learning process while you are learning new things about nutrition and health. Make it fun and exciting! The patterns of eating that children develop are based on their observations of how and what you eat. It's never too early to turn your children on to natural eating. Let them accompany you when you shop for food. If you can, spend some time in the produce area and show them the different fruits and vegetables. Make going to the supermarket a fun learning adventure!

A Saturday trip to a local farmer's market introduces kids not only to a dazzling display of the freshest foods, but it gives them a chance to meet the people who grow these foods with care and love.

The farmers usually will invite you to taste their delicious produce, which is a great way to introduce children to new varieties of fruits and vegetables. Make sure, however, that whatever you or your kids eat is thoroughly washed. Let kids taste for themselves the enormous difference between the flavor of a canned peach and that of a perfectly ripened peach picked fresh from the tree that morning. Explain the difference to them, and point out the additives in the ingredients section of the label on the can. Also point out that one peach is fresh and full of energy while the other is old, canned, and chemically preserved!

Establishing new eating habits can be fun for you and your family, especially when everyone is involved. The entire family can experience together how tasty healthful eating is. Remember, this is *not* about dieting. The changes you are making are for a lifetime of better health and ideal weight for you and your loved ones. Developing healthy eating habits for yourself and your children (or the children you care for) is important. It is a beginning, a beginning that, when taken collectively, can work against what I call our *nutritional crisis*.

This crisis can be overwhelming, especially for young girls. Simply, too many young girls succumb to obsessive dieting and worrying about their weight, even as early as age six. I call this the *sexy fashion doll complex*. Judith, a six-year-old girl, came for an office visit once, carrying with her a daintily dressed doll. As I spoke with her mother and examined the child, Judith chatted away with her doll. She was infatuated with the doll, petting her hair, praising her beauty, admiring her body. I couldn't help asking Judith why she liked the doll so much. She told me with her bright, innocent eyes, "Because she's skinny and beautiful, and I want to be just like her."

Now, it's just a doll, after all, so what's the big deal? I could see the power that the doll had over Judith. I also saw how a doll whose own body did not possess natural human proportions was shaping Judith's body image. Still, the doll enticed Judith, as it entices most young girls, teaching them to admire a physical form both unhealthy and unrealistic. From a very early age, young girls can develop a distorted image of their bodies, including an unreasonable weight for which to strive.

By the age of ten, most girls have already begun a career of dieting. A recent study of fourth-grade girls found that almost 90 percent of the girls were already on a diet. By high school, the numbers soar even higher. By the time young women reach college, this obsession with weight has often escalated to grievous levels. One out of every four young women is bulimic or anorexic.

You can keep your children from falling into the trap of obsessive dieting by helping them, at an early age, to increase their knowledge and change their mindset about food. If children develop healthy attitudes about food early in life, they will have a strong foundation for nutritional health throughout the rest of their life.

I cared for thousands of children in my pediatrics practice and observed that, except for those with metabolic disorders, the children who were overweight had parents who were also overweight. Research is inconclusive on how much obesity is genetically inherited. But while we're unsure about which parents pass on fat genes to their children, we have no doubt that children inherit their parent's attitudes, habits, and beliefs about food.

Low self-esteem and body hatred foster poor eating choices. With eating disorders, the food choices fueled by these self-deprecating thoughts can be disastrous. Why do children and adults fall into traps of obsession and body hatred? How do we become ensnared in dangerous webs of weight obsession? In addition to poor eating habits, many of us—especially females—have poor images of ourselves and our bodies. It's important to keep in mind that *good nutrition begins with body image*. Remember also that *you eat only as well as you think*. It's not just how you think about food, but how you think about *yourself* that influences what you eat.

Each of us has something we would like to change about our body—we crave longer legs, smaller feet, narrower hips. Many of us tend to take this desire to the extreme and develop distorted body images, which can drive poor eating habits. So take a moment to think about the questions in the following chart. Assessing your body image is just as important as assessing your body fat, cholesterol level, and blood pressure. Your thoughts and emotions about your body are the very thoughts that compel you to eat foods that raise your body fat, cholesterol level, and blood pressure. So, review each question below, as if you were having an honest, heart-to-heart talk with yourself.

ASSESSING YOUR BODY IMAGE

▶ When you look in the mirror, are you generally happy with what you see?

▶ Do you avoid looking in full-length mirrors?

▶ Looking in the mirror, do you focus on things you'd like to change?

▶ Is there a part of your body that you dislike?

▶ What part of your body do you like best?

▶ How do you think others see you?

▶ What would you like to change about your body?

▶ Can you look in the mirror and smile?

It's okay to want to change things about your body, okay to long for leaner legs, a flatter tummy, a trimmer waist. But too many of us let these longings spin into obsessions. A recent poll by a leading magazine found that among four thousand readers, 56 percent of women and 43 percent of men were unhappy with their overall appearance. Two-thirds of the women and over half of the men were specifically unhappy about their weight. Females between the ages of thirteen and nineteen felt the worst about their weight and appearance.

Even people who are not overweight often think they are in other people's eyes. In fact, thin girls often have the lowest self-esteem and most distorted body image. Sometimes a negative body image drives females to diet incessantly and to such extremes that anorexia or bulimia set in. Other men and women let a poor body image keep them from caring for their bodies by overeating. Becoming sedentary, overeating, and engaging in other self-destructive behaviors are frequent among people with severely negative body images.

If your body image gets in the way of your health and happiness, if it causes you to make poor food choices, then now is the time to take a small step toward improving your self-image. The information in *Balance Your Body, Balance Your Life* will help you do that. It begins with eating more fruits, vegetables, and grains, fresh foods for vivacity and vitality—and which will help generate more positive changes in your behavior and habits.

Aim for self-improvement, but don't let your body become an obsession. Accept who you are and how you are; be realistic about how you want to be. Go for it . . . you can do it! Fixating on your body image will likely fuel unhealthy eating habits, which in turn will reinforce your negative body image. When it comes to body image and food, it is easy to get trapped in an unhealthy cycle, where a negative body image fosters poor food choices that make you feel worse about your body.

It is easy to get off the deceptive merry-go-round. Eating wisely and naturally will generate a more positive body image, which will reinforce your new, healthy eating habits. The way you think and feel about your body will inspire you to eat healthier, and eating healthier will inspire positive thoughts and feelings about your body, building confidence and self-esteem.

Children develop their own body image mostly through the overt and covert values their parents give to them. How you feel about your body reflects outwards, and your children see it. A girl whose mother constantly diets and calls herself fat may very well learn to feel the same way about herself. Unless she learns otherwise, she may grow up to dislike her own body as well.

Food and emotions go hand in hand. In a phrase, food is emotional. Children, of course, learn from their parents what emotions to feel about food. Children can learn positive, healthy food emotions just as easily as they can learn the opposite. If children learn to criticize their bodies, they will develop a love-hate relationship with food. Food will become their enemy. And these feelings and emotions will grow deeper as children grow older.

When I was in college and medical school, I spent my summers as a camp counselor in upstate New York. I remember one summer in particular, when I was in charge of a cabin of eleven-year-old boys. From the very first day of the summer, Joshua isolated himself from the rest of the group. He was a chubby boy—not obese,

but very self-conscious about his body. He never wanted to participate in water activities because he was embarrassed to wear a bathing suit. When the other boys canoed or played on rafts, he would
sit under a tree, eating candy bars from CARE packages sent from
his mother back home. For Joshua, food was his comfort and companion, but it was also his enemy.

The more Joshua ate, the worse he felt about himself, and the
more he withdrew from social activities with fellow campers.
Ashamed of his belly, Joshua ate candy bars to feel better. Ultimately, it made him feel worse. As he grew more self-conscious
about his weight, he felt lonelier and lonelier sitting on the sidelines, as he did, during camp activities. His mother reinforced this
cycle by sending him weekly packages stuffed with sweets. Parents,
try always to remember: Take care of yourself and set the example!

The Myths of Infant Nutrition

As a family doctor and pediatrician for more than three
decades, I've seen how parents' nutritional mindset and body image
affects even young infants. It is what I call the *tube syndrome:* a
condition among infants whose parents begin to perceive them as
tubes that begin at the mouth and end at the anus. These parents
worry excessively about what goes into the child at one end, and
then worry excessively about what comes out of the child at the
other end.

I discovered the infant tube syndrome after noting skyrocketing
sales of prescription baby medicines. These baby medicines contain atropine, belladonna, hyoscyamine, phenobarbital, and alcohol, and are most commonly prescribed to treat gastrointestinal
problems and colic in infants. In my own practice, it seemed that
most of the gassy infants had mothers or fathers—often both par-

ents—who were insecure about parenting, stressed about their new responsibilities, and generally lacking in parenting skills.

These parents were caught in a maze of fear and worry over any sign of discomfort in their infant. To cope, they did what many people do; they turned to food for comfort. They began to feed their babies more and more, and with different kinds of food. They began to fret over what and how much food went into their baby, agonizing over the amount, consistency, flavor, smell, and temperature, as well as over the frequency and timing of feedings. When the feeding was over, they worried about the contents of their baby's diaper. And at that end, there was reason to worry. So many of the new foods introduced to the baby's system generally caused changes in stools: colic, constipation and diarrhea were common.

Parents who worry too much about their infant's diet and diaper content are not bad parents. They are like many people who associate food with love. When their baby was feeling bad, they showered him or her with love in the form of food. The best food, in fact, is served with love, but not in this way, and certainly not with worry, anxiety, insecurity, and fear. As adults, we characteristically turn to food for comfort when we are bored or need love. A pint of ice cream or slice of chocolate cake will do fine, the so-called "comfort foods" that soothe us when we are down. "Eat a little something and you'll feel better." How many of us learned this before we could even walk?

Moms and dads, worry less about what goes in and what comes out of your babies! He or she is not a tube, beginning at one end and ending at another. When you see your infant as a lively, thriving human being, love and nurturing will express themselves naturally, not through excessive feeding. This is the love and nurturing babies truly want. You see, in times of distress, babies swallow air, which causes colic and elicits loving attention from parents. Give your baby all the genuine love and attention he or she hungers for. You will all feel more comfortable and more at ease, and food will not be a problem.

Soon after birth, emotions about food and eating subtly register in a newborn's mind. The first taste of mother's milk establishes eating as one of life's most delightful pleasures. Infants eat for nutrition and nourishment, but also for comfort and pleasure. This emotion is carried with you throughout your lifetime, but as you grow, you can choose the wrong foods for comfort and pleasure. Instead of foods with the natural vitality and energy your body knew from mother's milk, you are guided by the demands of your taste buds.

Your eating experiences as an infant establish an emotional framework toward food that stays with you for the rest of your life. In those first months of life, food and eating can evoke joy, comfort, and nurturance. Or, like the tube syndrome babies I just described, meals can be stressful, even traumatic events. Imprinted in infants' memories, both experiences will influence the way they feel and think about food as they grow up.

Long before a newborn arrives in the world, the mother already thinks about how to nurture her baby. Contributing more to this anxiety than is healthy is the baby food industry. Who thrives most from creating and sustaining the impression that formula from a can or bottle has more nutrients than milk from a mother's breast, and that mashed, processed, refined food from a jar is nutritionally superior to food provided by Mother Nature?

Nothing in a can, bottle, or jar can match the nutritional power and nurturing force of breast milk—nothing. Science may indicate otherwise, but the value of mother's milk to nurture and nourish a baby cannot be seen under a microscope or measured in a test tube. Breast milk is all the baby needs. It is the natural source of infant nutrition and nourishment. If, however, you physically cannot breastfeed, for whatever reason, then an appropriate baby formula is quite acceptable.

The Myths of the Four Food Groups

It may be hard for you to digest the fact that our basic, earliest learned beliefs about food contribute to the weight and health problems we suffer. The good news is that you can change these beliefs and, with a little effort, revolutionize the way you think about food.

In school, one of the first things children learn about food is the story of the **four food groups:**

- meat, fish, and poultry
- grains
- dairy
- fruits and vegetables

On its own, of course, this division is quite benign. But as interpreted for us in 1956 by the U.S. Department of Agriculture (USDA), the four-food-group philosophy emphasized heavy meat and dairy intake. These foods, once the image of optimal nutrition, now embody all of our worst eating habits. Our belief in the need for daily doses of meat and dairy in our diets is literally making us sick.

Keep in mind that the four food groups were also promoted vigorously by the National Dairy Council. We now can understand that the four-food-group campaign was more a strategy to bolster the public's view of the dairy and meat industries than a public health message. As children learned to think of milk, eggs, and meat as pillars of good health at every meal, such eating practices, promoted as they were across elementary schools throughout the United States, were, in fact, advertisements that we taxpayers paid for then with money and now with poor diet. The result is clear: Americans—and American children, in particular—have become the most overfed, undernourished, and overweight people in the world!

Because of the eating habits instilled by the four food groups, Americans eat too many foods that diminish and not enough foods that boost health. Adhering to the four-food-group philosophy, Americans consume excessive amounts of:

- fat
- protein
- salt
- sugar
- calories
- red meat
- dairy products

Because Americans consume so much of these favorites from the four food groups, they eat too little of the foods that promote balanced health and energy, including:

- fruit
- vegetables

- fiber
- grains

For many children now, the four food groups seem to be candy, soda, potato chips, and cookies! A National Cancer Institute study discovered that only one in five children (just 20 percent) eats the recommended daily five or more servings of fruits and vegetables. What's more astonishing is that the leading source of vegetables for children and adolescents is deep-fried, fat-soaked french fries!

Now, you may be asking yourself, "Didn't the USDA recently launch a new food groups campaign, based on a pyramid emphasizing vegetables, fruits, and grains?" Absolutely. In 1991, under pressure to respond to the "New Four Food Groups" guidelines issued by the Physicians Committee for Responsible Medicine, the USDA launched a new campaign based on the Food Pyramid. Although the revised recommendations do emphasize eating more vegetables, fruits, and grains than the original four food groups, the USDA still advocates two or three servings of meat and two or three servings of dairy products daily!

Let's look more closely at the myths of nutrition underlying the four-food-group philosophy, and still influencing the new food pyramid. These myths take us straight to the heart of many health and weight problems suffered by Americans.

Because of the amount of saturated fat they contain, whole milk and cheese are two of the worst foods to drink and eat. (Joining them among the worst foods kids frequently eat is bologna.) Yet these foods are still promoted as staples of children's diets. The excessive amounts of dairy that children eat contribute greatly to the soaring numbers of cases of gastrointestinal illness, allergies, bacterial and viral infections, sore throats, and congestion seen by pediatricians every year.

At the same time, public awareness about the health hazards of consuming too many dairy foods is increasing. The dairy industry has responded with two recent ad campaigns that target adults more than children. The "milk" ads you see on street billboards and TV commercials, featuring celebrities wearing milk mustaches, are designed to restore adults' faith in milk. Here, drinking milk is good for your children and you, not to mention your whole family's image. These ads also acknowledge that concerns about reducing fat in our diets have lowered milk consumption. Does the dairy industry need, once more, to *milk* our nutrition?

Now these ads don't promote the health benefits of milk (for adults, there are actually very few that can't be more heathfully received from other sources). Rather, they project an image of happiness, hipness, beauty, and strength that has *absolutely nothing* to do with the product itself. The milk-mustache campaign, featuring sports heroes, models, and actors, plays on the popularity of the celebrity holding the empty glass. Drinking milk may not make you healthy, but the ads seem to promise that it can make you popular and cool.

The truth behind the promises promoted by celebrity endorsements is that *dairy products are the leading source of saturated fat in our diet*, with red meat a close second. Diets abundant in dairy products are high in fat, and are linked with certain types of cancer, especially of the colon and prostate. But the ads don't mention that.

From my more than three decades of medical experience, I do not believe that cow's milk is good for humans. It is good for baby cows. Only humans believe they should drink the milk of another species. Even adult cows don't drink cow's milk. And despite the dogma from the dairy board, children will develop and grow just fine without four servings of milk a day. Kids can get enough calcium for growth from other sources.

And women, who are now scared into drinking milk to prevent osteoporosis, should know that behind the milk myth is the fact that you can still get sufficient amounts of calcium from nondairy, plant-based sources. Women don't get osteoporosis because they don't drink enough milk. Osteoporosis develops as a result of calcium-robbing eating and lifestyle habits, *including over consumption of dairy products!* It's true: The very substance touted as essential to prevent osteoporosis can contribute to its onset when consumed excessively. The best sources of calcium don't come from dairy, but from green leafy vegetables, peas, beans, nuts, broccoli, and cauliflower.

Like the myth about milk, the national belief that you need meat to be healthy underlies some of the worst health and weight problems we suffer. Everybody needs protein, especially growing children. But, as a general rule, *our problem is not that we consume too little protein; we consume too much protein!* Few people have cause to worry that they are not getting enough protein in their diet. Most of us get much more than we require.

In the United States especially, the majority of protein in diets comes from animal sources. No other country in the world depends on animal protein as much as Americans do. It is a long-standing myth that you need meat for the protein that makes you healthy. A daily variety of plant foods can provide your body with an adequate supply of high-quality protein, as well as the iron and vitamin B_{12} that red meat supplies.

Recently, researchers at the National Academy of Science's Institute of Medicine announced that "there are no known benefits and possibly *some* risks in eating diets with a high meat content." What an understatement! There are numerous very well-known risks associated with a meat-laden diet.

For the good of your health, as well as that of your family, lower the amount of meat in your diet, especially red meat. Despite the National Academy of Science's hedging, evidence shows that meat consumption heightens the risks of developing a variety of diseases. At Harvard Medical School, researchers conducted a study of approximately forty-five thousand male health professionals and found that the men who ate red meat as a main dish five or more times a week had four times the risk of colon cancer compared to the men who ate red meat less than once a month. Men who regularly consume large amounts of red meat also double their chances of getting prostate cancer.

The good news is that simply cutting down on red meat in your diet will have tremendous health benefits. There are endless and delicious healthful alternatives to bring to the table, which you will discover as you read on. Medical research has shown that people whose diets contain little or no meat have notably lower rates of heart disease, hypertension, obesity, lung cancer, coronary artery disease, diabetes, and gallstones. Studies also have shown that a virtually meat-free diet lowers cholesterol significantly and, when combined with exercise and stress reduction, can actually reverse coronary artery damage.

It is not only the high rates of saturated fats in meat that contribute to health problems. Even *lean* red meat increases the risk of colon cancer. "Lean" labels on meat in the supermarket are misleading as well. For example, for foods to meet the USDA's "lean" requirements, they must not contain more than 10 percent fat by weight. The USDA allows the "lean" label on ground beef, however, that is up to 22.5 percent fat. The labels get even more confusing. The USDA allows claims like "85 percent lean" only on foods that are "low fat" (no more than three fat grams per serving). But the same regulations do not apply to ground beef. At some stores, you can find ground round labeled "85 percent lean" even though you learn that, upon closer inspection, one serving contains as much as fourteen fat grams. Ground beef is one of the fattiest meats available, yet it isn't held to the same "lean" standards as other kinds of meat. Ground beef labels are not even required to list "nutritional facts," which are now required on other foods.

If you want to improve your health, lower and stabilize your weight, and feel alive with energy and radiant vitality, then incorporate more and more vegetables and fruits into your diet. The healthiest diet you can eat is one based primarily on plant foods—fresh vegetables, fruits, beans, and grains—as opposed to animal muscles and organs. The evidence is so convincing that the chair of the nutrition department at the Harvard School of Public Health attests that "it's no longer debatable" that "largely vegetarian diets are as healthy as you can get."

Note the term "largely vegetarian." The health benefits are not only for those who eliminate meat entirely from their diets, but are enjoyed by people who just *reduce* their meat intake. Adopting the balance your body, balance your life eating habits will not require that you never eat meat, fish, poultry, or dairy products again. Simply eat less of the unhealthy animal foods and more of the fresh plant foods. It's really that simple!

There are many compelling reasons to eat less meat and more fruits, vegetables, and grains. I have already emphasized how eating foods containing less refined sugar and animal fat will help you lose weight and keep it off. But consider these other factors which favor a diet abundant in plant foods:

- Fruits and vegetables have protective properties against gastrointestinal cancers and even smoking-related cancers, including cancers of the stomach, mouth, larynx, colon, lung, esophagus, and bladder.

- People who eat a largely vegetarian diet have lower incidents of cardiovascular disease, high blood pressure, and noninsulin-dependent diabetes compared to meat-eaters.
- A largely vegetarian diet reduces the risk of osteoporosis, kidney stones, and gallstones.
- Women who eat less red meat have less breast cancer. Men who eat less red meat have less prostate cancer.

Limiting meat intake reduces amounts of saturated fats and cholesterol, but plant foods themselves have properties that protect the heart in other ways:

- The "sticky" soluble fiber in plants such as beans, peas, oats, and barley helps to lower blood cholesterol.
- Fruits and vegetables are excellent sources of folic acid, a B vitamin that can reduce the risk of heart disease.
- The antioxidants in fruits and vegetables can help protect the heart from cholesterol damage.
- Eating more fresh fruits and vegetables and less animal flesh will help protect you and your loved ones from food-borne illnesses. Fresh fruits and vegetables are safer than animal foods. The most common sources of food-borne illnesses are meat, seafood, and poultry. *E.coli* bacteria and salmonella occur in these foods much more frequently than they do in raw fruits and vegetables. In addition, emphasizing fruits and vegetables in your diet is better for the environment. Diets high in animal foods also take a tremendous toll on the environment, including three factors:
  - Stockyards and chicken factories cause catastrophic pollution of our water supplies with their waste, which is several hundred times more concentrated than raw domestic sewage.
  - Raising beef cattle depletes the water supply. It takes almost four hundred gallons of water to produce a pound of beef for consumption.
  - Producing and transporting livestock consumes about ten times more energy than growing and distributing vegetables.

From every angle, the nutritional scales tilt strongly in favor of a largely vegetarian diet. You don't have to give up all animal foods to reap the health benefits. Often, a strictly vegetarian diet is not reasonable, depending on geographic location and local food supplies. Improving your health and weight is as simple as shifting the balance of your eating in the direction of more plant foods and away from fatty animal foods. You will then be steering clear of perhaps the biggest roadblock obscuring your path to a healthy diet and permanent weight loss.

Now let's look at our nutritional evolution. There is very good evidence to suggest that man is not, as is commonly believed, a carnivore by nature. Archaeological studies indicate that the diet of our earliest ancestors was based primarily on plant foods. As hunter-gatherers, our ancestors passed most of their days searching the landscape for plants and only occasionally killed an animal for food. Early man, therefore, ate a very low-fat diet. Although we've evolved in many ways from our early ancestors, when it comes to nutrition, humans have been digressing for centuries!

The good news is that there are hopeful signs that this process of nutritional digression is coming to a halt. As more people move toward a low-fat diet, filled with vegetables, fruits, and grains, we are moving closer to the diet on which our ancestors survived and thrived.

Obviously, we are very different creatures than our ancestors, living in radically different environments, filled with creature comforts our ancestors never knew. When it comes to obtaining food as well, no longer are we hunter-gatherers. Our ancestors spent the majority of their time searching for adequate food; we don't need to. In 1800, 95 percent of Americans ate food fresh from their own or a local farm, or from the sea; today, however, 95 percent of all Americans eat food produced at a distance, then processed, preserved, and mass distributed to supermarket chains across the country.

As we navigate the aisles of the supermarket, we encounter an almost overwhelming range of foods from which to choose. The health claims that their bright packages and slick wrappings project are equally overwhelming. Learning how to sift through this jungle of offerings to find the foods that are best for us and our family does not come by instinct, however. For our ancestors, eating was a simple pleasure. Now, simply by taking a trip to the supermarket we enter a bit of a battleground, as packaging, displays, and brand names fight for our attention and the dollars in our wallets!

Your body naturally craves nourishment and nutrients. *Balance Your Body, Balance Your Life* will help you reawaken your body's wisdom. You can restore the natural cravings suppressed by decades of poor eating habits and the nutritional misinformation that promoted them. Your body has an inherent wisdom that is largely at odds with our food culture. But now is the time to turn the odds back in favor of your health and the health of your loved ones.

Our natural appetite for foods has been profoundly altered by a century of mass food production for mass consumption, by processing, refining, preserving, and packaging. If there are really only four food groups to which you need to adhere for good health, why in the world are there so many new kinds of foods appearing on the shelves of supermarkets every year?

It is the lifeblood of the food industry—the processors, marketers, advertisers, distributors, and retailers—to constantly create new tastes. Combined, they spend billions of dollars to sell us new foods, new flavors, and new categories of foods. In 1994, more than twenty thousand new food products made their appearance on grocery store shelves. Many of the products are not new at all, just dressed up in fancy new packaging. Examine the fine print on the nutritional label—the contents on the inside haven't changed; only the wrapping on the outside is different.

Is this progress? I don't think so. The food choices we are given are really not choices at all. In certain categories, all of the processed foods that line supermarket shelves taste exactly the same. They all have the same artificial flavors, textures, and qualities. Perhaps they taste the same because they have so many chemicals in common.

These foods take you further and further off the road to nutritional health and well-being. The same can be said of foods promoted for your convenience, foods engineered to save you time cooking and eating. These foods may or may not save you a few nickels and a few minutes, but convenience comes with hidden health costs. What these foods save you in preparation time is lost in both short- and long-term health benefits.

Food should make eating a simple pleasure for you to enjoy, not a time-saving convenience. Most people are willing to spend a few extra dollars for high-grade gasoline. Why cut corners when it comes to how you fuel your body? Eating healthy, the natural way, saves you more than time and money—it protects you from illness and disease, it inspires health and happiness, and it makes you feel more energetic and alive. Remember, *food is your energy!*

The wisdom of your body has been overshadowed by your senses, seduced by unhealthy foods. Supermarkets are designed, and the food on their shelves is displayed, to seduce your senses. Bright colors on packaging, attention-grabbing labels, and fancy wrappings capture your interest and tantalize your taste buds. Like everything else in our consumer culture, food has been turned into a fashion, with food styles changing as rapidly as clothing styles.

If you really pay attention to the refined and processed foods, if you eat them with awareness, you will find that they aren't so tasty after all. When the initial rush of fat, salt, and sugar on your taste buds subsides, you will be amazed to find that highly processed foods actually lack flavor. In the process of refining and processing, the natural flavors—the flavors from nutrients your body truly craves—have been stripped away.

Imagine making a salad from canned lettuce! The idea sounds ridiculous. You want your salad to be fresh and crisp, even freshly picked from the garden. Nobody likes wilted lettuce. Wilted lettuce is flavorless, lifeless, and unappetizing. Canned and processed foods are often *worse* than wilted lettuce. Processing, refining, and canning have reduced, even killed the natural energy of these foods. While the label on canned fruit salad, for instance, lists the nutrients it contains, read on—they aren't natural, they're added. Why would the food manufacturer need to *add* nutrients to naturally nutrient-rich fruits? It's because the manufacturing process destroys those nutrients, and then must replace them. But there is no substitute for nature's nutrients. A fresh fruit or vegetable salad satisfies and nourishes your body's natural cravings. You should expect the same from all of the foods you eat.

Processed, canned, dehydrated, and bottled foods have a uniform blandness. It's not really the flavor of the food that seduces your senses and tempts your taste buds. More seductive and appealing than the food is the image attached to it. Food advertisements and packaging work hard to create positive images that link foods to a sensual and beautiful lifestyle. But there is an enormous gap between the image of these foods and the reality of the life they actually help to create.

A romance brews between two thirty something professionals flirting over a cup of freeze-dried coffee. A grandfather and his grandson share touching smiles over a table at a fast-food restaurant and a box of chicken nuggets. A family comes together at breakfast to share a glass of "fresh" orange juice from concentrate, with the sun rising gloriously over the meadow in the background. These are all typical images used to sell processed foods. But how can something claim to be fresh after it has been boiled, dehydrated, crystallized, chemically preserved, and concentrated in a cardboard can? When you look long and hard at these images, they change; they become quite unbelievable. Now, we may not believe the images promoted in the name of foods they are not, but they do effect us emotionally. Supermarket sales tell us so. We continue to purchase such foods as fast as they hit the store shelves.

These foods never taste as good as their advertisements or packaging suggest. The promises of romance, happiness, or success, however, are simply promises—and promises can't be eaten. In a way, these promises are as empty as the nutritional value contained in a can of frozen, concentrated orange juice! Look where eating these foods has lead us: Our annual health care costs surpass the gross national product of every country in the world except for the eight major industrialized nations!

In reality, the general flavorlessness of processed foods found in supermarkets or fast-food restaurants actually contributes to overeating, undernourishment, and obesity. Researchers at Duke University Medical School, for example, found that the blandness characteristic of processed, packaged foods triggers you to eat more because, nutritionally speaking, you are satisfied less. When you learn to listen to the wisdom of your body, you will instinctively hunger for foods that are highly satisfying and you will eat less because you have met the needs of your appetite and your senses.

Our appetites have been cultivated by the multibillion-dollar food, diet, and advertising industries. Nor has the food industry lagged behind in response to our emerging public concern with health and nutrition. It has created whole new categories of foods designed to cash in on the dietary changes we are all desperately trying to make. Let's take a closer look at these so-called healthy foods.

Thousands of food products have been developed and marketed as healthy substitutes for the unhealthy foods we are trying to cut out of our diets. Sugar, fat, and salt are the main targets. Advised to reduce our intake of these substances, new products are chemically engineered to take their place. The seductive idea is that now you can have your cake and eat it, too. Or so it seems! These "healthy," "guilt-free" substitutes are filled with chemicals that may actually have side effects more injurious to your health than the products for which they are supposed to substitute!

Americans spend nearly $10 billion a year on products that claim to promote weight loss. Why do we spend so much money on these products? Why do we fill up our shopping baskets with "lite" salad dressings, "nonfat" frozen desserts, and "diet" shakes? There is good reason to be suspicious of claims that something is low fat or lite. In fact, some "lite" salad dressings contain 80 percent of their calories from fat. "Lite" may actually refer to the product's color!

How can you be sure anything is good for you? Forget all the fine print on the labels of these new products. The rule of thumb to follow is this: *It's generally best to stay away from foods that appear to be something they are not.* "Fake" foods have little or no nutritional value, and whatever flavor they provide is unnatural. Frozen orange juice from concentrate isn't fresh. "Fruit drinks" without fruit juice are not fruit—they aren't even juice!

Fake fats, fake meats, fake cheese, fake ice cream: These are foods produced in laboratories, not in nature. Even foods labeled "natural" are not necessarily natural at all, but filled with additives. "Food engineers" in white lab coats may say there is no nutritional harm in a chemical substance concocted to resemble butter. But just because a food does no *nutritional harm*—a claim you should always take with a grain of salt—does not mean it has any *nutritional value*. If it's fake, it's not fresh, and it does not nourish. *Fake*

◆

is fake! Ask yourself, "Would I rather feed myself and my loved ones food produced by a farmer or food developed by a 'food engineer'?"

It is vital that you learn to listen to your body's innate nutritional wisdom—because even science is not always a safe source of nutritional information. Some myths of nutrition come from the halls of our country's most respected and prestigious scientific institutes. Recently, a health newsletter produced by the esteemed Mayo Clinic asserted that *genetically engineered food is superior to what Mother Nature herself creates.* Wow!

High-tech tomatoes, *low-fat* french fries, *super* strawberries: Genetic engineering has produced fruits and vegetables that defy nature's seasons. How can tomatoes, a summer produce, be produced year-round? Can these tomatoes, engineered in laboratories, really be as fresh as vine-ripened tomatoes? Can molecular biology really produce foods that are healthier than those grown under natural farming conditions? Is food genetically engineered to have a longer shelf life really more fresh? (You might ask yourself this question: If it lasts that long on the shelf, how long is it going to linger in my body?)

These are the benefits touted by genetic engineering. But some things cannot be seen under a microscope. Tampering with the purity of food destroys its natural energy. New technology can add nutrients like vitamins C and E, as well as beta carotene, to fruits and vegetables. But if you eat a diet abundant in fresh fruits and vegetables, you will get these nutrients—in a form that ensures absorption and usefulness to your body—*naturally.*

The benefits of genetic engineering are often overstated, and it is downright misleading to claim that science is superior to Mother Nature! Good nutritional science has many lessons to learn from Mother Nature, and scientists are quite presumptuous to suggest it is the other way around.

When the wisdom of your body is in harmony with the wisdom of nature, that wisdom will be your guide and you will not be confused or misled by science gone astray. The ultimate nutritional science comes from the laboratory of your own body, which knows exactly what nutrients you need and where to get them. You can be your own expert on eating if you just learn to be guided by your natural hungers and not the seductions of your senses.

If I sound redundant, there is good reason. **Unhealthy ideas about food are so firmly ingrained within us, it requires repetition to break through those mental barriers.** Some points cannot be emphasized enough, since changing your mindset about the foods you eat, along with understanding what you have been exposed to, is absolutely essential to your successful journey to achieving your optimal weight and permanent weight loss.

Break the Mental Chains That Bind You to Poor Eating Habits Forever: Simple Mental Exercises

As you make your way through this book, you will learn how your thoughts and beliefs influence your health, weight, and energy. You will learn how, since the moment you were born, you have experienced myth after myth about food and eating. Years and years of exposure to such myths have created a mindset that is at odds with the good health, weight loss, and energy you are now striving for.

You will begin to build a new mindset about nutrition and weight loss, based on a clearer understanding of how and why your thoughts and feelings influence the food choices you make. Now that I have begun to help you separate the nutritional facts from the fictions still current in our society, you will understand why you must break the mental chains that keep your body's natural nutritional wisdom locked tightly away. The information you are now gaining will help you break these chains, one link at a time.

Are you ready to free yourself from these chains forever? Sound nutritional information is the first key. Since you have read this far, you already possess that first key. You are now prepared for the second, a simple method of mental relaxation that will help you obtain the discipline and determination to break free, once and for all, from the mindset that has kept healthy nutrition and permanent weight loss locked away from you. These simple mental exercises will speed your journey down the proper path and steer you safely on the road to abundant health, energy, and lasting weight loss.

Your mind is like a radio. Your thoughts, beliefs, and emotions about food and eating have created static. Radio static, for instance, distorts the sound of lovely music. Your impulse to reach for the dial and fine tune your radio so that you can hear the music as it's played is a sound one. Your mind works the same way. Unless you retune your mind, and *tune out* the static of misinformation and negative thoughts, the static will smother the feeling of good health you wish to be yours. Over time as well, that static in your mind will tend to make you ill and overweight.

You have read about some of the myths that cloud your understanding of good nutritional health. Depending on your own background, your own childhood, where you grew up, and so forth, you probably have other myths to add to this list. You have your own stories about the value and meaning of food told to you by your parents, your teachers, and your friends. Those stories are there, playing in the radio of your mind, shaping your attitudes and feelings toward food.

Now that you have a better idea about where these myths come from, and how they have influenced your health and weight throughout your life, here is your the next step: to reinforce this knowledge so that misinformation about food and eating will never again steer you off the road to well-being and weight loss. As you continue to read on, you will gain a tremendous amount of useful and accurate information that will help ensure your successful journey toward permanent weight loss. One of the most effective ways to develop new, healthy attitudes and feelings about food is through simple mental exercises. There is a method of mental relaxation that literally clears away the static of negative thoughts and emotions and retunes your mindset for well-being.

You may already be familiar with techniques of stress management, deep relaxation, or meditation. There are many, many varieties of meditation. When it comes to mental exercise, I promote the same approach I take to nutrition and physical exercise: *keep it simple*. In each of these arenas of activity—eating, exercising, relaxing—a simple approach is usually best. Of course, the tendency in these areas is to *overdo*. Among my patients, the simple method of mental relaxation I teach has been enormously effective. There are no fancy techniques to bog you down. You don't have to buy anything to do it, and it takes as little as ten minutes a day. Meditation is a simple and effective method for re-tuning your mindset and stimulating your body's internal pharmacy and healing forces to restore *homeostasis*—the medical term for internal balance. Restoring homeostasis, or your internal balance, is the key to achieving *Total Health Rejuvenation* and permanent weight loss naturally.

What happens when you practice these mental exercises? You help clear away the roadblocks. All of the confusion, anxiety, guilt, and fear about food that has created mental cobwebs in your mind are swept away. All of the thoughts and emotions about food that are keeping you off the road to weight loss disappear. You can build a healthy new mental outlook on food and your body. This retuned mindset will spark your self-esteem and guide you in making health-promoting food choices, in developing eating habits that ignite your energy and vitality, and increasing your physical activity.

On a deeper level, these exercises will allow you to quiet your thoughts so that you can listen to the voice of your own inner wisdom. Remember, the wisdom of your body is a perfect compass, always pointing in the direction of health, energy, and vitality. To follow that compass, you have to clear away the mental cobwebs, tune out the static of myths and misperceptions, and learn how to respond to your natural hungers.

◆

MENTAL RELAXATION EXERCISES

These exercises should be done every day, even after you feel secure in your new eating habits. Use them more frequently from time to time to reinforce your new mindset, especially when old habits seem hard to resist.

▶ *To begin, choose a comfortable, quiet place in your home. You will need at least five to ten minutes of privacy and silence, so take the phone off the hook, and if others are at home, just ask them to leave you undisturbed.*

▶ *Sit up with good posture, but do not be uncomfortable or stiff. Uncross your legs and ankles, and let your hands rest gently in your lap. After you know these exercises from memory, you may gently close your eyes and keep them closed until the end of your meditation. Until then, just relax, and be very calm, and read each step of the meditation.*

▶ *Begin to relax even more now and get ready to take several deep, full and long breaths. Every breath will relax you more and more, particularly as you exhale.*

▶ *While taking your first deep, long and even breath, relax all of the muscles in your face. As you exhale, let go of all traces of tension in your forehead and in the muscles around your eyes.*

▶ *Take a second long and deep and even breath now, and as you exhale, consciously relax all the muscles of your neck, your shoulders, your arms and forearms and hands.*

▶ *Take a third deep breath, and as you exhale, relax all the muscles of your chest, your abdomen and your back. Just relax.*

▶ *Take a fourth deep breath, and as you exhale, feel all the muscles in your buttocks, your thighs and your calves relax . . . all the way down to your feet and toes . . . relax.*

▶ *Take a fifth deep, full breath now and as you breathe in, scan your body for any tension. As you breathe out, let go of any tension and just relax. Breathe in, locate the tension; breathe out, let the tension go.*

▶ *Now just breathe normally, but slowly and calmly. Feel your entire body becoming even more and more relaxed. Be still and silent . . . just relaxing and breathing.*

▶ *Begin to imagine a warm healing golden light shining from your heart. Imagine this warm healing golden light filling your heart and radiating outward to fill your entire body with warmth . . . and healing . . . and relaxation.*

▶ *Imagine the warm healing golden light filling your lungs, your stomach, and your pelvis. Imagine the golden light flowing through your legs, feet and toes. Imagine the light flowing through your neck and your shoulders, and then down your arms, forearms, to the very tips of your fingers. Feel your fingers tingle with warm golden light.*

Imagine the warm golden light flowing upward, filling your mouth, your nose, your eyes, your ears. Imagine the warm golden light flowing through every cell of your brain. Imagine your entire body, from head to toe, radiating with warm . . . healing . . . golden light.

▶ *Now that your body is filled with warm and radiant light, silently and slowly say these words to yourself over and over and over again . . .*

I Have Strength . . . I Have Strength . . . I Have Strength

▶ *Repeat this empowering message to yourself at least a dozen times. Make sure to take plenty of time to pause and feel the strength flowing through your entire body. (If you wish, you may also say the following words too . . . over and over and over again . . .)*

God Loves Me . . . God Loves Me . . . God Loves Me

▶ *When you are ready, take a nice, slow, deep breath. Feel happiness and energy flowing through your body as you exhale. Now, slowly open your eyes and come back to your waking consciousness. Gently wiggle your fingers and toes. Just sit for a quiet moment, enjoying the stillness of your thoughts and the refreshed feeling throughout your body.*

How do you feel? What are your thoughts? Do they seem more quiet than usual? Do you feel less restless? Do you feel more energetic? How is your mood? You should feel relaxed but not tired, calm but energized. And you should feel a sense of mental clarity and satisfaction. Practicing these mental exercises daily will help to develop your new outlook on food and eating. You'll find that when you allow yourself to relax and your thoughts to quiet down and stop moving, a wonderful thing happens within you: *Your own natural healing mechanisms are ignited*. That is when the wisdom of your body can point your inner compass in the right direction. When you quiet your mind using these exercises, your inner compass will guide you to do exactly what is right to achieve *Total Health Rejuvenation* and a balanced, healthy weight forever.

Part Two

YOUR HEALTH PROFILE:

Profile Questionnaires to Help You Evaluate Your State of Wellness and Chart a Personalized Course to Lasting Weight Loss and Expanding Energy

Before continuing, I want you to understand that your health and weight are affected more by what you are willing to do for yourself than by what any doctor is capable of doing for you. The sophisticated tools of Western scientific medicine can tell you many things about your body. But you are the expert when it comes to assessing the habits of thought, belief, attitude, and action that underlie your current state of health. So now, let's do some personal evaluating and assessing to help prepare you for the tremendous knowledge that lies ahead.

The following sets of questionnaires are designed to help you assess your current health and weight profile. Please note that it is important for you to answer the profile questionnaires *at this point*, before you read any further parts of the book. Don't skip ahead and come back to the questionnaires later. The questions are geared primarily toward your *attitudes, thoughts, and emotions* about food, exercise, body image, and stress. Factors such as cholesterol level, blood pressure, body fat percentage, and body frame are very important. Your doctor or health professional can also help determine your physical health profile. But if you really want to understand your current health profile and, more importantly, *the reasons why you are where you are*, then your honest, insightful responses to the following questions are essential.

The questions are divided into four groups, dealing with four areas that contribute to your level of wellness and weight: body image, nutrition, exercise, and stress. Answer every question in each section and calculate your total points for each section. When you have completed the entire set of questionnaires, calculate the total points for all sections combined. At the end of the questionnaires you will be given a formula for interpreting your score and diagnosing your current level of wellness and weight. Determining this information will help you understand your needs and achieve your goals. Don't be nervous; there are no wrong answers. Just try to be as accurate as you can.

BODY IMAGE QUESTIONS

In Part One you read a brief survey about your body image. The following questions delve more deeply into this important area— for many people, it is the motor that drives poor eating habits. Answer all the questions. Be perfectly honest and direct with yourself. The more truthful you are in answering, the more accurate your assessment of your Health Profile will be. Keep in mind that your body image underlies many, if not most, of your eating habits and food choices. Before you restore balance to your diet, you need to restore balance to your self-image. Total your score at the end of the questionnaire.

1. When I look in the mirror I feel
   - (a) discouraged and disappointed   4
   - (b) critical of everything I see   3
   - (c) critical of some things, but accepting of others   2
   - (d) generally pleased with who I see   1

2. I compare my physical appearance to others
   - (a) constantly   4
   - (b) often   3
   - (c) sometimes   2
   - (d) never   1

3. My perception of my body is probably
    (a) very distorted   4
    (b) somewhat skewed   3
    (c) mostly realistic   2
    (d) right on target   1

4. When I see a model in a magazine or on television I
    (a) criticize myself for not looking like her or him   3
    (b) compare myself to her or him   2
    (c) don't give it any thought   1

5. What sets the standard of ideal weight, fitness, and beauty I aspire to?
    (a) fashion magazines   4
    (b) television and film   3
    (c) friends and family   2
    (d) my standard comes from within   1

6. My image of ideal weight, fitness, and beauty is
    (a) unattainable and probably unhealthy for me   3
    (b) possibly too ambitious   2
    (c) well within my reach   1

7. My thoughts about my body are
    (a) generally negative   4
    (b) sometimes negative   3
    (c) basically neutral   2
    (d) mostly positive   1

8. Does the way I feel about my body keep me from doing certain things (such as going to the beach, dressing up for a night of dancing, etc.)?
    (a) yes, I feel limited by my body   4
    (b) only sometimes   3
    (c) I do these things but feel shy or self-conscious   2
    (d) no, I do not feel limited by my body   1

9. When people comment on my looks, I feel
    (a) they must be lying   4
    (b) very embarrassed   3
    (c) slightly uncomfortable   2
    (d) appreciative and special   1

10. When the topic of conversation is weight, I
    (a)   disappear   4
    (b)   feel like all eyes are on me   3
    (c)   feel self-conscious   2
    (d)   am comfortable and secure   1

11. When someone gives me a compliment
    (a)   I completely dismiss it   4
    (b)   I generally feel undeserving   3
    (c)   I accept it but with embarrassment   2
    (d)   I accept it graciously and appreciatively 1

12. I haven't been happy with my body
    (a)   ever   4
    (b)   since I was a child   3
    (c)   in the last year   2
    (d)   I'm okay with my body now   1

Body Image Total: _____

NUTRITIONAL WELLNESS QUESTIONS

As you respond to the following questions, choose the answer that most closely fits you. You are not judging or criticizing yourself here, but identifying the eating habits and choices that you may take for granted. Now that you have decided to be proactive about bringing your nutritional energy back into balance, you need to know what food choices are disrupting that balance. When you complete the questionnaire, total your score.

1. I eat in my car
    (a)   most days   4
    (b)   when I'm running late   3
    (c)   almost never   2
    (d)   never   1

2. When I eat dinner, I am usually
    (a)   in front of the TV   4
    (b)   still at work   3
    (c)   in a restaurant   2
    (d)   at home, at the table   1

3. I usually eat my meals
    (a) alone   2
    (b) with family or friends   1

4. Meal times are
    (a) something I am usually too busy for   3
    (b) a necessary interruption from work   2
    (c) a pleasurable experience I look forward to   1

5. I eat while doing other activities
    (a) always   3
    (b) sometimes   2
    (c) never   1

6. In the grocery store, I spend most time
    (a) in the cookies and sweets aisle   4
    (b) in the butcher's section   3
    (c) in the canned or frozen foods aisle   2
    (d) in the fresh produce section   1

7. The following best describes my eating habits:
    (a) I am a meat-and-potatoes person   4
    (b) I eat whatever is convenient or around   3
    (c) I usually try to eat well   2
    (d) I am nearly a vegetarian   1

8. I eat fried or high-fat, greasy foods
    (a) at most meals   4
    (b) once a day   3
    (c) twice a week   2
    (d) I do my best to avoid fried and high-fat, greasy foods   1

9. I experience indigestion, heartburn, or other intestinal problems
    (a) regularly   4
    (b) a few times a week   3
    (c) once in a while   2
    (d) never   1

10. I am overweight by about
    (a) 50 or more pounds   4
    (b) between 25 and 50 pounds   3
    (c) 10 pounds or less   2
    (d) I am not overweight   1

11. I eat junk foods
    (a) daily   4
    (b) often   3
    (c) sometimes   2
    (d) rarely   1

12. In a restaurant, I'm most likely to order
    (a) a juicy steak   4
    (b) deep-fried chicken   3
    (c) pasta with chicken or fish   2
    (d) something vegetarian   1

13. I need to make some changes in my diet
    (a) but I'd rather enjoy what I eat than suffer   4
    (b) but my food habits are so ingrained   3
    (c) and I am moving in that direction   2
    (d) and I am ready now   1

14. The amount of water I drink each day is
    (a) less than a glass   4
    (b) one or two glasses   3
    (c) three or four glasses   2
    (d) at least six glasses   1

15. I eat _____ serving(s) of fresh fruit each day. (One serving equals one piece of fruit, one cup juice, or one cup fruit salad.)
    (a) zero   4
    (b) one   3
    (c) two or three   2
    (d) at least four   1

16. I eat _____ serving(s) of fresh vegetables each day. (One serving equals a half cup raw or cooked vegetables.)
    (a) zero   4
    (b) one   3
    (c) two or three   2
    (d) at least four   1

17. I eat _____ serving(s) of whole grains each day. (One serving equals a slice of bread, a half cup cereal, pasta, or rice.)
    (a) zero   4
    (b) one to two   3
    (c) three to four   2
    (d) at least five   1

18. I eat _____ serving(s) of dairy foods each day. (One serving equals one glass of milk, one cup of yogurt, two cheese slices, one scoop of ice cream.)
    (a) five   4
    (b) four   3
    (c) three   2
    (d) one or two   1

19. When I eat dairy foods
    (a) I eat regular, whole milk, full-fat products   4
    (b) I eat some low-fat varieties   3
    (c) I eat mostly low-fat varieties   2
    (d) I eat nonfat whenever possible   1

20. I eat vegetarian meals (without meat)
    (a) virtually never   4
    (b) once a week   3
    (c) two or three times a week   2
    (d) regularly   1

21. I eat fried foods
    (a) as much as possible   4
    (b) often   3
    (c) rarely   2
    (d) almost never   1

22. The amount of coffee (caffeinated and decaffeinated) I drink each day is
    (a) more than six cups   4
    (b) three or four cups   3
    (c) one or two cups   2
    (d) none   1

23. I drink alcoholic beverages
    (a) three drinks a day   4
    (b) two drinks a day   3
    (c) a few drinks a week   2
    (d) occasionally   I

Nutritional Wellness Total: _____

PHYSICAL WELLNESS QUESTIONS

Do you think that improving your level of exercise at the same time you are improving your nutrition is demanding too much? Now is the time to think again. Even moderate exercise helps prevent you from overeating or eating poorly. Determining your current state of physical wellness and your attitudes toward exercise will help prepare you for the information you will be reading later in this book. Total your score after completing this section.

I. In general, I lead a _____ life.
    (a) sedentary   3
    (b) moderately active   2
    (c) very active   I

2. When I think of exercise
    (a) I grimace at the thought   3
    (b) I feel guilty for not doing it   2
    (c) I look forward to doing it   I

3. My ideal weekend involves activities such as
    (a) sleeping and watching lots of TV   4
    (b) drinking and late-night partying   3
    (c) some outdoor activity   2
    (d) vigorous activities such as gardening, walking, hiking, cycling, etc.   I

4. The amount of physical activity I do at work is
    (a) none   4
    (b) minimal   3
    (c) moderate   2
    (d) vigorous   I

◆

5. My health and ideal weight are strongly influenced by physical activity.
   - (a) I don't believe this—genetics is everything   4
   - (b) I believe this but don't care   3
   - (c) I believe this but lack motivation   2
   - (d) I believe this and am motivated to improve   1

6. What keeps me from engaging in physical activity?
   - (a) Low self-esteem   4
   - (b) Too busy, and other things are more important   3
   - (c) It costs too much or the weather is bad   2
   - (d) Nothing keeps me from exercising   1

7. When I exercise
   - (a) I curse the bike I'm riding (weights I'm lifting, etc.)   4
   - (b) I'd really rather be doing something else   3
   - (c) I struggle but stick with it   2
   - (d) I enjoy myself and feel good   1

8. My confidence in my ability to stick with an exercise program is
   - (a) nonexistent   4
   - (b) low   3
   - (c) wavering   2
   - (d) I don't know if I can put my mind to it and stay with it   1

9. My motivation for exercise is best described as
   - (a) nonexistent   4
   - (b) low   3
   - (c) changes from day to day   2
   - (d) good to high   1

10. To raise my motivation to exercise, I am willing to enlist an exercise partner.
   - (a) no   3
   - (b) yes   2
   - (c) I'm already motivated on my own   1

11. How many times in the last month have I taken a walk?
   - (a) not at all   4
   - (b) once or twice   3
   - (c) once a week   2
   - (d) regularly; more than once a week   1

12. When was the last time an activity made me a little huffy and puffy and break into a slight sweat?
  (a) it's been so long, I can't remember   4
  (b) over a month ago   3
  (c) in the last month   2
  (d) in the last week   1

13. Does my present weight keep me from doing certain physical activities in which my body would be exposed (such as swimming, aerobics, joining a gym)?
  (a) yes   2
  (b) no   1

14. Sitting on the floor with my legs outstretched, I can bend forward and touch
  (a) my thighs   4
  (b) my knees   3
  (c) my shins   2
  (d) my feet   1

15. I engage in some aerobic activity (something that gets my heart beating faster and makes me a little sweaty)
  (a) hardly ever   4
  (b) a few times a month   3
  (c) a few times a week   2
  (d) almost every day   1

16. If I have a choice between the elevator or stairs, I usually
  (a) wait for the elevator   2
  (b) climb the stairs   1

17. If I have a choice between walking or driving, I
  (a) usually drive my car   2
  (b) usually walk the distance   1

18. In a parking lot
  (a) I circle the lot looking for the spot nearest my destination   2
  (b) I don't mind parking a distance away   1

19. When I climb a flight of stairs, I feel
    (a) I avoid stairs   4
    (b) exhausted   3
    (c) huffy and puffy   2
    (d) a little tired but energetic   1

20. My back
    (a) aches chronically and causes me to miss work   4
    (b) aches sometimes and limits my range of motion   3
    (c) rarely aches   2
    (d) is strong and flexible   1

21. When I look at myself in the mirror I think I look
    (a) unfamiliar to myself   4
    (b) tired and old   3
    (c) somewhat tired   2
    (d) healthy   1

22. My digestive health seems
    (a) poor, with frequent indigestion and constipation   4
    (b) fair, with occasional upset or discomfort   3
    (c) mostly fine   2
    (d) fine and regular   1

23. Overall, I consider myself to be in
    (a) poor shape   4
    (b) decent shape   3
    (c) fairly good shape   2
    (d) excellent shape   1

24. When it comes to getting into better shape
    (a) what's the use?   4
    (b) I don't think I can do it   3
    (c) it will be hard work   2
    (d) I can make the commitment because my health is worth it   1

25. It's too late to start exercising because
    (a) I'm too old   4
    (b) exercise is for other people, not me   3
    (c) I've tried but failed   2
    (d) it's never too late to start exercising   1

♦

26. Smoking is the number-one detriment to good health.
    (a) I don't care, I smoke anyway   10
    (b) I know, but it's too hard to quit   9
    (c) I smoke only occasionally   8
    (d) I don't smoke   1

27. I smoke
    (a) a pack or more a day   10
    (b) less than a pack a day   9
    (c) a few cigarettes a day   8
    (d) never   1

28. In the last year, after having several drinks, I have driven a car
    (a) several times   10
    (b) more than once   9
    (c) once   8
    (d) never   1

29. In the last year, drinking has interfered with a relationship or with my
    work
    (a) several times   10
    (b) more than once   9
    (c) once   8
    (d) never   1

Physical Wellness Total: _____

MEASURE YOUR STRESS

Review the following list of stressful situations and events and circle all that apply to your life now or within the past twelve months. Remember, stressors in and of themselves do not do the health damage; it is your harmful responses to stressors that eat away at your energy and well-being. After identifying the stressful situations in your life, proceed to the next set of questions, which will help you assess your current ability to respond to stress in positive, healthful ways.

Stressors

- death in the family
- job loss

- financial burdens
- conflict with a neighbor

- marital difficulty
- severe illness or health challenge
- sexual difficulty
- end of a relationship
- anxiety about a new relationship
- increased responsibilities at work
- new child
- going back to school

- buying a home
- mounting debt
- changes in workplace or job responsibilities
- moving or relocating to a new town or state
- problems with children
- irregular sleep patterns
- visit from family members
- deadlines at work

Total number of stressors circled: _____

How Many Stressors Do You Have in Your Life?

The more stressors you are dealing with, the greater the likelihood you will not be able to deal with them constructively and in a healthy way. *Stress is the leading cause of poor eating and overeating,* and the more stress in your life the greater the tendency to eat unhealthily. Use the following chart to determine your personal evaluation from the total number of circled stressors in your life.

(**Please Note:** Do *not* include the number of stressors you've circled when you calculate your total scores from the *Body Image, Nutritional Wellness, Physical Wellness,* and *Stress Resilience* questions.)

Number of Stressors	Evaluation
1–5	Your stress level is relatively low.
6–10	Your stress level, if not managed well, may easily spiral out of control.
11–15	You have a dangerously high level of stressors in your life and must become proactive in reducing your stress and managing your response to stressful situations.
16–20	The high number of stressors in your life could drain your energy to risky levels. This much stress, unmanaged, almost surely leads to illness.

◆

STRESS RESILIENCE QUESTIONS

Don't worry if the previous exercise revealed that you have many stressors in your life. Worry will only compound the stress. The most important factor is how well equipped you are to deal with these stressors. Answer the following questions to determine your strength in coping with stress. Once you have evaluated your present coping abilities, you will be ready to learn new strategies to improve your resilience against stress and stress-related illness. Total your score at the end.

1. In general, I think the amount of stress in my life is
   - (a) out of my control   4
   - (b) moderate but usually present   3
   - (c) minor but sometimes a problem   2
   - (d) inconsequential   1

2. Compared to those around me, my life seems
   - (a) like a nightmare   4
   - (b) fairly chaotic   3
   - (c) relatively calm   2
   - (d) fairly stress-free   1

3. I feel like other people seem happier than I am
   - (a) almost always   4
   - (b) sometimes   3
   - (c) once in a while   2
   - (d) never   1

4. The last time I felt truly happy was
   - (a) so long ago I can't remember   4
   - (b) within the last year   3
   - (c) within the last six months   2
   - (d) I'm happy right now   1

5. I would characterize my attitude toward life as basically
   - (a) pessimistic   4
   - (b) resigned   3
   - (c) hopeful   2
   - (d) optimistic   1

6. When I wake up in the morning, I feel
   (a) like I'd rather stay in bed — 4
   (b) nothing until I have my first cup of coffee — 3
   (c) on autopilot — 2
   (d) ready to face the challenges of the day — 1

7. My relations with people at work are
   (a) strained because I don't like my coworkers — 4
   (b) sometimes tense, but I mind my own business — 3
   (c) generally okay — 2
   (d) productive and positive — 1

8. When things feel really stressful
   (a) I fall apart — 4
   (b) I ignore them — 3
   (c) I sometimes face them — 2
   (d) I take it one step at a time and do the best I can — 1

9. Under pressure at work, I
   (a) get agitated and take it out on others — 4
   (b) panic but get the job done — 3
   (c) sometimes panic but manage to just get by — 2
   (d) ask for help when needed and do my best — 1

10. My temper is best characterized as
    (a) a short fuse — 4
    (b) occasionally volatile and unpredictable — 3
    (c) usually under control — 2
    (d) calm and reasonable — 1

11. I feel my friends and family
    (a) are a burden — 4
    (b) mean well but don't know how to relate to me — 3
    (c) are sometimes supportive — 2
    (d) support me and want the best for me — 1

12. My philosophy of life goes something like this:
    (a) life's difficult and then you die — 4
    (b) sink or swim — 3
    (c) we're all in this together — 2
    (d) everything will be okay because there's a purpose behind everything — 1

13. How often do I laugh?
    (a) I don't have anything to laugh about   4
    (b) rarely; I'm too busy   3
    (c) sometimes   2
    (d) I laugh frequently and heartily   1

14. Resentment and hostility are feelings
    (a) that eat away at me constantly   4
    (b) that sometimes get the best of me   3
    (c) that I experience on rare occasions   2
    (d) that are not part of my life   1

Stress Resilience Total: _____

INTERPRETING YOUR SCORE

Now that you have completed the questionnaires concerning your *body image, nutritional wellness, physical wellness,* and *stress resilience*, totaling all of your combined scores will enable you to evaluate your overall Health Profile. Add up your totals for each of the four questionnaires and mark your overall score below. Remember, DO NOT include in your total the number of stressors in your life that you have circled.

TOTAL SCORE: _____

Use the following guide to interpret your overall score:

Score	Evaluation
220–320	Your current health profile is extremely poor. Your energy is drastically out of balance and your beliefs are supporting poor nutritional habits. You are not getting the energy your body requires to burn fat, fight illness, and resist stress. But don't be discouraged. Help is on the way! The 28-Day Plan, presented later in the book, can help turn all of this around.
140–219	Your current health profile indicates that it is time to make changes. You are on the borderline of bad health and need to be proactive about taking steps that will increase your energy and bring it back into balance. High-energy nutrition, physical activity, and a strategy for coping with stress are essential to improving your health and weight.
78–139	Your current health profile indicates that you are on the path to wellness by taking personal responsibility for your health. It is important to continue caring for yourself, and this book will help you.

Part Three

TRUTH IS ON THE MARCH AND NOTHING WILL STOP IT

Are you stressed-out, out of shape and lacking energy? Do you suffer with headaches, neck aches, backaches, fibromyositis, or other pain syndromes? Are you short of breath or do you have high blood pressure, diabetes or heart problems? What about constipation, diarrhea, hemorrhoids, irritable bowel syndrome or colitis? Do you take antacids regularly? Does it take a long time for you to fall asleep or do you worry about things a lot of the time? If you answered yes to any of these questions, you have probably been accepting an invitation to illness. But as a person of strength and conviction who recognizes the power of your choices, you can just as easily turn down the invitation through *Total Health Rejuvenation*.

"Truth is on the march and nothing will stop it," was Emil Zola's battle cry a hundred years ago. "I accuse," he wrote in a public letter to the president of France. "Our nation has a stain upon its cheek and history will record that a social crime has been committed."

France's leading literary figure shocked the nation by standing up to the powerful forces leading the government and society. He had dared to denounce the widespread corruption and falsehood of his time. Captain Alfred Dreyfus, a Jewish military officer, had been convicted of treason for selling secrets to Germany and sent to prison on Devil's Island for the rest of his life. His trial had led to a vicious wave of anti-Semitism throughout France. But Emil Zola discovered that Dreyfus had been framed. The true facts were being covered up by the government, the generals, and the wealthy individuals who controlled society. Emil Zola was convicted of libel and exiled, then died in a mysterious manner. But in the meantime, Captain Alfred Dreyfus was exonerated and set free.

In ancient Greece, Socrates also dared to challenge the wisdom of the powerful leaders of society. He simply said they had no idea how much they didn't know. Socrates was proclaimed guilty of treason and forced to drink poison hemlock. Fortunately, Plato and Aristotle carried on his challenge by introducing the Socratic method of questioning so-called wisdom to the entire world. Many have since lived and died so that the truth could make others free.

How does all this relate to weight loss? In a nutshell, if you want to lose weight and be less sick and tired, then start questioning and stop listening to the so-called authorities who have led us to the perilous state in which we now find ourselves. Over half of all Americans are overweight, the incidence of childhood obesity has doubled in the last twenty-five years, and our country spends over $1 trillion a year on disease repair. That's $3,759 per person— substantially more than most people in the rest of the world earn in an entire year of hard work. So, if you really want to lose weight permanently and experience wellness, why would you listen to the same authorities? Why continue bothering with nonsense? As a wellness medical doctor, my challenge to the government, the food industry, and the media is this: *"I accuse you of committing the social crime of fattening and sickening the people."*

Physicians, Heal Thyselves

For what seemed like the thousandth time in my medical career, I was lecturing about weight loss to an audience of medical doctors, trying to teach them that what they learned in medical school about diet and nutrition was now largely irrelevant and doing their patients more harm than good. At the end of the lecture, I stressed again that deprivation and dieting were not effective means of permanent weight loss, that the only sure way to help patients lose excess weight was to encourage them to eat more foods that are full of life-energy and to engage in regular exercise. This combination, I explained, stokes the body's furnace and supplies it with the fuel it requires to burn off excess fat.

What did I mean by life-energy? Foods that are full of life-energy, I said, are provided by nature, *not* made in factories. Potato chips are not found under the soil. There are no fields flowing with *white* bread. Fruit does not appear floating in sugary syrups. Streams are not filled with soft drinks. Fruits, vegetables, nuts, and whole grains capture the energy of the sun to sustain the human lifecycle. They are steeped in starlight, infused with the elements.

I explained to the group of physicians that stress was the major virus of our time, affecting virtually every infant, child, and adult, causing obesity and many other illnesses. I also reminded my colleagues about something we had first learned in medical school: We had spent years studying the ways nature provides nourishment to sustain the lifecycles of every animal and plant species on earth. We had all graduated medical school believing that our task as physicians was to assist nature in her work. But sometime later we fell under the spell of technology, allowing high tech to replace the personal touch, care, and compassion that needs equal time for true healing to work its wonders.

I had hoped this group would be especially receptive to new ideas about permanent weight loss because they were the types of physicians that patients rely on for sound nutritional information. These were pediatricians, general practitioners, internists, and obstetricians—the primary care doctors who work in the trenches of everyday patient care. Each doctor who came up to me afterwards, however, could only share his or her unsuccessful experiences in trying to help patients lose weight. More disturbing still, most of the doctors were overweight themselves!

What stunned me even more, though, was hearing the doctors admit they no longer had the time or energy to consult with overweight patients who wanted help. They complained that all they could do was tell patients to eat less food, particularly less fat, and exercise more, suggestions already obvious to patients trying to lose weight. Or they could prescribe the latest diet pill and cross their fingers that no irreparable side effects would result.

Finally, I asked Dr. Frank Thomas, an old friend who started a practice next door to me over thirty years ago, why he and the other doctors weren't more interested in what I had just said regarding food as energy. After all, I thought, they must realize that healthy food contains a life-force patients need to sustain, and possibly extend, their natural human lifecycle. Moving closer, he looked me in the eye and replied, "Of course I'm interested. But I'm also a physician and I can't let my personal beliefs or intuition cloud my scientific judgment." Then he added that there was a more practical issue to be considered. "How can you expect practicing doctors to take the huge amount of time that's necessary to convince our patients to take better care of themselves, much less teach them that what they think they know about nutrition is totally irrelevant?"

On a sadder note, he continued: "For those of us who are still in medical practice, everything has changed. Under managed care and HMOs, we can't prescribe what we want to prescribe. We can't order the tests we think our patients need. We can't even send our patients for consultations we believe are necessary. But the worst thing is that we have to see forty to fifty patients a day just to survive. That's just a few minutes per patient! And that doesn't count all the paperwork and phone calls for prior authorization for just about everything I do except go to the bathroom! It's a jungle out there. It's not about patients anymore. It's about profits. So maybe you'd be better off teaching 'energy nutrition' directly to all the people out there who want to lose weight, because we doctors have too much else to worry about right now."

Dr. Thomas's response was absolutely typical of most Western medical doctors. They tend to maintain a very rigid scientific division between their work as physicians and their lives as ordinary people who realize food is basically life-energy that nature provides to sustain our human lifecycle. In my lecture, I had informed my colleagues that the health of our patients is primarily determined by personal responsibility, self-value, and reverence for life. I then reminded them that the deepest purpose of our profession is to empower our patients to unleash their own internal, pharmacy-powerful healing forces that are capable of reducing weight and reversing disease.

My own belief is one thing; convincing other medical doctors to put such beliefs into their own practices is entirely different. That is why I address and dedicate this book to patients themselves—to everyone who finds him or herself stuck on the path to permanent weight loss and good health. It is my genuine attempt to help heal my noble profession and patients across the United States (and perhaps the world). This book is for everyone who is sick and tired of being sick and tired. It also is for everyone who is well and wishes to stay that way. It is a carefully-thought-out scientific plan for *Total Health Rejuvenation* and permanent weight loss.

The Expert Conspiracy

Do you remember the story of the emperor's new clothes? All the subjects in the kingdom pretended that the emperor was wearing beautiful garments but, in fact, he was naked. Just like the emperor, the nutrition establishment in the United States has no clothes on. You are being fattened without questioning its wisdom. Entire industries depend on you to be sick and overweight. Did you know that more money in the United States is spent on repairing illness and reducing weight than on our military and defense budget? In fact, about 15 percent of this country's gross national product is spent on disease repair. Actually, in the United States we spend more money repairing bodies than all of the countries in the entire world produce in an entire year, combined, except for the eight major industrialized nations.

Wake up! Misinformation has caused you to lose sight of the fact that nature provides you with food that contains the life-force you require to nourish your body. You have been brainwashed. Your taste buds have become enslaved and your appetite has been inflamed. Your mind is being managed by powerful people and institutions making enormous profits by fattening you, as well as by causing you to become ill. So-called orthodox nutritional science has become a sham, and your food information is coming from the very companies and people who prosper most by your becoming overweight. You are being inundated with so much refined, processed, fake, factory-made food that it is often difficult to find food that still has some of nature's life-force left in it.

Being chronically overweight is a disease, but you can determine your own health destiny and lose weight far more effectively than you have been taught to believe. But to do so, you must stop giving yourself to the same people and industries that caused your problems in the first place. Approximately half of all Americans are overweight and the major reason is clear: the industries and people we depend upon for nutrition and weight loss information are the very ones that prosper most by our unhealthy eating habits. That's why it's time to stop putting the foxes in charge of the chicken coops!

The people and institutions of great wealth and influence can't afford to speak the truth about health or weight loss. Neither can the politicians and industry-funded scientists, nor the food, tobacco, and alcohol industries; ditto for the drug, for-profit hospital, and managed care industries. They, along with the advertising, radio, television, and newspaper industries, are all singing in unison, from the same sheet of unhealthful music, while living off the fat of the land—yours!

Just look around at all the overweight adults and children who are joining what I call the legions of the worried well and walking wounded. There are tens of millions of people who are stressed out, tired, and easily fatigued. These are the people who don't have the symptoms that indicate a specific disease, but who nonetheless lack vitality and don't feel well.

Americans are the most atherosclerotic, hypertensive, hemorrhoidal, diabetic, ulcer-ridden, arthritic, cancer-, stroke- and coronary-prone people on the planet. We also are the most overmedicated, overtested, overradiated, and oversurgerized people since the very beginning of recorded history. Yet we are still getting sicker and sicker. We are also getting fatter than ever before, and we should be asking ourselves the following question: *Why do we continue to rely on the same old information, from the same politicians, scientists, industries, and media that have been responsible for fattening us in the first place?*

If so many are overweight, why should you believe that the guidelines of the so-called nutritional experts are applicable in the real world, when it has been reported that only one percent of our children ages two to nineteen follow the governmental guidelines for nutrition? If virtually everybody who goes on a diet gains back their lost weight (and usually more), why should you continue looking to "diet experts" for help?

Telling the Truth

In George Orwell's classic novel *1984*, powerful leaders of society programmed people's minds to believe "war is peace." Orwell wrote the novel to demonstrate the horrors of a society in which mental habits were so programmed into people that all other modes of thinking were made impossible. New words and phrases were invented to replace unacceptable ones, which were outlawed. "War is peace" replaced the term "Love thy neighbor."

In America, we have been programmed to believe that refined, processed, irradiated, genetically engineered, fake food is real. Recall the advertising slogan for a cola—is chemically flavored, syrupy sugar water really the "real" thing?

The truth is that the food industry has committed a travesty against the natural food chain—and against our health—by inundating us with refined, fake, or dead foods to enhance its profits.

The first scientific paper on coronary artery disease and myocardial infarction was not even published until 1912. The first description of a heart attack due to a blocked artery was published in the *Journal of the American Medical Association* during this century. Since then, coronary vascular disease has become a major killer, and autopsy studies of even young adults reveal that their coronaries are typically slathered with fat! We are being killed by what we eat.

A recent study, *Chronic Care in America: A 21st-Century Challenge,* reported that there is a vast army of people, nearly 100 million, who suffer from chronic ailments such as heart disease, cancer, and diabetes—all diet-related diseases. For the sufferers and their families, the hardships associated with these diseases are all too real. Add to that army the legions of the worried well and walking wounded, those who lack energy and zest for life, and you begin to discern the enormity of the problem we face.

My professional and ethical commitment to my patients is to tell them the truth, blunt and undisguised. I find this necessary because they, as you, have been so thoroughly deceived that I must, so to speak, flatten your old ideas—so that new ideas can rise up and take their place. Consider the once vibrant houseplant whose leaves suddenly begin to droop and decay. You can give it plant food or cut it back. Or you can place it in a new pot with fresh soil, move it to a new spot where it receives more sunlight, and give it water. Under better conditions, it will more than likely sprout new buds and return to good health. Just like the plant, if you change the way you eat and live, your body can restore itself to optimal health—and that is the miracle of homeostasis.

The Broken Contract

Staying healthy is a matter of keeping your energy in balance. This is the wisdom of Hippocrates, the Greek physician known as the father of Medicine. He believed that medicine should work to build the patient's strength through appropriate diet before taking more drastic steps. He also recognized the link between environment and disease. Unfortunately, Western medicine is based almost exclusively on repairing the human body with drugs and surgery, instead of stimulating the will to be well. Since the average doctor's office visit is only twelve minutes long (and declining rapidly!), how can physicians devote even five minutes to helping overweight patients lose weight if there are only seven minutes left over to deal with other issues of infection, pain, and degenerative diseases?

As flawed as Western medicine may be, however, there has always been an unspoken contract for the public to rely upon. Two shining attributes have never failed patients. First, for patients in need of medical care or surgical repair, there is no more advanced technology available anywhere in the world than that which we possess in the United States. Second, there is the medical profession's underlying ethic: *primum non nocere*—first do no harm. We have, indeed, been fortunate to depend upon such an unspoken contract—until now.

Our present misfortune is this: The huge for-profit managed care industry has broken the first part of the contract. It has locked out approximately 50 million people, mostly middle-class citizens who are not eligible for insurance through their place of employment and cannot afford to pay for it themselves but are not poor enough to qualify for aid. Even if those patients were able to access the system, what good is advanced technology such as MRI machines when doctors are denied authorization to use them because stock prices rise on the basis of how little, rather than how much, can be done for patients? That's called the bottom line . . . *profits!*

Furthermore, it is extremely troubling to observe that the managed care industry does not support traditional charitable care for patients without insurance or money; nor does it support the efforts of non-profit teaching hospitals, which are our primary means of advancing medical research. Profits, not quality of care, come first now.

Corporate profit-seekers have also broken the second part of the unspoken contract with physicians, their pledge to practice ethically. The best and most outspoken doctors have their hands tied when profit, not care, is the new priority.

A Call to Action

The following example of the broken contract with the American public was published in the December 3, 1997, issue of the *Journal of the American Medical Association*. This call to action was signed by 2,300 medical doctors and nurses who were protesting being bribed and punished by corporate profit-seekers.

> *We are Massachusetts physicians and nurses from across the spectrum of our professions. We serve patients rich and poor, in hospitals and clinics, private offices and HMOs, public agencies and academia. . . .*
>
> *Mounting shadows darken our calling and threaten to transform healing from a covenant into a business contract. Canons of commerce are displacing dictates of healing and trampling our professions' most sacred values. Market medicine treats patients as profit centers. . . .*
>
> *The time we are allowed to spend with the sick shrinks under the pressure to increase production, as though we were dealing with industrial commodities rather than afflicted human beings in need of compassion and caring. . . .*
>
> *Doctors and nurses are being prodded by threats and bribes to abdicate allegiance to patients, and to shun the sickest, who may be unprofitable. Some of us risk being fired or "delisted" for giving, or even discussing, expensive services, and many are offered bonuses for minimizing care. . . .*
>
> *Listening, learning and caring give way to deal-making, managing and marketing. The primacy of the patient yields to a perverse accountability—to investors, to bureaucrats, to insurers and to employers. And patients worry that their doctors' and nurses' judgment and advice are guided by the corporate bottom line. . . .*
>
> *Public resources of enormous worth—non-profit hospitals, visiting*

nurse agencies, even hospices—are being taken over by companies responsive to Wall Street and indifferent to Main Street. . . .

Communities find vital services closed by remote executives; savings are committed not to pressing health needs, but to shareholders' profits. Not-for-profit institutions, forced to compete, must also curtail research, teaching and charity, or face bankruptcy . . . A single HMO president nets $990 million in a takeover deal; and insurers' overhead consumes $46 billion annually. . . .

At the same time, the ranks of the uninsured continue to grow, while safety-net public hospitals and clinics shrink and public health programs erode. Even many with insurance find coverage deficient when they need it most; care or payment is too often denied for emergencies or expensive illnesses. . . .

The sick are denied skilled nursing care, rushed out of hospital beds and hurried through office visits. Increasingly, the special needs of the elderly, infirm or disabled are ignored if they conflict with the calculus of profit. . . .

The shift to profit-driven care is at a gallop. For doctors and nurses, the space for good work in a bad system rapidly narrows. For the public, who are mostly healthy and use little care, awareness of the degradation of medicine builds slowly; it is mainly those who are expensively ill who encounter the dark side of market-driven health care. . . .

We criticize market medicine not to obscure or excuse the failings of the past, but to warn that the changes afoot push medicine further from caring, fairness and efficiency . . .

The headlong rush to profit-driven care has occurred . . . through a process largely hidden from public scrutiny and above citizen participation. This must be replaced by an open and inclusive process that is not dominated by the loudest voices—those amplified by money and political influence.

Integrative Medicine

Perhaps the best thing that can be said about the whole HMO and managed health care mess is that it may have done us a great favor by pointing out how important it is for us to take more responsibility for our own health and well-being. Wise physicians already know that the spiritual, physiological, and mental resources of their patients are a crucial part of any total treatment strategy, along with the best that modern medicine has to offer.

We are not overweight because we aren't receiving enough medical care. We are overweight because our homeostasis is suppressed and our energy is out of balance. Until we move away from a medical system based on disease repair to a system based on stimulating our body's natural will to be well, we will continue to suffer with the highest levels of stress-related illness in the world.

Throughout world history, except for Western medical science, almost all other healing traditions are based on the concept of life-energy. They share a common understanding that this vital force is responsible for life. Chinese medicine calls it *ch'i*. Indian medicine calls it *prana*. Plato envisioned it as the Ideal Good, breathed into us at the very moment of conception. Aristotle understood it as simply the Breath of God.

We seem to have forgotten the three-thousand-year-old wisdom of Hippocrates, who taught us that health is a matter of balancing our physical, mental, and spiritual energies. Western medicine is based on repairing disease, instead of stimulating the will to be well. The understanding of illness and excess weight as energy imbalance has evolved for nearly three millennia. In each century, however, the essential idea that health is a matter of energy balance has been refined and filtered through the beliefs of a given culture at a given historical moment. In our own medical culture, governed by a profit-driven health industry and the mechanical logic of disease repair, this belief has become so diluted as to almost be forgotten. But just because medicine has forgotten about the healing power within us does not mean it no longer exists.

Be very alert because even Integrative Medicine is now being diluted by marketing hype for all sorts of "holistic" treatments for diseases from arthritis to cancer. I developed and first presented Integrative Medicine to the Institute of Medicine in Washington, D.C., in 1982, in a paper entitled: "A Scientific and Spiritual Approach to Health." *Anything less is not Integrative Medicine.*

Living Downstream

The following fable illustrates why I believe Integrative Medicine is so important for the twenty-first century.

> *The town of Downstream is located just where a stream of sparkling waters enter into a river. It used to be rather idyllic, with townspeople peacefully raising their families and making a decent living, mostly as farmers, shop owners, and workers at the town's button factory. One day, much to everyone's amazement, a few weakened and ill people, clearly not from this town, were found floating in the stream. Exhausted and in need of assistance, they were rescued by kindly townspeople, who nurtured them back to health.*
>
> *Soon, hundreds and then thousands of similarly sick people, desperately in need of care, were found floating in the stream every day. New ambulance companies, paramedic companies, laboratory companies, medical supply companies, and insurance companies (housed in skyscrapers) were formed to service new nursing homes and hospitals employing respiratory therapists, occupational therapists, physical therapists, dietitians, social workers, X-ray technicians, and nurses, all of whom were under the command of an army of physicians led by very important surgeons and specialists who were overseeing legions of family doctors.*
>
> *The people of Downstream have become so very busy, and gainfully employed, that to this day, no one has the time, or perhaps the insight, to stop and wonder for a moment: What in the world is going on upstream?*

We are finally stopping and wondering. There is a moral imperative for offering better health care, particularly to children, families, and senior citizens. Furthermore, to save Medicare from bankruptcy, as well as to help balance the federal budget, Congress wants the elderly to enroll in managed health care plans. This will be a decade of destiny for the health care industry. The political power structure has created an unprecedented opportunity for preventive medicine and wellness services. Managed health care is supposed to reduce overall costs via a prepaid scheme in which consumers pay a set monthly bill, whether or not they need care, and providers are paid, whether or not they deliver care.

Although health maintenance is the basis of this scheme, its reality is somewhat different: the established medical system has no traditional means of maintaining health. Prevention is not merely the early detection of disease after it has started. Pap smears and mammograms, for instance, are for early detection, not prevention, of disease. Because nearly 80 percent of diseases, including cancer, are related to lifestyle, and therefore need to be addressed *before they occur,* the current situation is no longer economically tenable. Integrative Medicine helps turn patients into partners with their physicians. It is dedicated to helping people control their own health destiny.

Twenty-first Century Health Care

Wise patients can become partners in their health care by combining the best that modern medicine has to offer with other means of care that seek to strengthen and balance the energies of the body, mind, and spirit. Your health is much too important to leave up to science, but it's also much too important to be unscientific about.

Your body is a complex, self-repairing energy system comprised of ever-replicating DNA, an exquisite healing force and a biological clock. Unfortunately, in the prevailing medical system with its focus on drugs, surgery, and radiation, such concepts are very difficult to deal with. To do so requires a shift in consciousness—from a sickness paradigm to a wellness paradigm.

The Integrative Medicine approach to permanent weight loss is based on the following simple and easy-to-understand precepts:

- *Homeostasis* is the medical term for energy balance. Hippocrates called it the *"Vix Mediatrix."*
- If you are well, your energy is in balance.
- If you are ill or overweight, your energy is out of balance.
- Your natural healing force remembers wellness; thus, it strives always to balance your energy. However, it requires life-energy to do its work.
- There are basically two types of food: food filled with life-energy and food that is relatively dead.
- Your body requires clean and efficient fuel to nourish and sustain it through its cycle of life.
- Food filled with life-energy provides efficient fuel for the body's metabolic requirements.
- Your body uses any life-energy in excess of daily metabolic needs to burn off excess fat and attain a healthful balance.
- Food comprised mostly of dead energy fuels the body's metabolism like cheap, low-grade gasoline runs in a high-powered car—with knocks, pings, poor starts, and dirty emissions.
- Leftover dead energy is converted to fat, which first drenches the blood and organs, then is stored in the larger blood vessels, abdomen, thighs, and buttocks.

Wellness Genetics

DNA is the substance of human genes. It contains billions of bits of ancestral information, including the templates of disease that we have been inheriting from our family since time immemorial. The information encoded in our DNA appears to date back over 60 million years. Your own gene pool is as vast as the stars. It carries your mental characteristics, including your temperament; your physical characteristics, such as hair color; and an inborn biological clock to signal adolescence, adulthood, menopause, even the time for hair to grow in your ears!

In the first half of life, your genes strive to keep you healthy and to enable you to pass on your DNA to preserve our species. During the second half of life, your genes strive to keep you alive for as long as possible to enable you to pass on your intellect, love, skills, and devotion, to protect our species. Nobel laureate physicist David Bohm pointed out that even the very atoms of a human being are invested with meaning and purpose. Although most people believe it is difficult to establish a sense of higher purpose or mission in life, it's much easier than one would think. We are all part of the very fabric of life. What touches others touches us.

The major function of your genes is to transmit health and the inborn resolve to remember wellness. In the sickness paradigm, we are taught that disease-carrying genes determine our destiny. This is a false and life-threatening view. If we were truly destined to live by such genes, we would suffer from the thousands of diseases experienced by our ancestors for as long as we lived, which would not be very long at all. Fortunately, our ancestral templates, or blueprints of disease, are influenced by factors well within our control. Disease-carrying genes are not our destiny because they must answer to our inner compass, our healing force, which remembers wellness and keeps templates of diseases safely stored away in vaults within our cells. Even if the vaults containing the templates have already been unlocked, it is still possible to summon our healing forces to fight for wellness. Our physical, mental, and spiritual vitality stimulates our natural internal pharmacy of biochemical healers.

Everything in Moderation—Including Moderation

How do you get motivated to lose weight permanently? Others cannot or will not do it for you. Motivation requires setting realistic goals, like a 5 to 10 percent (of your total weight) weight loss for the first year. Motivation also requires understanding life-energy versus dead energy. Finally, motivation requires developing a reverence for life through understanding the beauty and power of the human lifecycle.

It is truly remarkable that the decline in coronary vascular disease and stroke in the United States during the past twenty-five years has not been accompanied by a decrease in obesity. Actually, the prevalence of excess weight has doubled during that time period. Although the majority of medical and nutritional scientists believe that the incidence of coronary vascular disease and stroke has declined because we have become more cholesterol-conscious, this may not actually be the case because of two other phenomena: in the past twenty-five years 60 million Americans quit smoking and the diagnosis and treatment of hypertension improved dramatically.

Despite all the complicated theories about why we gain weight and all the scientific terms that describe what we eat—calories, saturated fats, trans-fats, polyunsaturated fats, monounsaturated fats—we are still getting fatter. New weight-loss drugs won't help; you can't tinker with your metabolism and expect to be all right. Fad diets won't work, because they disobey natural laws (which we will discuss later on) and ignore the fact that obesity is largely a symptom of inaccurate information, stress, and inner dis-ease. Your inner works—the mind and soul—need fixing before your body can look good and feel better. It would be impossible to underestimate the magnitude behind this shift in vision. Nor does such a discovery diminish present nutritional science. Instead, it shapes it into a clinically effective field that allows people to lose weight permanently. Remember: The triumph of one scenario over another does not necessarily mean the loser must be discarded. In fact, good nutritional science means using past nutritional science in a more accurate manner.

Attitude and weight are inseparable. Your body and your mind are a complete ensemble. From this viewpoint, it is obvious that fat begins and persists in the mind. It is no wonder, then, that the idea of changing the mind's appetite for food has been the impetus behind thousands of diet books. After all, it seems so obvious: Eat well, exercise, and just kick the habit! The problem is that this simple idea never works in practice for very long. Why? When we are stressed, we forget or ignore our resolve. This is the *stress disinhibition effect,* which I will revisit throughout this book. Practically, it means that our food urges and cravings are so strong that, once we get stressed, we obey them.

What does it mean if you make a resolution to eat more appropriately and then don't do it? Is it a matter of copping out, giving up too easily, not having the courage of your convictions, being weak-willed or looking for the easy way out? Absolutely not. If you are stressed, you can actually forget or ignore your resolve. If the desires of your taste buds are unfulfilled, you become further stressed. It's a vicious cycle that causes dieters to always lose—their hope, that is, but unfortunately not their weight.

While sitting at my computer for seemingly endless days and nights writing this book, a personal problem began looming larger and larger for me. I was developing a powerful for craving chocolate. And I also gave into it, big time! I tried to stop my chocolate cravings mentally but couldn't. My mind said to me, "Eat the chocolate," and I did. I began to pay more attention to my craving for chocolate and tried to ascertain the feelings behind them. I remembered my early childhood, and Grandma showering me with incredible love by letting me lick the warm chocolate pudding right out of the pot. This was exactly the type of comforting feeling I was now getting from eating chocolate when I overworked.

How could I block out that warm memory, along with the quivering feeling it caused in my stomach? Certainly not by using my very same chocolate pudding–drenched desires to make a resolution to break my habit. Chocolate pudding goes a long way toward soothing the savage beast called stress!

We can combine good science and effective stress management to forge a brand-new frontier for lifelong healthy weight. But the journey there can only be accomplished by building a *new path of least resistance*. This is a matter of human nature and good common sense. Unhealthy eating habits begin in the mind, where stress and misinformation create "mental malnutrition." The overweight person's mind is deficient in mental nutrients such as love, serenity, and self-esteem. Once we repair such deficiencies, the mind naturally hungers for food with life-energy. Then, and only then, the process of natural weight loss begins.

Imagine the mind as a mental pantry whose shelves we must clear out. First we take inventory, then we clear out the thoughts and feelings that cause weight gain. Finally we restock the pantry by filling the shelves with essential ingredients for permanent weight loss: self-respect, stress management, enjoyable exercise, and food filled with life-energy.

My chocolate habit? There was one basic fact that was so obvious that even my chocolate-drenched thoughts could not obscure it: Everyday joys of youth, especially candy, may have little effect on a body that is mostly intent on passing on its DNA to the future. Those same youthful pleasures, however, become the potbellies of middle and older age. More regular meditation and exercise helped me overcome my urges and cravings. It was amazing how some simple steps enabled my brain to search for different meanings and make new connections to bypass my inflamed appetite, building a *new path of least resistance** to a much healthier frontier.

My chocolate habit is still there, but it's safely tucked away in the vaults of my memory. Fortunately, *"Moderation in all things— including moderation"* is an unspoken tenet of Integrative Medicine. I only remove my craving from its safety-deposit box when I go to the movies, where I enjoy chocolate-covered raisins. It's not a

---

*Robert Fritz addresses this general concept very well. See bibliography.

problem I can readily solve, because my pleasurable memory is always there, perhaps a part of my very being. Instead of solving the problem, I created a new result.

Looking for Help in All the Wrong Places

The troubling paradox of modern medical science is that doctors, with so many years of schooling, find it hard to accept that the natural healing abilities of the body are more intelligent than medical science. But don't let your mind become prey to the tempting notion of medicating away the results of your misguided eating habits. The most inspiring resource we have to overcome obesity is within ourselves. Our own natural healing force is equivalent to an inner pharmacy. It is like a biological compass within our cells that always remembers wellness.

Only in the past century have our natural healing forces been so neglected by technology and diminished by stress. Yet they still struggle to maintain our energy balance and health against all odds. My 28-Day Plan will help get you on track. It is a strategy for *Total Health Rejuvenation*—unleashing the power of your healing forces so that the spirit of wellness reigns throughout your body and mind.

Your healing force is like a sacred song echoing through the chambers of your heart and the deep spaces of your soul. It is the music that drenches your spirit, calms your mind, and gives your body the strength to shed its excess fat. Your healing force is like an eternal flame, still burning even in those people who have forgotten its soothing light. It is your inner biological compass that stimulates your body's will to be well. Let us embark upon a healing journey to lose weight comfortably and permanently.

A Special Note From Me To You

Now that you have completed Parts One, Two, and Three of this book, it is very important for you to understand what I have been trying to help you accomplish. I consider this book a "gift of life" from me to you.

Now you will be so much more knowledgeable and discriminating about what you put in your body. For the rest of your life, every time you watch a television commercial about food, you will be able to think, *What audacity! Does anyone have the right to suggest to me (or my children) that I eat something that is not good for me?* You will be able to look at food advertisements with a skeptical eye and say to yourself, *No way!* And, with an inner laugh, you can add, *Don't insult my intelligence.*

When you are in the supermarket, don't be fooled. You know the advertising game, so ignore all the fancy packaging. Now that you are beginning to understand the myths and advertising images created to sell food to you, be alert and discriminating. Be sensible . . . be healthy . . . and you will achieve your optimal weight. Whenever you are in doubt, think about what you have learned in Parts One, Two, and Three. Just feel good about yourself and read on! Remember, *you have strength!*

Part Four

ENERGY NUTRITION AND THE CYCLE OF LIFE

How do you feel about what you have read so far? I wish we were face-to-face so we could discuss weight loss one-on-one. For the moment, at least, that's not possible, but books are a helpful medium; they allow physician-authors to talk to so many people in a thorough and complete manner.

Isn't it amazing that we can go through life with our eyes open, yet miss so much of what's around us, especially when our environment so totally influences our health and life? Unfortunately, with our busy lifestyles, heavy workloads, and two-income families, we don't take the time to take care of ourselves. Yet it is so easy and possible to do. Once you have a new mindset about the food you eat, you will develop new healthful eating habits, along with many other wonderful and healthful benefits. It requires no more time or work to eat and live the *healthy balanced way*, as opposed to the *out-of-balance way*.

Did you know that you are one of trillions of components of nature? Your own personal human lifecycle regulates and guides the sequence of events occurring in your body from the moment of your conception until the time of your death. Beyond that, who knows? Perhaps we humans are just like animated star dust, hur-

tling through time and space until we return to the heart of God.
What the caterpillar calls the end of the world, nature calls the butterfly.

The cycle of life is represented by the following stages:

- Prenatal
- Infancy
- Childhood
- Adolescence

- Young Adulthood
- Middle Adulthood
- Maturity

Throughout your entire lifecycle, you require proper fuel to
nourish and sustain each stage of the cycle. Your body derives the
necessary fuel by extracting energy from the earth, air, water, and
sun. Your human lifecycle is clearly an endangered entity. Most of
us drink more soft drinks than water, and most of our food is refined or artificial, stripped of its life-energy. The air is so polluted
with dirt and particulate matter that millions of us develop asthma
with each passing month. The sun's rays cause cancer because
much of the ozone in the atmosphere has been depleted.

What can you do to better sustain your own lifecycle? You must
truly glimpse the truth for yourself. Only in that way can the information in this book give birth to wisdom. It is essential that you
read about each stage of the human lifecycle. I am going to teach
you about certain aspects of human biology, psychology, and natural laws in a deeper, more profound manner than even physicians
learn in medical school. Please do not skip over the parts of the
book that you believe are not relevant for you. Even if you are over
fifty years old, it is essential that you understand the prenatal,
childhood, and adolescence stages of your human lifecycle. And
even if you are twenty-five years old, it is essential that you understand the maturity stage of the human lifecycle. Each stage of the
lifecycle is part of nature's entire cycle of life, and it is essential for
you to understand the truth. You are a component of nature.

In the Beginning

Let me take a moment to give you a brief definition of DNA. Simply put, DNA is the basic building block of life. The scientific chemical name for DNA is deoxyribonucleic acid. Now here's a more in-depth definition:

> Each of our trillions of cells contain genes that are made up of our DNA molecules. These molecules consist of two long strands that are twisted together to form a double helix. DNA molecules contain the intelligence, information, and instructions that are required for our cells to function well and stay alive.

Your personal human lifecycle encompasses more than just the length of time between your conception and death. Your DNA is comprised of your parents' DNA, and their parents', and their parents', and so on. It is said that there is a species of bamboo tree in China which, in twelve months, grows more than one hundred feet from its initial sprout. But its seed, buried deep in the soil, requires weekly watering for thirty years before sprouting to the surface. Does this tree grow one hundred feet in one year, or did it take thirty-one years? Did the prenatal stage of your personal human lifecycle take nine months, nine generations, or nine millennia?

Every human lifecycle is rooted in one common ground—an inexhaustible universal storehouse of energy that initially breathes life into every living thing. Therefore, let us begin by considering your own personal human lifecycle. The initial breath of energy that ignited the spark of your own human lifecycle occurred as the sperm of your father united with the egg of your mother. Your human lifecycle began at the moment of fusion between their DNA, ancestral genetic matter that had been accumulating for millions of years. Then, in the moment it took for your mother's fertilized egg to divide into two cells, you were transformed into a microscopic pre-embryo.

What an incredible chain of events had to occur before your human lifecycle could actually begin! Did you know that your mother had all the eggs she would ever have in her life already present in her ovaries at the moment of her own birth? As many as a quarter of a million eggs lay quietly in her ovaries, awaiting the adolescence stage of her human lifecycle so that she could start yet another human lifecycle: yours!

Examining the various stages of the human lifecycle will allow you to understand the normal changes you should expect during the seasons of your time on earth. More importantly, it cannot help but cause you to be in awe of your body. From the time of fertilization right up to the present moment, your human lifecycle has been persistent and resolute, conquering almost any obstacles that you may have raised along the way. Your body is like a bird that flies. If you allow it to, it will flourish.

Your own human lifecycle began when one particular egg in one of your mother's ovaries, responding to some dim message, perhaps in phase with the moon, began a migration for which it had been preparing for a lifetime, or even longer. This solitary egg began moving slowly toward the thick, fibrous coating of her ovary. Finally, the egg burst through the ovarian wall in a splash of blood. Free-floating in your mother's pelvis, a wave of energy propelled the egg through a space which, in terms of the egg's tiny size, was equivalent to jumping across the Grand Canyon.

Arriving safely at its destination at the opening to one of your mother's fallopian tubes, the egg began to roll down almost one-third the length of this tube. It did this slowly, through forty-eight hours, to await the arrival of one particular sperm from your father's ejaculate of over 50 million sperm. That's how you were born. Now that's energy!

Until recently, we believed that tens of millions of your father's sperm engaged in furious battle with each other to conquer your mother's egg, enter it, and close it off to all competitors. Alas, the warrior's tale is no longer told! Yes, it is true that millions of sperm in your father's ejaculate were propelled toward your mother's uterus with an explosion of energy that allowed them to burrow through the thick plug of mucous in her cervix, then climb vertically upward along her inner uterus wall, find the tiny opening to the correct fallopian tube and climb further upward to meet her waiting egg, into which only one sperm would penetrate and enter.

However, it now appears that your mother's egg chose that particular sperm that made you. In a sense, your mother's egg invited this one special sperm to fuse its DNA with hers in order to give birth to you. This one special sperm had to race at top speed, over a distance that, for its tiny size, was equivalent to running a race nonstop from Los Angeles to New York City, before entering into your mother's waiting egg, then rolling down her fallopian tube while dividing into a sixteen-celled pre-embryo that had to be embedded in the wall of her uterus within seventy-two hours in order to prepare you to be nourished by your mother's life-energy for the first nine months of your human lifecycle. Now that's energy, too!

How, Why, and When Obesity Begins

A serious mistake has been made that continues to harm us later in life. The most basic nutritional standards for keeping infants and children in energy balance are wrong! A growing body of evidence shows that the food requirements of the infancy and childhood stages are a good deal lower than previously estimated, up to 20 percent lower for infants and 25 percent lower for children from one to ten years of age. We have been mistakenly encouraged to overfeed our babies and children from the very beginning.

What happened? It's really very simple. The old testing methods used to measure food intake data were inaccurate. Weighing foods, keeping records of food intakes, then submitting personal diet histories to researchers do not produce objective data. In fact, we now realize that such subjective methods produce grossly inaccurate data. When questioned, adults generally misrepresent their own food intake patterns because less makes them feel better. On the other hand, adults tend to overestimate the food intake of their infants and children because more makes them feel like they are better parents.

New testing methods with nuclear isotopes can now measure the actual energy requirements of infants and children directly. These tests demonstrate that the food energy requirements of infants and young children are significantly lower than scientists once thought. That's too bad, because human fat-storing cells (adipocytes) develop to handle excess energy during infancy and childhood, and then tend to hang around for life.

Another reason why current recommendations for food energy are too high is that food intake data collected during the 1970s are not very relevant to the 1990s. The reason? Today children exercise less and less often. Physical activity burns up about a third of a child's food energy intake, yet current food intake standards fail to account for the huge decline in exercise in children. If children continue to consume the same amount of calories suggested since the 1970s, while continuing to watch more TV and exercise less, then childhood obesity will continue to skyrocket. So will the incidence of diseases associated with being overweight, including cardiovascular disease, diabetes, and many types of cancer.

If you really look fat, then you probably are fat. This is a fairly workable measure of excess weight during the adolescent and adult stages of the human lifecycle. The same is definitely not true, however, during infancy and early childhood, because most chubby babies and kids are fine. If they are truly overweight, then adjusting their food intake or exercise patterns will help them. During the early stages of the human lifecycle, the only real obstacle to predictable weight loss may be overweight parents who are unable to recognize the need to make healthful changes.

Time is a friend for chubby infants and young children. Six- to twelve-month-old babies normally accumulate more body fat than at any other time in their human lifecycle, until puberty ensues. This is why the "little Buddha" appearance is so common during the early months. As the human lifecycle progresses, plumpness diminishes because children start growing two to three inches in height every year, while their body fat remains stable.

Most children appear rather lean by the time they reach their fifth or sixth year. After that time, however, muscle mass as well as body fat begin to increase dramatically until the growth spurt at puberty. As a result, many boys and girls appear a bit chubby or husky just before they enter adolescence.

It is important to understand these earlier stages of the human lifecycle. Remember: The number of overweight children has doubled in the past twenty-five years. Nearly 40 percent of overweight seven-year-olds and 70 percent of overweight adolescents will turn into overweight adults. Although heredity is a powerful factor, it's important to realize that heaviness in the adulthood stages of the human lifecycle is not related to birth weight. If one or both parents are heavy, however, there is greater likelihood that an overweight infant or child will grow into an overweight adult. When it comes to heaviness, the type of adult we become is largely determined by our childhood habits.

What can parents do to prevent their children from becoming overweight? What is the best help parents can provide for children who are already overweight? It's relatively simple during the early stages of the human lifecycle. Breast-feed infants for at least six to twelve months. Avoid giving solid foods until six months. Never use a baby bottle as a pacifier. During the childhood stage of the human lifecycle, a more holistic approach is very helpful. It involves the entire family's eating habits, assuring regular exercise, building self-esteem, and controlling the amount of time that children watch television.

The Prenatal Stage of the Human Lifecycle

Your mother's fertilized egg divided into two identical cells within twenty-four hours of your conception. In the next twenty-four hours, the two cells divided into four cells, which also began to divide. By seventy-two hours, a sphere consisting of your first twelve cells began to form. It rolled down your mother's fallopian tube to enter her uterus and then implanted itself in the wall, where it would grow, over the next 265 days, into what would ultimately become you.

Do you ever wonder whether you were really meant to be alive? Albert Einstein answered the question by saying, "God does not play dice with the universe." Here are the approximate odds and the obstacles you had to surmount in order for you to come into this world: One special sperm out of 50 million had to reach one special egg from out of a quarter of a million that had been awaiting its arrival since the very day of your own mother's birth. Now, consider the fact that less than 20 percent of fertilized eggs ever reach the uterus, and that less than half successfully implant themselves within the uterus wall. What odds you overcame! What obstacles you transcended! But that was not the end of your early journey.

Once you were implanted in your mother's uterus as a microscopically small pre-embryo, a massive organization began to occur among your dividing cells. They became thousands, then millions, then tens and hundreds of millions of dividing cells. Within six weeks, your dividing cells formed islands of cells to create a primitive brain and spinal cord, then a rudimentary heart and circulatory system, and then an early type of skeleton. It is estimated that just 10 percent of all embryos are able to survive this very complex growth period.

After six weeks within your mother's uterus, your body developed very rapidly and became an embryo. Tiny outgrowths of cells became the beginnings of your arms and legs. Other groups of cells coalesced to start forming your esophagus, stomach, and intestines. Islands of other cells began growing into your eyes and ears. Miraculously, by the tenth week, your sex was evident and you were transformed into a tiny humanlike fetus, about one inch in length. By eighteen weeks, your brain had most of its cells, your mother felt your first movements, and you were well on your way to becoming a viable baby with a life expectancy, as a girl, of almost eighty years, and, as a boy, of seventy-five years.

In the womb, through a placenta and an umbilical cord, you received from your mother sufficient life-energy to sustain your human lifecycle. About ten days after implantation into her uterine wall, your mother's fertilized egg began developing into the marvelous structure called a placenta, to which you were attached via your umbilical cord. The placenta has two components—one from your mother and one from yourself. The maternal component was rich in blood vessels that delivered nourishment to you. Yours also was rich in vessels that carried blood to your organs and heart. These two circulatory systems do not normally mix with each other. They are separated by a thin layer of cells through which nutrients pass from mother to baby. Can you imagine how much life-energy your mother had to supply for you to sustain the first stage of your human lifecycle, driving your growth from a one-inch fetus at twenty-eight days to a twenty-inch infant at 270 days?

During the prenatal stage, it is impossible to overestimate the importance of good nutrition. Pregnant women need abundant amounts of fresh fruit, fresh juice, fresh vegetables, nuts, beans, lentils, and complex carbohydrates. They also require large amounts of water. How much? At least five servings of fresh fruit, five servings of fresh vegetables, and six to eight eight-ounce glasses of water a day. It is wise either to boil tap water or use bottled water if the chemical content of the local water supply is reported to be high.

Additionally, even if a pregnant woman eats well, it is crucial for her to take a daily multivitamin-mineral supplement. Recent studies indicate that the incidence of premature births is lower among women who take a daily supplement. Moreover, taking four hundred micrograms of folic acid daily helps to prevent up to 80 percent of the congenital spinal cord malformations called spina bifida.

By a true miracle of nature, even mothers suffering with malnutrition can produce healthy full-term babies. Certain hormones released within them cause their bodies to supply sufficient nourishment to the growing fetus, even when it detracts from their own survival.

It is the mother who can also help to resolve the major problems facing the prenatal stage of the human lifecycle, including infection, diabetes, alcohol, drug, and tobacco use. Exposure to second-hand smoke is dangerous, too. Even if only the father smokes during pregnancy, nicotine can be found in his newborn's hair. Radiation and exposure to environmental toxins also can be disastrous to the growing fetus. Consider what small doses of X-rays or toxins might do to a tiny bundle of cells undergoing rapid growth.

The current trend of using ultrasound to determine the sex of a fetus is also cause for concern. Routine ultrasound for an unborn baby is unnecessary. Why should a new growth industry influence prenatal care while we still don't know conclusively the effect of high frequency sound waves on the fetus? We may one day look back on such casual use of ultrasound with the same concern that we physicians experience when we look back just forty years ago, when it was common to use X-rays in shoe stores to fit shoes.

The amount of sunshine, fresh air and exercise that an expectant mother gets is important. So is her attitude. A fetus who shares his or her mother's body also shares her feelings and emotions. In fact, there is a new science called, Psycho-neuro-immunology, which actually demonstrates the ways that feelings and emotions affect all the cells of the body. What is on your mind and in your heart can help keep you well or make you sick. The intricate network of mind-body connections in pregnant women affects their babies, too. Growing humans in the prenatal stage experience their mother's stress as well as her gladness and joy.

Let's review some of what you have learned about the prenatal stage of the human lifecycle. First there was the cross-country race of sperm while the egg was jumping the Grand Canyon. Then there was the tumultuous six-week growth period, during which 90 percent of human lifecycles fail to survive. Thereafter, very many more human lifecycles could also come to an end during the remaining months of pregnancy. Surely you were meant to be!

You are already a winner. Despite all the obstacles, the mighty healing force within you has sustained your human lifecycle. Knowing this empowers you to take charge of the present stage of your life, no matter how old you are, including losing excess fat. You control your own health destiny to a far greater extent than you have ever been led to believe.

Total health rejuvenation ignites the healing force present in all your cells, which remembers wellness. What Hippocrates called *vix mediatrix*, the French call *le mileu interieur* and the English call homeostasis. It doesn't really matter what we call the force; perhaps it is just God's presence in each of your cells. What matters is that your body is a marvelous, self-repairing, complex energy system. Yes, you may have been overweight for a very long time, but your inner healing force has infinite patience. It is merely awaiting your resolution to *take charge of your own health destiny.*

The Infancy Stage of the Human Lifecycle

Babies require breast milk for optimal health. There's nothing like it. Unfortunately, generations of medical doctors, mostly men, have been trained not to urge mothers to breast-feed too much for fear of making them feel guilty if they don't breast-feed. Additionally, billions of dollars have been spent by the baby formula industry to offer subtle enticements to women not to breast-feed. There is a loud and clear message attached to the sample bottles and cans of baby formula given out freely by the most prestigious hospitals, even to contented breast-feeding mothers. "This is good. This is convenient. This is scientific. This is best."

The truth is that the benefits of breast-feeding for your baby's health go far beyond that which scientists can measure. We know that breast milk passes a mother's antibodies on to her baby, as well as nutrients that cannot be reproduced in formula. Through her breast milk, a mother helps protect her baby against infections during infancy. But how can scientists measure the vital emotional, psychological, and physical bonds that emerge between mother and baby during breast-feeding? How can science measure the positive, comforting feelings toward food and eating that are communicated to a breast-fed baby?

Breast milk is easier to digest than formula, and babies fed on breast milk are less likely to experience the gastrointestinal problems so common among "tube syndrome" babies. In a study of twenty thousand babies, those who were bottle fed experienced twice as many infections as their breast-fed counterparts. Some bottle-fed babies tend to sleep longer, because formula takes longer to digest. But the benefits of a baby who rests more are not as important as the health benefits a baby derives from breast milk. Breast-fed babies grow up to have lower cholesterol levels and lower rates of heart disease as adults; iron deficiency is less frequent in breast-fed babies; certain enzymes in breast milk have the power to lower the incidence of allergies, diarrhea, upper respiratory infections, otitis media, sinusitis, pneumonia, blood poisoning, meningitis, botulism, urinary tract infections, enterocolitis, and sudden death syndrome in both infants and children.

Overall, breast-fed babies become ill nearly half as frequently as bottle-fed babies. And finally, recent surveys indicate that breast-fed babies are less prone to becoming overweight adults. There is also strong evidence that breast-feeding decreases the incidence of diabetes, Crohn's disease, ulcerative colitis, and lymphoma during adulthood.

The energy in breast milk is live and pure, compared to the so-called high energy of artificial baby formulas. Along with added minerals and vitamins, baby formulas contain whey, nonfat milk, lactose, palm olein oil, soy oil, coconut oil, high oleic sunflower oil, carrageenan, monoglycerides, diglycerides, sodium chloride, potassium hydroxide, adenosine 5-monophosphate, cytidine 5-monophosphate, disodium guanosine 5-monophosphate, and disodium uridine 5-monophosphate. Not a single one of these ingredients possesses life-energy. Not even a mixture of one hundred times more of all of them could direct an ant's leg to move or a butterfly's wing to flutter. That requires life-energy.

Each stage of the human lifecycle benefits from the life-energy in breast milk. Breast-feeding definitely protects the mother by reducing her blood loss after birth and by improving her bone mineralization so that risk of hip fractures during menopause decreases. It also appears that the mother's risk of ovarian and breast cancer is lessened. When it comes to nutrition and nourishment—for babies as well as adults—nothing manufactured in a laboratory can ever match, let alone surpass, the goodness and vitality of food made by nature. This same principle applies to what we eat throughout our lives.

I am not suggesting that bottle feeding is wrong, or that mothers who bottle feed are bad, or that their children are doomed to a lifetime disadvantage. Many women are unable to breast-feed, and in these cases, commercially available formula is an adequate substitute for breast milk. But the healthiest nutritional beginnings come from breast milk. Like fast and convenience foods for adults, the makers of formulas promote their product not only as a way for a mother to save time, but as an anxiety-free way to keep track of how much a baby eats. It is an anxiety that they, the formula makers, have helped to create! It is simply not necessary to monitor exactly how much your baby eats. The breast-feeding mother and her baby develop a natural code of understanding as to when the baby is hungry and when the baby has had enough. Nothing is more assuring and comforting to a mother caring for her newborn than the knowledge that her baby is thriving and growing naturally.

Every physician should take a strong position on behalf of breast-feeding and work toward eliminating the standard hospital practice that discourages breast-feeding by giving away free infant formula packs at discharge. Dr. Oliver Wendell Holmes (1809–94) aptly noted: "A pair of substantial mammary glands has the advantage over two hemispheres of the most learned professor's brain in the art of compounding a nutritious fluid for infants."

The natural rate of growth during the infancy stage of the human lifecycle is about six ounces a week for the first six months. Birth weight then doubles at about four months of age and triples by about a year. Cow's milk should be particularly avoided during infancy. Soy milk, fresh juices, and even nut milk are good alternatives when the breast-feeding days are over. Solid foods do not need to be a part of a baby's menu until six months or later.

When it comes to solid foods, just remember that the later the better, the fresher the better, and the least amount of variety the better. Nutritionally, it's impossible to match the energy of foods prepared in your kitchen to that of the factory. Preparing fresh baby food is easy and convenient, and it saves money. Be sure to wait at least seven days before introducing another new food. Steaming food helps to preserve its vitamins and minerals. Parents can even feed their baby some of the food they are serving for their own meal if it's free of added salt, sugar, other spices, and fat.

Babies don't have an inborn preference for spices or fat. Nor should you encourage them to develop an early taste for salt, sugar, and other additives. Try a single grain cereal such as home-prepared rice cereal, or mash up some potato, squash, string beans, sweet potato, pumpkin, green peas, pear, apple, or banana, then serve it to your baby knowing that the food is free of the additives, spices, chemicals, and fillers found in factory-made baby foods. Making your own baby food, full of life-energy, doesn't require a lot of equipment: a clean pot to steam, boil, heat, simmer, or sauté food; a fork for mashing food to a soft, easy-to-swallow consistency, and a simple strainer to remove seeds and lumps is all you need.

The Childhood Stage of the Human Lifecycle

Toddlers want to eat more and more like Mom and Dad. This is the perfect time for parents to involve children in food preparation, from helping to mash a banana or a baked apple to shopping together to pick out the reddest tomato. Now is the time to educate children as to what is good for them and what is not, before television does the job for you. Teach them the difference between good and not-so-good bread by having them squeeze the soft white kind and saying "Yuck!" and the firm dark variety while saying "Yum!" Teach them how good it is to drink water instead of soft drinks, tell them about the goodness of fresh fruit juice. Mostly, don't instill in them the idea that if they eat more, you will love them more. Don't bring junk food into the house. Your children are what they eat, and they will emulate their parents' eating preferences—what to eat as well as how to eat.

Good childhood nutrition is a holistic adventure comprised of equal parts nurture, nourishment, and nutrition. Besides good food, it's about sunshine, love, family, fresh air, cleanliness, prayer, and self-discovery. Parents can teach children as young as two or three years old that food is energy that makes them happy, healthy, and strong. You can show them colorful apples, bananas, carrots, or tomatoes, then explain that they all give us strength because they grow on trees or underneath the soil, outside in the sunshine, and in nature. You can show them a potato that comes from the soil and a potato chip that comes from the factory, then explain that one contains life-energy and the other does not. You can show them a glass of water and a glass of cola, explaining how one flows healthily in rivers and streams, while the other does not. You can compare the feel and texture of a slice of grainy whole wheat bread with that of a slice of white bread containing dead energy.

Everyone talks about the need for five servings of fruit and five servings of vegetables a day. How realistic is that? As it turns out, not very! According to recent surveys, only 20 percent of our children and teenagers have five servings of fruit and vegetables per day. Moreover, only one percent follow the general governmental guidelines for nutrition. It is realistic, though, not to buy junk food, and to continually reinforce how wonderful fresh fruit and vegetables are. Serve lots of carrots, sweet potatoes, and green peas. Have fun with spaghetti squash. Make a meal out of a baked potato. But keep in mind: french fries should not be counted as a vegetable serving!

Fish and poultry can be introduced after the first year. Red meat is just not necessary and should be eaten sparingly, if at all. Buy good food that is full of life-energy, insist on family meals, complete with conversation, and don't serve food while watching television. Everyone should be sitting while they eat, taking care not to gobble down their food. Make eating healthy and fun; your children will remember this throughout all the later stages of their human life-cycles.

Celebrate summer with watermelons. Don't forget to introduce special foods such as pumpkins when autumn approaches. Make sure to call attention to ordinary foods when they are at the height of their season, so that your children can understand the taste of a really special tomato in summer as compared to the bland, genetically engineered variety. Always point out to growing children how much they are helping themselves to become healthy and strong by eating foods from nature as close as possible to the way nature first offered them.

Encourage your children to eat what you serve, but never coerce them to eat by pleading or showing anxiety or annoyance. Never, ever broadcast the subtle notion that you would love your children more if only they would eat more. The childhood stage of the human lifecycle is initially associated with a decrease in appetite, as the natural growth rate slows to about one and one-half ounces weight gain per week during the second year of life—just about 30 percent of the growth rate during the infancy stage of the human lifecycle. As iron deficiency commonly occurs about this time, consider iron supplementation as a solution.

The nutritional needs of babies and children change as they develop through the human lifecycle. Foods containing life-energy support the ability to develop clear vision and fine movement, so that a growing baby can begin to use its fingers, then its hands, to grasp objects, and soon will be able to pass a toy block from one hand to the other. The baby will start to lift its head, sit up unsupported, roll over from front to back and back to front, crawl and, finally, walk. Hearing and speech develop as the baby babbles away, imitates sounds, says a few words like "ma-ma, da-da," and even links words together to form a simple sentence: "I love you." Social awareness develops as the baby smiles or cries, behaves in uneasy or friendly ways with strangers, makes eye contact, gurgles, laughs, and grows more alert.

The concept, *we are what we eat*, along with my recommendations for proper nutrition during the early stages of the human lifecycle, are also crucial to understanding weight loss, no matter how old you are.

Older babies and toddlers need a wholesome, single grain (not mixed) cereal, a few fresh fruits and some vegetables, not milk from a cow, food from a jar, or complicated main courses. Why spend a dollar on a jar of organic mashed carrots when you can mash less expensive, fresh carrots yourself? Toddlers thrive on a variety of whole grains, including breads, cereals, rice, and pasta, along with many kinds of fresh fruits and lots of vegetables. Older children thrive (and stay lean) by eating plenty of fresh fruits, vegetables, whole grains, and complex carbohydrates like good breads, pasta, rice, and potatoes.

By all means, it is important for parents to avoid turning mealtime into a battleground. Forcing children to be "clean-platers" only backfires later in the human lifecycle. Many children are picky eaters but still grow well despite that fact. During the early stages of the human lifecycle, nutrition doesn't really get a whole lot more complicated than this.

The natural growth rate of the human lifecycle slows down during the childhood stage, until puberty begins. During this time, children build strong food preferences as they increasingly develop more control over what they will or will not eat. Because the eating patterns established in childhood will last forever, a holistic approach here is vital. Believe it or not, osteoporosis, irritable bowel syndrome, diabetes, and atherosclerosis are pediatric diseases; this is when they begin.

For a growing child to achieve increasing degrees of independence for the next stages of the human lifecycle, he or she will experience tremendous physical and emotional changes. Obviously, it is important for these changes to occur in an environment of love and security. Quality time between children and parents is essential, particularly talking, eating, playing, and reading. The basic holistic approach to raising healthy children who are not overweight, and preparing them for the next phase of the human lifecycle, requires good sense. It's all about instilling healthy habits. Get children outside to play when it's daylight and the weather permits. Hats, scarves, boots, and mittens help to stretch the limits of "permissible."

Don't use the television as a baby-sitter. Limit watching TV to an hour or two at most on any day, and make sure that the show is not violent or sexual in content. Better still, get rid of the TV. Children who spend a lot of time sitting on the couch watching television are more than likely to be overweight. Actually, in the last three decades, TV has been the leading factor in weight gain among children. Kids and teenagers now spend on average more time sitting in front of the television than they do in school. Being sedentary most of the day, instead of running around and burning off excess energy takes its toll. *Energy that is not burned is converted to fat.*

A landmark study published by Dr. Steven L. Gortmaker and his colleagues at the Harvard School of Public Health examined the relationship between the amount of time spent watching television and the prevalence of obesity among ten- to fifteen-year-olds. The results were startling. There was more than a 500 percent increase in the rate of obesity among youths watching more than five hours of television per day, compared with those who watched for two hours or less per day. The study found that the average child watched television 4.8 hours per day, or thirty-four hours per week. Only 11 percent of the youths watched television for less than two hours per day.

This Harvard study was conducted in 1990. Now, a decade later, the numbers are considerably higher. Each hour spent sitting in front of the television means one less hour of hopping, skipping, jumping, running, playing tag, baseball, or just hide-and-seek. The lack of vigorous physical activity in kids is as alarming as their generally poor nutrition. To add insult to injury, while they are sitting in front of the TV, kids are bombarded with thousands of commercials that seduce them into making poor food choices, forever.

Believe it or not, the most important thing that parents can do to prevent obesity in children is to *turn off the television!* The Harvard study also showed that if your child or teenager is already overweight, each hour he or she spends watching television increases the odds of remaining overweight by 130 percent. Although the American Academy of Pediatrics recommends that television be limited to no more than two hours per day, I believe even less would be good. And none is best.

Spending half an hour at bedtime or an hour during the day reading to a young child is rewarding for child and parent alike. Children fondly remember reading time, and time spent playing games with parents, throughout their entire life. Reading should be fun, not a task; make it interactive by letting your child read to you, too. These are the times that become ingrained memories that enhance self-esteem and begin to pay big dividends as young people enter adolescence. Here's a fun poem to share, especially at bedtime:

> The more you read,
> the more you know;
> the more you know,
> the further you go.

Whatever happened to playing cards, chess, or checkers during quiet times? What about hobbies—collecting stamps, baseball cards, or coins? What about jigsaw puzzles? Jumping rope? What about reading a book? If your kids are not in school, then they should be outside playing and running around as long as there is daylight. If it's too cold out, visit the local library or be active indoors.

Make no mistake about it, obesity is the most significant childhood disease of our time. More than a third of children and teens are overweight, and the numbers are rising. While genetics may predispose some kids to plumpness, most are getting fat because they don't exercise and eat too much of the wrong kinds of foods. Fifty years ago, most plump kids would have outgrown their weight problem because they would be outside playing tag or climbing trees, but that is not happening today.

Another major reason children become overweight is because of malnutrition. I'm not talking about the malnutrition that comes from starvation or famine but its modern form that comes from overeating, eating too much dead food, or both. Being overweight is a terrible disease for kids. Besides the fact that it sets them up for many adult diseases, it detracts from the very joy of childhood. Many overweight kids are called lazy, but it is really their excess fat that limits them. In other words, they easily lose their breath and suffer from all sorts of discomfort.

Also, there is the emotional trauma of being ridiculed and called names. As a result, kids withdraw, become depressed, and fall behind in school. Losing weight, however, can have a dramatic effect. Not only do children feel better and become more physically agile, they gain self-esteem, improve in school, and develop more friendships. Diets can help kids lose weight, but they are rarely successful in keeping the fat off later on.

Cow's Milk Is for Baby Cows

I am sure the following paragraphs will surprise you, since you have been taught to believe that cow's milk is essential for your good health. One of the major causes of malnutrition, however, is cow's milk. Don't get me wrong: Cow's milk is wonderful food; that is, if you are a baby cow. Facing this issue during the early stages of the human lifecycle is the key to preventing a terrible disease that occurs in the last stage of the human lifecycle: osteoporosis. In fact, osteoporosis is a pediatric disease, because it is during childhood that we are trained to believe in the necessity of cow's milk.

Cow's milk should be kept to an absolute minimum, especially after the first year of life. Many prominent medical doctors have tried to inform the public that dairy consumption contributes to acne, allergy, anemia, asthma, bronchitis, dental cavities, diarrhea, ear infections, eczema, sinusitis, osteoporosis, and atherosclerosis. Flip through the pages of many major medical journals and you will find research linking cow's milk to sudden infant death syndrome, childhood cancer, and diabetes mellitus. Contrary to what the commercials tell you, cow's milk is not good for your health.

Doctors have been all to slow to recognize and accept the truth about milk. Frank Oski, M.D., the late director of the Department of Pediatrics at the John Hopkins University School of Medicine, devoted a major part of his career to trying to inform physicians that the consumption of large amounts of cow's milk is unhealthy. Dr. Oski had his hand in over twenty medical textbooks, including several that are still the standard at most U.S. medical schools. Yet, at the time of his death, in 1996, too many medical doctors still ignored his concern about cow's milk. The story is similar to the experience of Dr. Ignaz Semmelweiss, who pleaded with physicians to wash their hands before delivering babies or conducting surgery . . . a plea that was widely ignored until the turn of the 20th century!

We have been taught to believe that children need cow's milk for health and strength. Adults believe they need cow's mild to prevent bone weakness. The marketing here is so successful that one dollar of every seven spent for food in the United States goes for milk and dairy products. Indeed, we now regard milk ads almost as public service announcements. These ads don't tell us that the milk of humans, cows, elephants, camels, wolves, walruses, and yaks are different. The milk of each mammalian species differs a great deal in its content because nature designed each type of milk to provide optimum nutrition for the young of that species. This is why in many parts of the world, particularly in East Asia, Africa, and South America, people regard cow's milk as unfit for human consumption.

Before we can absorb lactose into the bloodstream, the primary sugar in cow's milk, it must be broken down by the lactase enzyme. Far more people are unable to digest lactose than are able to digest it because most children gradually lose the lactase in their intestines by the time they are four years old. This is a normal process that accompanies the progression of the human lifecycle. As many as 75 percent of people at every age with low levels of lactase will experience cramping pain, gas, or diarrhea after drinking just one glass of milk. The worldwide prevalence of lactase deficiency according to Dr. Oski, may surprise you:

- Japanese 85 percent
- Chinese 85 percent
- Arabs 78 percent
- Ashkenazic Jews 78 percent

- African-Americans 70 percent
- Peruvians (as representative of South Americans) 70 percent
- American Indians 50 percent
- American Caucasians 15 percent

It is no wonder that Dr. Oski wrote, "Being against cow's milk is equated with being un-American. Yet, the milk of each species appears to have been specifically designed to protect the young of that species. Cross-feeding does not work."

He continues: "Since the human infant was never supposed to drink cow's milk in the first place, it is not surprising that they are most vulnerable. And since no other animal drinks milk after it has tripled its birth weight or has been weaned (except perhaps domesticated house cats), it is not surprising that the drinking of cow's milk after one to two years of age will produce disease. What is surprising is how frequently cow's milk does produce disturbances and how long it has taken for the medical profession to recognize this factor."

Preventing children from becoming unhealthy and overweight during the early stages of the human lifecycle requires a comprehensive, holistic approach—changing the ways kids think, move, and eat, not just for a few months but for life. Parents can make a tremendous investment in their children's health by reducing the role of dairy products in their life.

The Adolescent Stage of the Human Lifecycle

The onset of puberty in American children is occurring earlier than ever. Adolescence now begins in girls between the ages of eight and ten, and in boys between nine and eleven. Times are changing!

Developing breasts and a dramatic growth spurt are most often the first signs of puberty in girls. Pubic hair tends to appear about a year later as the uterus, ovaries, and vagina grow progressively larger. Menarche, the time of the first menses, usually occurs between 11 and 13 years of age. For boys, the first sign of puberty is an increase in the size of their testicles, which double, even quadruple, in size. At the same time that their testicles are growing, the skin of their scrotum reddens and wrinkles. Pubic hair appears soon thereafter. About a year later, the penis enlarges and, during the next year or two, facial hair starts to grow and the voice deepens.

Until this century, the menstrual cycle was thought to relate to the twenty-eight-day lunar cycle. Women in most other parts of the world still believe this to be true. Scientists now know that hormones regulate the menstrual cycle. Interestingly, groups of women living or working together often synchronize their periods. Scientists say this is because the primitive part of the female brain unconsciously detects almost imperceptible changes in the body odor of surrounding females and adopts accordingly.

A girl's growth spurt usually occurs at the very beginning of puberty, peaks at around twelve years old, then continues until about sixteen. A boy's growth spurt generally begins about two years after the onset of puberty, when his penis is already well developed and his testicles are producing sperm. Male growth peaks at about fourteen years old, then continues until about seventeen years old.

During no other time in the human lifecycle, other than the infancy stage, is growth so rapid. Visible growth usually begins with the hands and feet. Then there is rapid growth of the legs and spine. Energy requirements increase dramatically. This explains why teenage boys are seen so often with their heads in the refrigerator, trying to eat everything in sight.

At this stage, girls are gaining fat, as they are supposed to. It is also at this time that girls are bombarded with social messages to closely monitor their weight and fear fat. At the beginning of the human lifecycle, boys and girls are born with the same amount of body fat. But by six weeks, girls normally develop more body fat than boys, so that by one year girls have about 10 to 12 percent more body fat than boys. This normal body fat difference is fairly constant until early adolescence, when girls' normal body fat percentages begin to rise to 30 percent to 35 percent more than boys', and then stay at that level during the height of their reproductive stage. Female body fat does not normally lessen until about the age of thirty, when it levels off to about 20 to 25 percent more than men.

Junk food and adolescence have become synonymous. The best thing parents can do is to take control over what is served at meals and what is available at home for snacks. They should also do whatever they can to encourage physical exertion. It's important to have already prepared the groundwork for healthful eating *before* adolescense sets in. Otherwise, hot dogs, hamburgers, colas, french fries, and pepperoni pizza may be as good as it gets. In any case, this is the ideal time to strengthen the amount of healthy fiber in the diet by having plenty of fresh fruits and vegetables around the house.

Dramatic changes in body shape and composition are primarily controlled by male and female sex hormones, androgens in boys and estrogens in girls. The most obvious changes in boys are the increase in muscle mass, the widening of the shoulders, the growth of the heart and lungs, and the decrease in body fat, allowing boys to better adapt to more strenuous work. Indeed, by the end of adolescence, boys are about 50 percent stronger physically than girls. In girls, the hips widen, body fat increases, and breasts develop, as preparations for renewal of the cycle of life through yet another generation.

Infants sleep about sixteen to eighteen hours a day. Children younger than five years old sleep about twelve to fourteen hours a day, and then about ten to twelve hours until puberty. At puberty, both boys and girls experience a marked decrease in their sleep requirements, to about only eight hours a day. Additionally, boys begin ejaculating sperm while they sleep, as if they, too, are preparing to do their part in the renewal of the human cycle of life.

Nature's Code

Before continuing on with the adult stages of the human lifecycle, it is important for you to gain a deeper perspective on how the human body functions—especially the ways that it uses and stores energy. This is the key to achieving permanent weight loss. Examining the natural human lifecycle allows you to understand the normal changes you should expect during the stages of your time on earth. More importantly, it cannot help but cause you to be in awe of your own body.

Your mother's and father's fused genetic material, DNA, has controlled the phases and rhythms of your body from your conception up until now, no matter how old you are. From the time of your conception to the present moment, your inner healing force has been so resolute that it has conquered untold numbers of obstacles you may have encountered along the way. This is because your personal human lifecycle is an integral component of nature's code, which controls everything under the sun . . . and under other suns!

Nature's code is so vast and incomprehensible that we cannot even begin to conceive of where it all begins and where it ends. Apparently, our galaxy alone contains over 400 billion suns, and the entire universe contains at least 600 billion galaxies, with that many more suns. We have no idea how big infinity might be. The entire universe that is familiar to us might be equivalent to just one mere atom, with planets orbiting around suns much as electrons of atoms orbit around their nucleus. Nor do we know how small the smallest object might be. The infinitesimally tiny quarks present in atoms may themselves contain a universe of even smaller objects.

The infinitesimal and the infinite elude us. But however big or small the universe is, nature's code regulates all of its components.

Science has actually measured some of these components, which are called natural laws. If you are overweight, then you have thwarted certain natural laws. The information contained in this book will help you work with nature's code rather than against it. The fact that there are so many thousands of failed diet strategies is a testimony to the power of what we call the *Natural Laws of Thermodynamics*.

Everything Is Energy

The First Law of Thermodynamics is based on the conservation of energy. This law states that energy can neither be created nor destroyed. Albert Einstein discovered that energy constantly transforms into mass while mass constantly transforms into energy. In a phrase, everything is energy, or can be converted into energy. The energy in food is converted into the actual substance of your body. Thus, according to this natural law, *you really are what you eat*.

Any food you eat in excess of your body's energy needs is stored—and mostly as fat. It is an exercise in futility to try to avoid this law; energy cannot be created or destroyed. If you consume too much food energy, or too much of the wrong type of food energy, your body must either (1) burn off the excess energy with exercise; (2) eliminate the excess energy through its lungs, skin, kidneys, or intestines; or (3) store the excess energy as fat.

You are a complex energy system. Did you know that once your body stores excess energy as fat, it then attempts to conserve the fat for some future time of famine or starvation? Is this a defense mechanism that came into play during evolution, when famine and starvation for our cave-dwelling ancestors were common dangers? At the moment we do not know for sure. But we do know that the body tends to burn away its healthy muscle before it burns away its stored-up fat.

The purest type of fuel, that which contains life-energy, can by-pass your body's natural defenses to conserve its fat. This is why deprivation and dieting are not effective means of permanent weight loss. The most effective way to lose your stored-up fat permanently is to consume foods bursting with life-energy and to engage in regular exercise. This is the combination that stokes your body's internal furnace and gives it the fuel it needs to burn excess fat.

Life-energy is highest in foods that are grown in the soil, that are fresh, and are as close to their natural state as possible. Processed, refined, irradiated, microwaved, and fake foods are stripped of fat-burning life-energy. The Food Energy Ladder, described in Part Six, will help you understand which foods are dead energy.

Everything Falls Apart

The Second Law of Thermodynamics is based on entropy. Simply stated, the law of entropy means that everything eventually falls apart. Entropy is the force that makes all energy systems fall apart. This is why everything in nature, including the human body, breaks down with age.

Everyone who has reached the middle adulthood stage of the human lifecycle, especially those over age fifty, will know what entropy means. Entropy causes the human body to experience its natural decline in concert with all of nature, so that nature, can replenish itself. Just as leaves fall from the trees in autumn so that new leaves can come back in spring, entropy causes the physical substance of your body to eventually return to the vast storehouse of universal energy from which it came.

The plant kingdom captures the life-force of the sun to help human bodies slow down entropy. Nature sustains the human cycle of life with plant-based foods that are steeped in sunlight and infused with the energy of the soil and rain—pure life-energy. We know that plants utilize the energy of sunlight in a process called photosynthesis to create the oxygen that is crucial to the very survival of the human species. It is not surprising that nature also sustains the human lifecycle by offering it the very essence of its life-energy through vegetables, fruits, nuts, lentils, beans, and grains.

Animal-based and artificially created foods contain little sunlight. They have poor life-energy and tend to hasten entropy. Of course, flesh food and animal products are essential for humans living in less temperate climates, such as extremely hot or cold places, where the availability of plant-based food is limited.

We can slow down entropy by eating foods that are full of life-energy. How and when we eat is also critically important. The added ingredient to every meal must be patience and care in its preparation, as well as in its consumption. Believe it or not, when we eat with calm and appreciation, it helps our body change food into healthful energy that can then be used to burn up excess fat. Slowing down and being aware of what we are eating also helps us eat less, because we realize when we have eaten enough, instead of rushing to stuff as much food as we can into our stomachs.

Just think of the fact that your food enables you to see, hear, touch, breathe, grow, and love. Surely eating deserves a moment of wonder! I first realized this while wandering through the farmers' markets near Bellagio, Italy. There, local farmers and gardeners rent booths to sell their fresh foods daily. The fruits and vegetables are so fresh, in fact, that the ripe soil still clings to the tomato vines. In these markets, the colors are overwhelming; neon green apples still attached to their stems, tomatoes a brilliant orange-red, onions purple and sweet enough to eat like fruit, peaches dripping with juice. Combining these foods together in a bowl is like serving up rainbows.

Body Time

We have been discussing *what* to eat and *how* to eat, but learning *when* to eat is equally important. The human body processes its food in certain ways to best extract and utilize its energy. This means that it naturally gathers, assimilates, and eliminates its energy in rhythm with the rising and setting of the sun. All three of these bodily functions mix together to some degree, but they are most natural and most intense during three distinct phases of the day.

After all, the human lifecycle is part of nature, in which such rhythms occur in all living things. Your body thrives by ingesting the food it requires for energy from about noon until 8:00 P.M. Your body functions best by assimilating its food and extracting its energy from about 8:00 P.M. until 4:00 A.M. From about 4:00 A.M. until noontime, your body's natural inclination is to eliminate yesterday's waste products and food debris as well as take in high-energy fuel to start the day. Let's look at these phases more closely.

REJUVENATING AND REPLENISHING
(Noon–8:00 P.M.)

You can slow down entropy with foods that are full of life-energy. The best time to supply your body with the fuel needed to sustain the human lifecycle is between noon and 8:00 P.M. These are the healthiest hours of the day in which to eat substantial meals. It is best to have at least one meal consisting almost entirely of life-energy during this time; for instance, a lunch of vegetables in a salad or a soup, or both, perhaps with some good bread. If you are still hungry, it would be good to have a heartier meal of life-energy by combining complex carbohydrates like rice, pasta, or potatoes, with vegetables. Americans usually prefer to eat their heartier meal at dinner. Europeans prefer it at lunch.

Remember, dead foods actually deplete your body of its own life-energy. This occurs because your body must use its life-energy to get rid of and excrete dead food. Unfortunately, this energy is no longer available to your body to help bring itself into healthier balance and to burn off excess fat. If you are overweight, your body needs all the life-energy it can get to retain its balance and burn off its fat.

RESTING AND REBALANCING
(8:00 P.M.–4:00 A.M.)

During the later part of the evening, from about 8:00 P.M. to about 4:00 A.M., your body assimilates what you have eaten by absorbing it into its cells and fluids to sustain your metabolic needs. Depending on the type and amount that you eat, food can remain in your stomach for about four hours, so it is important to finish eating by 8:00 P.M. to give your body the chance to do its work. For proper absorption, food needs to leave your stomach and enter your intestines.

During the night, as the body goes into its natural fasting pattern, people can go without eating for almost twelve hours without feeling hunger. Bodily rest is important during this phase of the day. If you feel you must have something to eat after 8:00 P.M., it is best to limit your choice to fresh fruit or vegetables. If your work schedule necessitates it, eat at least two hours before bedtime.

Finally, if you have an occasional evening out for fine dining (or even some not-so-fine dining), it's okay! Remember, *everything in moderation—including moderation.* You will find, however, that as you age and the force of entropy builds in your body, the pleasures of the past become the pains of the present. Haven't you noticed that the later you eat and the more you eat, the more lethargic and muddle-headed you feel in the morning? In any case, just following the natural daily cycles of your body is a wonderful strategy for becoming healthier, happier, more energetic, and leaner.

REAWAKENING AND ELIMINATING
(4:00 A.M.–Noon)

Eat mostly fresh fruit and drink mostly fresh fruit juice from the time you wake up until noon. You may eat as much fresh fruit and drink as much fresh juice as you wish. If you remain hungry, some foods are more suitable than others, as discussed later.

Having only fresh fruit and fresh juice from the time you wake in the morning until about noontime is the single most important way to kick-start yourself to a healthier, happier, more energized, and leaner future. Fresh fruit and fresh juice demand the least amount of energy for digestion because they are filled with so much life-energy. While the typical American breakfast leaves you stuffed and ready for a nap, fresh fruit will give you a lasting surge of energy to help your body eliminate its wastes and burn its excess fat.

From about 4:00 A.M. until noon, your body processes the wastes and debris of the food you consumed the day before by eliminating them. Digestion, of course, takes more energy than any other bodily function. Most foods that people eat during their natural morning elimination cycle also tend to deplete their energy; for example, bacon, eggs, and toast slathered in butter. These foods seriously interfere with the orderly process of your body's elimination cycle. Couple this with the slow production of digestive fluids such as saliva, stomach acid, pancreatic secretions, and bile—our fasting nighttime metabolism—and you will see why you can interfere with your body's waste removal mechanisms—if you continually eat outside of the general guidelines that are best for your body's natural functioning.

We are consuming more food that nourishes us less and leaves behind much more residue and debris in our intestines. People who eat food full of life-energy tend to be healthier and leaner. People who don't are, among other things, constipated! It seems as if having regular bowel movements is an old-fashioned concept, but it's isn't. A major function of our intestines is to process our food into a firm, well-formed, mildly odorous stool and then expel it from the body daily. Constipation is one of the most prevalent conditions that contributes to lethargy, moodiness, and disease.

The body eliminates waste products in a variety of ways, including breathing through your lungs, perspiring through your skin, urinating via your kidneys, and discharging leftover food debris in your stools. One of the very best things you can do to move the waste process along is to limit your intake of flesh foods to no more than once every three days. Why? It takes the body about seventy-two hours for the debris from the last consumption of flesh to pass through your intestines.

Constipation contributes to obesity, lethargy, moodiness, sexual dysfunction, backache, irritable bowel syndrome, colitis, and other diseases. Dairy also causes constipation, especially after age and entropy set in. Substitute sugars, particularly in diet soft drinks, cause constipation. Excess animal protein causes constipation. Plant food is steeped in sunlight; it's as if you're eating and absorbing the very rays of the sun. Flesh food captures very little sunlight, which is why it quickly rots, outside as well as inside your body. George Bernard Shaw quipped: "Think of the force concentrated in an acorn. You bury it in the ground and it explodes into a great oak. Bury a sheep and nothing happens but decay."

All sorts of refined, processed, irradiated, factory-made, and genetically engineered foods cause constipation. If you feel like napping after you eat, it's probably because your meal actually drained your body's available energy to digest food that is so poorly digestible. It also depletes the energy the body needs to discharge its wastes. The human body, which has survived countless generations of evolution, is apparently stymied by products such as diet colas.

Our grandparents were right when they said it was important to stay regular. The body is a complex and integrated energy system; what affects one part of the body affects its other parts. It is ludicrous to think that years of constipation—the buildup of residue and waste in the intestines—is of no serious health consequence. Regularly accumulating several pounds of solid waste that stagnates in the colon is not compatible with performing daily activities with a great deal of zest!

The best ways to avoid or overcome constipation while supporting your body's elimination cycle are simple:

- Get regular exercise
- Ingest more fiber-containing food or take a fiber supplement

- Drink at least six to eight glasses of liquids a day, preferably water, juices, and herbal teas
- Eat mostly fruit until noon

Hippocrates Would Agree

Health, as Hippocrates knew, and as modern medical scientists must know again, is a matter of energy, of energy in balance. Being overweight in this regard, is an illness, a sign that energy is out of balance. Your body is a complex energy system that seeks to maintain its healthy equilibrium at all times by staying in energy balance. *Your body remembers wellness.*

Your body requires food for energy. If you consume more food energy than your body needs, it must either burn it, eliminate it, or store it. It naturally burns foods that contain pure life-energy. It stores up the impure energy of other foods in its attempt to maintain energy balance. *Your body tries to stay well.* When you store up too much fat there comes a time when you begin to look and feel overweight. Eventually, your body is no longer able to maintain its energy balance and dynamic equilibrium. *Your body becomes ill.*

But how many extra pounds does it take before your body becomes unhealthily overweight? Unfortunately, current weight standards are notoriously inaccurate and overly restrictive. They don't take into account perfectly normal, sex-related, and age-related weight gain!

Considerably lower weight standards have arbitrarily been proscribed to women, without any evidence proving that women stay healthier or live longer by weighing so much less than men of the same height and stature. Men's current visions of female attractiveness, rather than true science, have decreed that women should be so much slimmer than men. Furthermore, normal fat accumulation during the later stages of the human lifecycle in both men and women has been roundly ignored by the accountants and actuaries who helped to develop the standard height and weight tables— standards based on life insurance company statistics that measure longevity rather than health and quality of life values.

Traditionally, obesity was defined this way: as 20 percent or more above the optimal weight for height derived from life insurance company tables that correlate with the lowest death rates. New numbers that account for some normal weight gain with aging are partially replacing those statistics. Currently, it is also believed that where your extra fat is located is more important than the actual total amount of extra fat in your body. Hip and thigh fat is thought to be healthier than abdominal fat, because the former travels through the general blood circulation to take care of your metabolic needs, while the fat in a potbelly goes straight to the liver and interferes with its ability to clear insulin from your bloodstream. Higher levels of blood insulin can then cause cells to become insulin-resistant, which results in elevated blood sugar level. Supposedly, in response to the elevated blood sugar, your pancreas secretes more insulin, which prompts your autonomic nervous system to produce adrenalinelike chemicals, which then sets the stage for you to develop diabetes, hypertension, and heart disease.

Sound like gobbledygook? All or some of the above theory may or may not be true. I try to be skeptical about such scientific statements. I began studying the history of science at a very young age and was taught early on to maintain a state of permanent doubt. All we truly know is this: when our body's energy is in balance, we are generally healthy and well. Conversely, when our energy is out of balance, we are generally sick and tired or overweight.

Because each of your fat cells can balloon up to more than ten times its original size and then divide, when necessary, to make new fat cells, your body has an immense capacity to store extra fat. That is why the human body can get bigger and bigger, as well as heavier and heavier. Perhaps it's an evolutionary holdover from the days when our ancestors huddled together in cold caves, ready at all times to use stored-up energy in order to outrun saber-toothed tigers.

Furthermore, *obesity* and *overweight* are arbitrary terms. There is no absolutely standard definition for either, and there probably never will be. It's all relative because every added pound of body fat is not a threat to health. Actually, in otherwise healthy individuals, there is a relatively healthy "safe zone" of about ten to fifteen pounds above their "best common sense weight when looking in the mirror." Fat cells also become less metabolically active as the levels of our sex hormones change, particularly in women. This means that excess fat becomes a lot more difficult to burn off, even with exercise. Fortunately, the human body adjusts and allows us to gain weight with age and still be healthy. Carrying around some extra pounds as we age is perfectly normal!

The definition of obesity should expand to meet two important new criteria. Healthy weight standards should increase steadily throughout the stages of the human lifecycle. In the real world, gaining one-half to three-quarters of a pound a year (five to seven-and-a-half pounds a decade), from age twenty-five years to sixty-five years, is usually within healthy limits (unless, at twenty-five, you are already overweight). So if, as a woman, your "youthful weight" was 120 pounds at age twenty-five, you might healthfully weigh as much as 150 pounds by the time you turn sixty-five. A man who weighed 160 pounds at age twenty-five could healthfully weigh as much as 190 pounds at age sixty-five.

Furthermore, there should be an approximate 20 percent increase in the healthy weight standards for women throughout adulthood when compared to men of the same height. In other words, most of the current height and weight tables should be adjusted, so that if a woman's ideal weight is listed as 130 pounds compared to 160 pounds for a male of the same height, then the thirty-pound difference should be increased by six pounds, to make 136 pounds the more ideal weight for the woman.

The National Institutes of Health recently announced a new set of numbers defining healthy and unhealthy body weights. According to the federal government, 55% of Americans or about 97 million American adults are overweight. The numbers are calculated by using a formula known as the body mass index (BMI), which measures weight in relation to height. The announcement also noted that obesity leads to more preventable deaths than all other causes, except smoking.

The new governmental guidelines are a mixed blessing. On the one hand, the numbers remind us how serious the epidemic of excess weight is in the United States. In response to the announcement, researcher James O. Hill at the University of Colorado, blamed the American environment: too much food available, too many people who eat too much of the available food, and too much technology making it too easy to avoid exercise. The negative side of the new guidelines is that they do a clear disservice to women in general, and to individuals who are in the later stages of the human lifecycle. The BMI is a single number that represents height and weight without regard to gender or age. Clearly, we are not all young male athletes!

Being overweight, then, is related to heredity, environment, attitude, how much we eat, what we eat, and our age, gender and level of physical activity. Heredity is an exceptionally important determinant of how much we weigh as well. Some people are simply more prone to weight gain than others, even when their food intake and levels of physical activity are the same. In the last decade, I have watched my wife eat more than I do and exercise less, yet maintain her weight exactly as it was ten years ago, while I have gained about seven pounds during that time. Many other people are even less fortunate, those who seem to gain weight simply by looking at food. Here, genetic factors, apart from diet or lifestyle, strongly influence how much a person weighs. How much does the genetic factor contribute to being overweight? Approximately 25 percent.

Because nutritional science teaches that all calories are created equal, it is crucial for you to understand the heredity factor as well as some simple arithmetic. For instance we have believed that approximately four thousand excess calories will convert into one pound of fat, and that's that! We are taught that the human body has certain basal metabolic needs that require a certain amount of calories for fuel. Beyond such metabolic needs, we commonly believe that the body requires extra calories to fuel any unusual physical activities. However, every four thousand extra calories consumed is supposed to result in a one-pound weight gain. Conversely, every four thousand fewer calories consumed is supposed to result in a one-pound weight loss. The standard thinking is as follows:

- Assume that an individual requires about two thousand calories a day to maintain his or her healthy weight, with neither weight gain nor weight loss, during a day of routine physical activity.

- Therefore, if the individual eats an extra four hundred calories a day, without an increase in physical activity, he or she will gain an extra pound of fat in ten days (400 calories × 10 days = 4,000 calories = 1 pound of fat).
- Conversely, if the person eats just 1,600 calories a day, in ten days he or she will lose one pound of fat.

This simple notion and arithmetic is the basis for most standard nutritional teachings, diet books, and medical treatment plans to lose weight. Over the years, this formula has misled me into counseling thousands of dieting patients (mostly women) that if they weren't losing three pounds a month by eating 400 fewer calories than the daily requirements, they were just not telling the truth about how much they were really eating. I'm embarrassed by how bad I must have made my patients feel before I knew better. The whole theory is wrong!

The theory is wrong because heredity plays an influential role and all calories are *not* created equal in terms of their effect on your body. Identical twins have the exact same genetic makeup, whereas fraternal twins do not. Studies of fraternal twins eating large amounts of food show that in three months, some will gain ten pounds, while others will gain more than twenty pounds. On the other hand, the weight of identical twins, even when raised apart from each other, varies hardly at all. There may even be a recessive obesity gene. This means that a strong tendency to gain weight could occur if a child gets the same gene from each parent.

Furthermore, calorie counting, doesn't work—not all calories are the same once they enter your body. Three hundred calories from a piece of fresh fruit is *not* equivalent to three hundred calories from a slice of factory-prepared dead bologna. Restricting food intake to 800 or 1,200, or 1,500 calories a day in order to lose weight doesn't work either, because your body will do just what it is "programmed" to do. As a marvelous, self-adjusting energy system, once its food intake is limited, the body will just lessen its metabolic rate to burn fuel more slowly. Once your body begins losing weight, it begins to protect its stored fat by producing certain chemical substances that actually promote more fat deposition in the very fat cells that have already shrunken through dieting.

Apparently the more weight you lose, the more your body fights to regain it. That is why people trying to lose weight by calorie counting fall into a yo-yo pattern of weight loss and weight gain. Your body is able to defend itself very well from the danger of starvation, but it is not evolutionarily equipped to handle the eating opportunities of modern civilization.

Consider the fact that 60 to 80 million Americans are dieting right now. Most of them are women, and only a few will ever achieve, at risk to their health, the image of slimness projected by the advertising industry. Adding to this injustice is the fact that fat cells in a woman's thighs and buttocks are used for long-term energy storage, while fat cells in the abdominal area of men release their contents more easily for quick energy needs.

According to current medical science, being overweight is associated with diabetes, gallstones, gout, hypertension, heart disease, varicose veins and osteoarthritis, as well as colon, rectal, prostate, breast, uterine, and ovarian cancer. But being overweight is so much more than that. It is an illness itself, and a signal that the excess fat in and on your body may have gone beyond the limits of good balance and good health. Despite this, it has recently become more fashionable, and even politically correct, to believe that being overweight is just a normal and acceptable part of modern life. This is truly an amazing public relations feat accomplished by the economic interests that thrive on fattening us.

An editorial published in the prestigious *New England Journal of Medicine* in December of 1997 provides a perfect example of how nutritional nonsense can become widespread belief, even among physicians. The editorial informed medical doctors in no uncertain terms that their ongoing efforts to encourage their patients to change their behavior and lose excess weight were probably misguided. The editorial claimed that such efforts may be causing more harm than good because they were making patients feel bad. As predicted, the article received widespread publicity, with front-page headlines in major newspapers and lead features in syndicated television news programs.

A few years ago, the same journal accepted no drug advertisements whatsoever. The edition of the journal containing the "forget about encouraging weight loss" editorial comprised eighty-two pages of scientific articles and ninety-four pages of drug advertisements, many of which are directly or indirectly associated with diseases related to obesity. Most stunning of all was the fact that the April 2, 1998, edition of the *New England Journal of Medicine* contained a full-color, eight-page advertisement for Meridia, the latest weight-loss drug! Advertising money taints editorial choices.

Permanent Weight Loss Anyone Can Achieve

The ultimate goal for virtually all of you who are overweight should be a weight loss of 5 to 10 percent of your total weight, over a period of between eight and twelve months. It's crucial to be realistic about your weight loss goals. The *vast majority* of overweight people need to lose only five to twenty-five pounds in the first year to look good and feel great, as well as to counter the most serious effects of being overweight. Trying to lose more weight at a faster rate, through dieting, only creates temporary illusions of success. Dieting causes most people to ignore their natural biological signals of hunger and satiety. Then, once people stop dieting, they don't know when to naturally stop eating. That is why various studies indicate that approximately 90 percent of dieters who lose weight gain it all back, and often even more.

In this book, I will show you how to *safely* lose up to 10 percent of your excess body weight in eight to twelve months, and keep it off *permanently*. For those who want to lose much more weight, this is attainable by allowing more time. The secret is simple: eat more food containing the life-energy that allows your body to regain its balance and burn its excess fat.

You will lose excess fat *steadily and permanently* by climbing the

Food Energy Ladder presented in this book and staying on its upper rungs. This means eating less flesh, fewer eggs, less dairy, less refined sugar, and less junk food. But more importantly, it means eating more fruits, more vegetables, more whole grain breads and cereals, more beans, more lentils and legumes, more rice, pasta, and potatoes.

Your excess fat is directly linked to the proportion of animal fat and sugar in your diet. Many studies show that limiting total fat intake to 10 to 20 percent of total calorie intake helps people lose weight, even though they have failed to do so on a variety of calorie-reducing programs. But why bother? By staying on the top five steps of the Food Energy Ladder, you will not feel deprived and you will not have to bother with counting calories or multiplying, then dividing, to determine the percentage of fat calories. Just restrict your use of oils to olive oil and canola oil, and make sure to use them in moderation. You don't have to be a rocket scientist either to know how to eliminate 95 percent of the fat in your diet: *Eat less animal flesh and animal products!*

Perhaps you were surprised to learn that scientists consider all calories equal. In a laboratory, a calorie is the amount of heat that it takes to raise the temperature of one kilogram of water by exactly one degree centigrade. Thus, science doesn't differentiate between calories that come from fat, carbohydrates, or protein. In a laboratory, one hundred calories produced by burning carrots is the same as one hundred calories produced by burning chocolate!

This calorie measurement has led us, scientists and public alike, to accept a major delusion. What happens in a test tube does not happen in the same way in a human body. Carbohydrates, fat, and protein are burned differently in the human body than they are in a test tube. They are also used differently by the body. Furthermore, different bodies use the same calories differently because of heredity. It's as if there were some absurd "Dieter's Law of Thermodynamics" which states that, calorie for calorie, pork chops and milkshakes are no more responsible for weight gain than carrots and peas, as long as the amount of calories they contain are the same.

It gets even sillier. A gram of fat produces nine calories when it's burned in a test tube or a calorimeter in the laboratory. But a gram of carbohydrate or a gram of protein produces only four calories. Therefore, it is assumed that for the same number of calories an individual can choose to eat more than twice as much protein or carbohydrates than fat. Also, if the fat in a gram of avocado contains the same amount of calories as the fat in a gram of bacon, why not have the bacon? The reality is that the energy of an avocado is different than the fat from a pig's belly. One contains life-energy, while the other is dead!

Potato Chips Don't Grow Under the Soil

There are no easy gimmicks to make you lose weight. Fat-blocking pills, fat-burning pills, whole meals in a glass—in the long term, they just don't work. It's also absurd to spend money on commercial weight-loss programs that eliminate normal food choices by offering prepackaged meals. Almost all these dieters slide back into their old eating habits when they go back to the real world of eating. Additionally, it is dangerous to depend on drugs for losing weight. Amphetamines and their derivatives, as well as new drugs that affect your serotonin levels, have serious side effects.

So-called diet drugs make billions of dollars for drug companies, but their effects are short-lived once the drug is withdrawn. Both patients as well as doctors should stop deluding themselves into thinking that diet pills are an answer to permanent weight loss. It is an ethical travesty for scientific medical journals to accept millions of dollars from drug companies to feature eight-page, colorful advertisements that lull physicians into prescribing diet drugs without reading the small print.

It's disingenuous to claim and naive to believe that advertising dollars do not taint the editorial content of the scientific journals that physicians rely upon for their up-to-date information. These journals are currently publishing more articles about diet drugs, based on even skimpier information, and highlighting positive rather than negative results. Diet drugs are dreadful science because we just cannot tinker with the human metabolism and not expect serious side effects. There really is no such thing as a free lunch!

Another spectacular full-color advertisement for Meridia, the latest diet drug, appeared in the February 14, 1998, *Journal of the American Medical Association*. The following are some of the adverse reactions that were listed in very small print at the very end of the ad:

ADVERSE REACTIONS OF MERIDA

Headache	30%	Tachycardia	2.6%
Dry mouth	17.2%	Sweating	2.5%
Anorexia	13%	Vasodilation	2.4%
Constipation	11.5%	Taste	
Runny nose	10.2%	perversion	2.2%
Insomnia	10%	Hypertension	2.1%
Increased		Palpitation	2%
appetite	8.7%	Nervous system	
Back pain	8.2%	stimulation	1.5%
Flu syndrome	8.2%	Emotional	
Dizziness	7%	lability	1.3%
Nausea	5.7%	Rectal	
Nervousness	5.2%	disorder	1.2%
Sinusitis	5%	Joint	
Dyspepsia	5%	disorder	1.25%
Depression	4.3%	Vaginal	
Painful		moniliasis	1.2%
menses	3.5%		

This small print goes on to report additional adverse events occurring in patients using Meridia in less well-controlled studies: flatulence, gastroenteritis, tooth disorder, peripheral edema, arthritis, leg cramps, abnormal thinking, bronchitis. Finally, again in small print, the following warning appears: *"The safety and effectiveness of Meridia, as demonstrated in double-blind placebo-controlled trials, have not been determined beyond one year at this time."*

Shockingly, Meridia has been introduced to the public less than six months after one of the largest drug disasters in history. Tens of millions of patients may have been put at risk for heart valve disease because of the popular diet drug Redux, which was recently removed from the market. Even though Wall Street analysts are hailing the introduction of Meridia as a well orchestrated 500 million dollar national marketing campaign, I call it a glaring example of irresponsibility and undisguised greed in the weight-loss marketplace. *Are you awake yet?*

It should be obvious to you that advertising money taints so-called scientific editorial choices. Medical journals are also printing second-rate articles while accepting research support or advertising dollars, in glaring conflicts of interest. For instance, the *Journal of the American Medical Association* (January 1998) published an outrageously poor lead article about fat-free, fried potato chips. The article was based on research funded by the manufacturer of this so-called miracle fake fat!

A few hundred people of unstated age, attending a movie of an unstated nature, were given free potato chips and some soda to wash them down. Half of the people received potato chips made with fake fat, while the other half received "normal" potato chips, and no one knew which was which. The participants were called a week later to ascertain whether there was any difference in gassiness, indigestion, or anal leaking between the fake-fat potato chip eaters and the real-fat potato chip eaters. The article concluded that there were no reported significant differences. This conclusion was then widely reported in most of the major news media as a green light for dieters to enjoy their fake-fat potato chips. *Is this any way to conduct science?*

The study itself was supported through a grant from the manufacturer. Ironically, an April 1, 1998, editorial in the *Journal of the*

American Medical Association concludes that one-third of grant donors request prepublication reports of any articles and that grant
recipients frequently believe grant donors place restrictions on
their work and expect certain returns. Clearly, if researchers hope
to tap into more funds in the future, it makes sense that their natural bias would lead to positive results for the company that funded
their research.

The real bottom line is this: Potato chips made with fake fat are
not the answer to permanent weight loss. Potatoes are found under
the soil, not potato chips of any kind. There is no free lunch—only
lots of not-so-free advertising money!

The Seasons of Our Lives

Imagine the human lifecycle as a slowly spinning wheel.
Scientific concoctions like diet pills and faddish meals in a can—
these are like sticks poked through the spokes of that wheel. They
disrupt the natural flow and balance of energy in the body. We've
now looked extensively at the first four stages of the human lifecycle: prenatal, infancy, childhood, and adolescence. These are
foundational stages in the development of your nutritional habits
for life. *For life!* That is why it is so important, before going on to
the adulthood stages of the human lifecycle and a permanent solution to weight loss, to revisit some basic concepts.

We have seen how nature functions according to predictable cycles with beginnings and endings. Thus, the human lifecycle and
your own natural body cycles are in tune with the daily rising and
setting of the sun, the monthly phases of the moon, and the seasonal cycles of the earth's tilt on its axis. To everything there is a
season. Spring and summer—growth and reproduction—define the
early stages of the human lifecycle. Autumn and winter—maturity

and aging—comprise the times for nurturing ourselves and others, then letting go. This wisdom allows you to move through your cycle of life as normally and effortlessly as leaves drop from trees.

A major focus of this book centers around the biological differences during the stages of the human lifecycle. To understand why we gain excess weight and how we can lose such weight, however, it is important also to understand the psychological aspects involved. It is particularly important to consider the influence of social and family roles during the various phases of our life. Modern studies, by such esteemed scholars as Erik Erikson and D. J. Levinson, indicate how each stage of the human lifecycle is organized around specific mental and social issues.

What are the psychological and emotional characteristics of the early stages of the human lifecycle? During these foundational years, the feelings and thoughts that enter our hearts and minds are just as vital as the foods that enter our stomachs. During the prenatal stage, a mother's feelings of gladness, sadness, fear, or happiness effect her infant in as yet unmeasured ways. It is also important to realize that in good science, absence of measurable or quantitative evidence does not mean evidence of absence.

The infancy stage lasts until the time a baby is able to walk and be naturally independent of mother's milk. Infancy is a time for babies to receive nurturing and develop trust or mistrust of themselves as well as others. Babies who are comforted by loving and nurturing parents grow up to be more trusting than those whose parents do not behave that way.

The childhood stage lasts until boys and girls can pass on their DNA to the future. Childhood is a time for gaining autonomy and acquiring values. Thus, the "terrible twos" are marked by stubbornness and a child's exclamation of an emphatic *no*! This is why school-age children explore and experiment. Parents who encourage and support appropriate behaviors teach children to become autonomous. Parents who are critical and punishing teach children to feel shame and guilt.

During late childhood, just before puberty, humans develop a sense of being either industrious or inadequate. This sense tends to develop according to how productive children are in school, how well they get along with other children, and how much quality time their parents spend with them. These are the crucial years for parents to be actively listening to their children, helping them to understand their experiences at school, reading to and with them, and helping them with their homework.

Adolescence is a time of psychological turmoil, during which the growing child decides which mental and emotional "clothing" he or she wishes to wear as an adult. Social approval from friends is often more important than pursuing good physical or mental health. Developing a well-balanced adult identity, including the inclination to serve others, doesn't develop automatically, and experimentation is often the painful key to choosing well. Adolescence is marked by the human lifecycle coming of age into a reproducing, autonomous adult. Spring arrives in every sense of the word.

Reviewing the early stages of the human lifecycle is crucial for you to fully appreciate your present and future potential for *Total Health Rejuvenation* and weight loss. In the remainder of this book, I will turn my attention to adulthood, when entropy slowly begins to reign supreme.

To understand why you gain excess weight and how you can lose such weight, it is important to recognize the physical as well as the mental and social aspects of the human lifecycle. It is also crucial to realize how different the male and female human lifecycles are from each other. Men and women are as different internally as they are externally. All the egg cells females need to produce offspring are present at the time of their own birth. They are there until the time is right for them to develop into mature eggs that might be fertilized. Also, even though a woman's reproductive system stops functioning during the middle stage of her life, the woman still remains strong and full of vitality. In contrast, a man's testicles do not begin creating sperm until puberty, but then they keep producing sperm continuously, often into their eightieth or ninetieth year, despite the loss of overall strength and vitality.

Yet women generally live longer than men, because of their physiology as well as their lifestyle. Estrogen gives premenopausal women some built-in protection against heart disease, and men more often engage in high-risk behaviors. On the other hand, men are naturally leaner. The comparison between males and females leads to many intriguing questions. Why is there such a remarkable sex difference in the normal physiology of reproduction across the entire human lifecycle? Does this account for the marked behavioral differences between males and females throughout life? Are men normally leaner than women, regardless of chronological age, because of evolution? Perhaps only the fittest and leanest of our male ancestors survived their testosterone-driven "warrior mentality" to continue to reproduce the species. Is this the reason why, on average, men are 50 percent physically stronger than women as young adults?

I doubt if we will ever answer such questions. Immortality, as well as the keys to staying young forever, are not available to the human lifecycle. And yet we truly are immortal, because our DNA has been passed down to each of us from our ancestors, and lives on in the future. Bearing children is not required for immortality though, because our family's DNA thrusts toward the future through our siblings, cousins, nieces, nephews, and other blood relatives.

Understanding the stages of life is a wonderful way to gain a true perspective on the human condition: how we are conceived, how we grow from an infant into an independent adult, how we reproduce, how we mature and grow older. The deterioration of time takes its toll on the human body, but it is counterbalanced by growth in character and wisdom. This perspective has the power to propel you to change your eating habits in order to keep making progress in your life. Let's continue now with the adulthood stages of the human lifecycle.

The Young Adulthood Stage: Mating, Reproducing, and Testing Values

The young adulthood stage (about eighteen to forty years old) is a time of active human reproduction. High levels of estrogen and progesterone maintain the female shape, with a narrow waist, in spite of the worst eating habits imaginable. Raging testosterone levels in males bulk up their muscles, lower their voices, and cause hair to sprout all over their body, as they don the plumage of much of the animal world in a search of their mates during the summer of their lifecycle. During young adulthood, a need for intimacy develops, which propels both sexes toward marriage, childbearing, and childraising. A healthy, growing sense of intimacy results in the development of enduring relationships that allow us to embrace compromise and sacrifice. Establishing a career is paramount as well, at this time, which is also marked by learning to serve society and testing values.

Often, and amazingly, neither beer nor grease nor sugar nor the worst food excesses imaginable seem to have much of an effect on either sex until after age thirty. Then, young men and woman notice an extra pound or two of fat appearing, and remaining, on their bodies each year until nature, as well as society, begins ushering in the autumn of the human lifecycle.

A difference in the normal amount of body fat between men and women becomes very evident during this stage of the human lifecycle. During adolescence, the average amount of fat in growing boys is 18.5 percent, compared to 21 percent in growing girls— about a 12 percent difference. During young adulthood, between the ages of eighteen and thirty, the average male body is 16 percent fat and the average female body is 22.5 percent fat, almost a 30 percent difference!

Before the age of thirty, women tend to experience more urinary infections and vaginal discharges. Both sexes contract sexually transmitted diseases. Asthma, hay fever, and allergies begin to occur or worsen. Men experience more strains and sprains and are involved in more accidents. During these years, when accidents are the main threat to life, seven out of each thousand men will die, compared to just three out of each thousand women.

Aging happens. We begin to age the moment we are conceived. Then a complex combination of genetic, biological, cultural, and environmental factors come together to determine how many years we will live and how well we will live. The force of entropy increases throughout the entire human cycle of life and, with the force of life, we are in a state of constant balance and interplay.

The force of entropy begins overtaking the force of life toward the latter half of young adulthood, between ages thirty and forty. Hypertension, lung infections, stomach ulcers, enteritis, ulcers, and neuropsychiatric disorders, such as schizophrenia, begin occurring more frequently. Fourteen out of every thousand men will die during these years, compared to ten out of every thousand women, with cancer, heart disease, and accidents as the main culprits here.

Today's adults in their mid-thirties are likely to notice that their eyesight starts to worsen, hearing begins to deteriorate, gum disease becomes common, and facial wrinkles appear where before there were none. Women experience the effects of gravity and fat deposition as their breasts and buttocks sag. Men suffer with new sore spots in their ligaments and joints. Staying out late at night takes more of a toll and hangovers take on a new meaning for both men and women.

More excess fat begins accumulating now, which becomes more difficult to burn off. Both men and women have to work harder to stay in shape. They notice that their bodies don't seem to be able to take the same punishment. Those who are more likely to be leaner start to realize, as they age, that their bodies require a little more respect.

Perhaps you are somewhere in this stage of the human lifecycle, between eighteen and forty years old. This is the ideal time for you to take more personal responsibility for your overall health and weight loss. By now, you have lived long enough to know the direct consequences of your actions. Also, your raging sex hormones may finally be waning, while your ability to make adult decisions is rising. If you don't do it now, it will be more difficult to do it later. Health and weight during the next stages are very much a reflection of the habits you have acquired during the earlier years of young adulthood, while your biological clock was still ticking slowly toward autumn.

Right now, you have a great opportunity to launch a preemptive strike against the major enemy of your later years. Atherosclerosis is most likely building up in your body right now—fatty deposits building up in your blood vessels that could trigger heart attacks and strokes down the road. But why would a magnificent self-regulating and self-protecting energy system such as the human body persist in slathering the inner lining of its crucial blood vessels with fat?

It makes no sense whatsoever, yet the current scientific understanding of atherosclerosis is based on the simplistic notion that the cholesterol we ingest is somehow deposited on the walls of our heart and brain arteries, causing eventual obstruction and possible heart attack or stroke. But there is a better explanation. First, the inner linings (endothelium) of our blood vessels suffer injury from stress. Then the fatty deposits that lead to heart attacks and strokes begin to occur.

It wasn't too long ago that scientists also believed that maggots were the major cause of rotten meat. It was only when enough people observed that meat having become rotten allowed maggots to flourish, that scientist changed their tune. Now scientists believe that a bacterial infection, rather than stress, is the major cause of duodenal ulcers. Wrong again! It is more likely that the bacteria found growing in duodenal ulcers only begins flourishing after the stress-induced ulcers start to develop.

How do such examples relate to atherosclerotic heart disease and stroke? It's simple. The health of our heart and brain vessels is first compromised, then plaque builds up and creates obstructions. Keep in mind that the human body isn't so poorly constructed that it would just deposit excess fat on the inner linings of the very blood vessels that support life by nourishing the brain and heart. Indeed, mounting scientific evidence supports the notion that the fatal buildup of atherosclerosis occurs *after* the inner linings of our arteries have become thickened and damaged. Moreover, I believe that the deposition of fatty material upon these injured cells represents our body's ill-fated attempt to protect the injury and halt the damage. I call this the *inadequate Band-Aid effect*. I will discuss this later on in the book insofar as it relates to elevated homocysteine levels, and the importance of taking a well-balanced nutritional supplement each day.

The Middle Adulthood Stage: Applying Values and Facing Entropy

Middle adulthood (about forty to sixty-five years old) marks the beginning of many not so subtle emotional and physical changes. Individuals face the challenge of being creative and productive so they don't become stagnant and complacent. The so-called midlife crisis commonly arises, and many people begin to ask themselves, *What does it all matter?* The common thread in finding the answer to such a question rests on *how well you have made the successful passage from each stage of the human lifecycle to the point you are at now.*

In our forties, the growing force of entropy begins taking over; by fifty, it is in full swing. As we age our muscles atrophy while our body fat rises. Thus, both men and women find themselves developing larger bellies but smaller arm and leg muscles. With each new year it becomes easier to gain a few excess pounds of fat, and much more difficult to lose them.

Before menopause, estrogen and progesterone maintain the female shape, with narrow waist and rounded hips. In middle age, women find their waists thickening and their curves lessening, while deposits of fat settle around their abdomen, buttocks, and thighs. Women then also begin to catch up to men in the incidence of cardiovascular disease.

Men begin losing considerable amounts of hair on their scalps while growing more and more hair in the ears and nose. By age fifty, half the hairs on an average person's head, male and female, will be turning gray. The nails, especially the toenails, thicken and develop ridges. Wrinkles in the skin begin to form. The lenses of the eyes lose elasticity and cause difficulty in focusing on objects

♦

close up. Ligaments become less flexible and joints become stiffer, causing new aches and pains.

Weight gain as well as a variety of stress-related disorders begin to occur with greater frequency: migraine, hypertension, backache, indigestion, irritable bowel syndrome, depression, and chronic fatigue syndrome. The incidence of breast and lung cancer increases sharply, too.

Remember that encoded in your DNA are the templates of most of the diseases of your ancestors. Diabetes has two forms: insulin-dependent and non-insulin dependent. Insulin-dependent diabetes tends to develop in overweight people during this stage. Very often, the disease can be controlled simply by balancing the diet and losing weight. If diabetes is not well controlled, a decline in kidney function and eyesight loss may occur as the individual ages, along with atherosclerosis, cardiovascular disease, and stroke.

Hiatus hernias are also much more common in overweight people, especially if they smoke, suffer constipation, or are stressed. The opening through which the esophagus goes through the body's diaphragm is called a hiatus. Sometimes the lower part of the esophagus, and even part of the stomach, is pulled up through this hiatus and causes severe pain and discomfort.

Also remember that very few templates of diseases inherited from your ancestors are ever meant to appear during your personal lifecycle. Guarded by the force of homeostasis and your body's will to remember wellness, they will not manifest. On the other hand, when your energy falls out of balance you are at risk. And during middle adulthood, that risk usually relates to diseases caused by stress.

Surely the digestive system shows the effects of aging and the cumulative effect of decades of eating a poor diet. As a result, an estimated 30 percent of Americans suffer from irritable bowel syndrome (IBS). This condition affects mostly women, beginning in their thirties and becomes more bothersome to them in their forties. People with IBS have mild to severe abdominal pain, flatulence, chronic constipation, or sometimes diarrhea. Although IBS is generally thought to involve only the large intestine, it actually affects the esophagus and small intestines, causing nausea, heartburn, and dyspepsia.

Additionally, many patients with IBS have urinary tract complaints that are presumably caused by bladder irritability. Gynecologic symptoms, often including pain with sexual intercourse, are probably related to pelvic irritability. Other associated problems include depression, anxiety, insomnia, chronic fatigue, and migraine. Interestingly, a large proportion of patients with IBS also have symptoms caused by lactose intolerance, particularly abdominal distention, flatulence, and diarrhea.

Stress control, along with dietary adjustment, is the key to treatment of IBS. The overall systemic imbalance is a prime example of how a template of disease affects not only the target organ, which in this case is the gut, *but the entire body and mind.*

The typical human body, formerly able to tolerate myriad lifestyle indulgences and dietary indiscretions, cannot do so any longer. As entropy takes a firm hold during middle adulthood:

- gassiness and flatulence commonly occur after drinking milk and eating dairy products.
- constipation results from too little fiber, too few liquids, and too many diet colas. It leads to crankiness, lethargy, and decreased sexuality.
- heartburn, indigestion, and dyspepsia are caused by eating fried and greasy foods.
- alcohol starts to cause tiredness and irritability.
- coffee leads to headaches, heartburn, jitteriness, and frequent urination.
- refined sugar (pastries and candy) cause mental fuzziness and sleepiness.
- salt becomes a stimulant, leading to mental edginess and water retention.
- cellulite forms on the thighs, hips, and buttocks of women as they gain more weight.
- backache occurs with stress, lack of physical activity, and failure to stretch.
- sleepiness occurs sooner at night, while awakening occurs sooner in the morning.
- hormonal variations of menopause lead to hot flashes, sweats, irregular bleeding, and mood changes.

- an enlarging prostate gland begins causing men to wake at night to urinate.
- depression, panic disorder, anxiety, and despondency become common.
- widespread gum disease loosens the teeth.

Much misunderstanding surrounds middle adulthood. For example, it is common to say that people who cannot tolerate milk are "lactase deficient." This means that they have inadequate amounts of the lactase enzyme required to digest lactose, the sugar in cow's milk. That's nonsense! The vast majority of the world's adult population can't digest lactose very well, especially in the later stages of life. Humans lose their ability to manufacture lactose because nature never intended lactose-containing foods, such as milk, to be consumed after infancy or childhood.

We cannot fool Mother Nature, and perfectly normal people who were able to consume lots of milk and ice cream during their youth begin to experience gassiness, flatulence, constipation and irritable bowel syndrome during middle adulthood.

Osteoporosis is characterized by a serious loss of bone material and predisposes us to softened, easily broken bones. Osteoporosis affects as many as half of all adults, especially women over the age of fifty. The key to preventing osteoporosis is to initiate preventive measures earlier in life. You know, when I was in medical school, just thirty-five years ago, osteoporosis was a relatively uncommon and not very serious condition.

Today, however, nearly 50 percent of women over age sixty experience broken bones from osteoporosis, especially broken vertebrae; approximately 30 percent of men experience broken bones, mostly vertebrae, as well. But will milk consumption help stave off osteoporosis, as we are encouraged to believe? A recent analysis of the diet of nearly eighty thousand nurses tracked by Harvard Medical School certainly challenges this prevalent assumption. In fact, the study found no evidence that women who consume more milk or dairy products reduced their incidence of hip fractures, which is the standard measure of osteoporosis.

Calcium derived from cow's milk is not the key to preventing osteoporosis. A Cornell University study demonstrated that osteoporosis is exceptionally rare in Chinese men and women, although they consume little, if any, dairy products. Instead, the Chinese tend to eat lots of green vegetables and stay physically active.

A study in the *Journal of Clinical Nutrition* (March 1983) also demonstrated that vegetarians have stronger bones than meat-eaters. Indeed, the study showed that by age sixty-five, meat-eaters had five to six times more bone loss than vegetarians. Clearly, calcium is essential to building strong bones and preventing osteoporosis later in life. Supply your body with the calcium it needs, by reducing your consumption of flesh and animal products and increasing your consumption of fresh green vegetables, including a daily calcium and vitamin D supplement. Stopping smoking, drinking less coffee, and staying active, are also important here. Later in this book, I will discuss the importance of exercise in building strong bones.

During middle adulthood, it is particularly crucial to eat more foods filled with life-energy. Other simple steps to smooth out this autumn of your lifelong journey, and prepare the way for the final season of your lifecycle include the following:

- Know what happens to you physically at your age. For example, women are usually healthier after menopause, even if they are about 10 percent heavier than they were in their twenties, and about six to eight pounds heavier than they were just before menopause. In other words, don't worry about maintaining your youthful figure at this stage of the lifecycle; it could be injurious to your health!

- Drink more water. The amount of water stored in the human body dwindles as it ages. When the body is dehydrated, it is more vulnerable to disease. The body normally loses about twelve glasses of water each day through the skin, lungs, kidneys, and feces. Half that amount of water is usually replaced by water in the foods we eat, particularly fruits and vegetables. Carrots are 88 percent water and bananas are 76 percent water. The rest must come from drinking at least six to eight glasses a day.

- Exercise. Just a brisk, twenty-minute walk will substantially change the way you look and feel about yourself before you enter the final season of the human lifecycle.

Keep in mind that even cancer is a preventable illness if you start now! According to the *Harvard Medical School Report on Cancer Prevention*, published in 1997, approximately 50 percent of all cancers are preventable through better diet, increased exercise, decreased alcohol use, smoking cessation, and using common sense with the sun. Nearly two-thirds of cancer deaths in the United States are linked to tobacco, diet, and lack of exercise.

Prevention is clearly the best hope for reducing suffering and death caused by cancer. It can be your hope, as well, but only if you stay informed about what places you at risk. The following measures will help you to reduce your cancer risk:

1. **Exercise at least 20 minutes a day.** The evidence is overwhelming that physical activity helps protect against breast and colon cancer. Physical inactivity is associated with a twofold increase in the rate of colon cancer, which is the second largest cause of death due to cancer in the United States. In a recent study of nearly twenty-five thousand Norwegian women in the *Journal of the American Medical Association*, the rate of breast cancer decreased by 37 percent among those who exercised approximately four hours per week; there was a 52 percent decrease in breast cancer among women engaged in heavy physical labor at work; and women exercising four hours per week who were also lean had 72 percent less breast cancer!

2. **Avoid excess alcohol intake.** It is important to realize that consuming two alcoholic drinks a day increases the risk of breast cancer by about 25 percent.

3. **Be responsible in the sun.** Use sunscreen with a sun protection factor (SPF) of at least 15. Avoid sunburn and exposure to midday sun. Almost all skin cancer, including melanoma, is caused by sun damage.

4. **Don't smoke.** Lung cancer, at least 25 percent of colon cancer, and a significant amount of uterine cervical cancers are attributed to cigarette smoking. Fortunately, within five years of quitting smoking, the ex-smoker's risk of cancer decreases by half. Within ten to fifteen years, the ex-smoker's risk is comparable to people who have never smoked. More than sixty million Americans have already quit smoking.

5. **Eat more fiber, fruits, and vegetables; eat less animal fat; avoid being overweight.** Overweight women have a 50 percent greater chance to develop uterine, breast, colon, and gallbladder cancer. Simply eating more vegetables is associated with a 20 percent reduction in breast cancer. Women living in the same country in Europe who consume or cook with olive oil have less breast cancer than women who use little olive oil. This raises the intriguing possibility that monounsaturated fats, such as olive oil, may actually help protect against cancer.

Overweight men have a 40 percent greater chance of developing colon and prostate cancer. The risk of prostate cancer, the most common cancer among men in the United States, increases considerably in men who eat more red meat. In both men and women, high consumption of red meat doubles the risk of colon cancer, a type of cancer rarely seen in vegetarians. Evidence suggests that reducing your intake of red meat to less than one serving per week, and increasing your intake of vegetables and fruit, is likely to reduce your risk of colon cancer.

Truly, the major task of the middle adulthood stage of the human lifecycle is simply to make entropy smooth sailing for the final season.

Maturity: Offering Leadership and Becoming Dependent Again

Maturity (ages sixty-five to eighty-five and beyond), the last stage of the human lifecycle, is marked by individuals offering leadership and sharing knowledge and values—at home, at work, and in society. We all want to leave a legacy behind us. In the United States, the average life expectancy is about seventy-two years for men and seventy-nine years for women. With so many people now living to advanced ages, however, the later years can also be marked by a dependence upon others—in a way, similar to our earliest years.

Nature renews and sustains herself on schedule. It is not surprising, then, that our lifecycle also functions on schedule. Nature supplies us with the necessary life-energy to sustain us healthfully for eight or nine decades. Your body extracts its life-energy from the sun's rays, air, water, and food.

With each decade after young adulthood, it is common to lose about seven pounds of muscle and, to double the amount of body fat in proportion to muscle. This rate of muscle loss usually increases during maturity, but it can be reversed. By age sixty-five, the body's ability to use oxygen efficiently decreases by 35 percent, but this, too, can be reversed. So can the steady loss of bone and rise in blood pressure. The Surgeon General has estimated that two-thirds of the illnesses during this stage of life are preventable.

At no time during the human lifecycle is it more important to exercise than during maturity. Before the twentieth century, most people were intensely active and would have scoffed at the idea of exercise. But at that time, human labor accounted for 80 percent of the work needed just to till the soil on a farm. Human labor now accounts for only one percent of the energy needed to work the land. Cars, stores on every corner, and all sorts of labor-saving devices have caused a dramatic decline in physical activity for city dwellers. Regular exercise, proper nutrition, and an enhanced sense of well-being are keys to energy balance and weight loss during maturity. Your body strives to remember wellness.

If we do not care for ourselves properly, entropy overcomes us and can unlock many of the disease templates stored within us. Atherosclerosis and hypertension begin to predominate and lead to heart attack and stroke. Bone and joint disorders, such as osteoporosis and arthritis, occur. Neoplastic diseases develop as colon, prostate, and uterine cancers. Also, about 35 percent of adults over age sixty, mostly women, develop diverticulosis, or small sacs within the walls of the colon. Many will then develop painful inflammations. Diverticulosis is found most often in people who eat too little fiber. Insufficient dietary fiber also contributes to a near 50 percent higher rate of cancer in the gastrointestinal tract.

For most Americans, dietary fiber intake in general is much too low. Fiber, also known as roughage or bulk, is important for preventing as well as reversing unhealthy weight gain. High fiber foods are bulky, take longer to chew, and cause feelings of fullness after eating. Obviously, fiber also keeps the bowels moving because it passes quickly through the digestive system. To increase fiber, eat more vegetables, fruits, whole grain breads, bran muffins, and bran cereals instead of processed baked goods and cereals. Baked beans, kidney beans, and green peas are also very good sources of fiber. You may also wish to take a fiber supplement.

The following list features some of the best high-fiber foods:

- apples
- apricots
- baked potatoes
- bananas
- blueberries
- broccoli
- cabbage
- cantaloupe
- zucchini and zucchini bread or cake
- carrots and carrot cake
- corn
- dates
- dried figs
- nuts and seeds
- oatmeal
- oatmeal cookies
- oranges
- peanut butter
- pears
- popcorn
- prunes
- raisins
- raspberries
- spinach
- strawberries
- sweet potatoes
- turnips
- whole wheat cereals

There are many unhealthy obstacles that are disruptive during maturity. We need life-energy from the sun, but the sun's rays now cause more cancer than ever before due to our depleting ozone layer. Since people spend fewer and fewer hours outside, about half of the people over sixty-five tend to be deficient in vitamin D as well. Recall that our bodies require sunshine to manufacture vitamin D, which is crucial for building strength in our bones and preventing osteoporosis. Moreover, genetic reengineering of foods and leaching the soil of vital nutrients is resulting in widespread B$_{12}$ deficiency and the potential of undiagnosed pernicious anemia.

Pollutants have befouled and depleted the life-energy of our air. Air is so dirty that more than 10 million children a year develop asthma in our smoggiest cities. We are also destroying our rain forests, which supply up to 80 percent of the oxygen in our air. Our water supply is widely contaminated with deadly mercury and other toxic chemicals, which extends to the fish we eat. Our soil is depleted of crucial minerals necessary to produce food filled with life-energy, and most of the food that does manage to grow we refine, process, pulverize, radiate, and genetically reengineer.

A Wakeup Call

What can you do about this? First you can wake up! Just like cows, pigs, and chickens, you are being unnaturally and artificially fattened for profit. Pick up any newspaper and look at the supermarket ads for fake food, artificial food, convenient food, salted food, and seductively packaged food. Where's the *real* food? Our ancestors may have been deprived of supermarkets, with its tens of thousands of items questionably called food. Nevertheless, they were exposed to healthy sunshine, inhaled pure air, thrived on clean water and uncontaminated fish, consumed meat without hormones and antibiotics, and valued fresh vegetables, homemade soups, and whole grain bread. On the other hand, we eat genetically reengineered and microwaved vegetables, our soups come in cans and contain whopping amounts of salt, nitrates, and chemical preservatives, and our bread is white, fluffy, and full of lard.

Do you see why it is time to take more control of your own health destiny? If not for your sake, then for the sake of those you love and care for, especially for children who look to their parents as role models.

We have seen how the human lifecycle encompasses different biological cycles and rhythms that change dramatically with each phase of our human season. The rhythms of our brain waves, the frequencies of our heartbeats, the pressures in our blood vessels, the transit times through our intestines, the cyclic appearances of the human egg, and the ebb and flow of human sperm all create an endless symphony.

Underlying this symphony is the complex living entity called the human lifecycle. Spring blooms with your conception. Summer arrives with your reproductive years and stays until the autumn of middle adulthood. We have to be reminded to take better care of ourselves, so that when winter arrives we have time to savor the fruits of our lifecycle's past as it transforms into the roots of our future. In *Leaves of Grass*, Walt Whitman reminds us of life's healing force and its never-ending quest for energy balance and *Total Health Rejuvenation*.

> *You will hardly know*
> *Who I am or what I mean,*
> *But I shall be good health*
> *To you nevertheless,*
> *And filter and fiber your blood.*
> *Failing to find me at first,*
> *Keep encouraged,*
> *Missing me one place, search another,*
> *I will stop somewhere waiting for you.*

Part Five

BUILDING A NEW PATH OF LEAST RESISTANCE

After reading Parts One through Four, I hope you have gained a greater understanding about life-energy, permanent weight loss, and your personal "Cycle of Life." This is all part of the process of changing your mindset about the food you eat. When you can successfully achieve that goal, then—and only then—will you attain *Total Health Rejuvenation* and your optimal weight.

As I told you earlier in this book, there are no quick fixes. The healthy way is the *only way*! Can you think of any materialistic thing you own that is more valuable than your health? I can't! And please remember: In addition to bettering your self-image, reaching your optimal weight through *Total Health Rejuvenation* will have *many positive benefits*!

Begin by asking yourself the following questions: Have you ever lost weight and shortly thereafter gained it all back? Do strong urges or uncontrollable cravings cause you to eat too much food, or too much of the wrong type of food, or both? If so, you are not to blame. Urges and cravings have been cunningly programmed into your mind by the advertising industry to create eating habits that help support sales. Profits, not your health, is the priority.

Most overweight people regain their lost weight after dieting because their bad eating habits were merely temporarily overcome, not transformed. Unhealthy habits are continually reinforced— even by the so-called health care industry.

Recall that Americans suffer from the outset simply because we require less food energy than we are taught to believe. Even the nutrition information on food labels misleads us since it depends on an inflated daily energy requirement of two thousand calories for a "typically healthy adult." Potentially, that's a whole lot of dead food.

The 28–Day Plan to Take Advantage of a Perfectly Natural System

My 28-Day Plan takes you step-by-step through the simple processes that allow you to overcome food urges and cravings by establishing a new mindset. The plan literally kick-starts your body into burning its excess fat. Why does the 28-Day Plan work? Because it takes full advantage of a perfectly natural system.

Psychologically, it's called "cognitive restructuring" and "conscious reprogramming." In layman's terms, this means uprooting ideas and thoughts about food, and planting healthful seeds in their place. The bottom line is that once you reconstruct your mindset, you can lose up to 10 percent of your present excess weight in eight to twelve months. And you will keep it off for life without ever feeling deprived. If you have more than 10 percent excess weight, you will simply need more time and more effort, especially exercise, to lose the weight. Your new mindset will enable you to comfortably lose another 5 to 10 percent of your weight during the next year and perhaps another 5 percent during the third year.

This treatment plan is so flexible, it works for the slightly overweight, the very overweight, and for those who are close to their naturally optimal weight and just want to stay healthy. What do *you* want to lose? Your excess weight or your time? If you want to lose weight, then don't waste your time on crash diets and crazy diet pills. The 28-Day Plan uses your time efficiently to lose weight effectively—and for good!

Don't discourage yourself by setting unreasonable expectations. It is realistic to aim for a 10 percent to 15 percent total and permanent weight loss. Here is a letter from a patient who lost 20 percent of her excess weight over four years after attending my Voyage to Wellness program on a transatlantic crossing of the *QE2*. Once she lost the weight, she never gained it back.

> *Dear Dr. Taub,*
>
> *I just finished reading your* Rx For Life *book and I'm so happy that you have not veered from what you taught all of us on the* QE2 *during our memorable voyage to wellness. It's difficult to believe that ten years have already gone by since my half-century struggle to lose weight ended. I had tried so many diets before attending your seminar that I felt like a yo-yo going up and down most of my life. I was depressed, obsessed, and possessed—until you helped me change my mindset about food, exercise, and attitude.*
>
> *I lost fifteen pounds that first year—I went from 160 to 145 pounds—but better yet, I went from a size 12 to a size 10 dress. Then I lost about six pounds a year for the next three years—about a half a pound a month, just like you said I would. So here I am ten years later, now weighing 125 pounds and wearing a size 7 dress. I'm happy as can be with my new habits and my new life—loads of fruit all morning, lots of veggies all day, baked potatoes or pasta whenever I want, and walking at least a half-hour a day, no matter where I am, in virtually any kind of weather. Thanks again for giving me a new life.*
>
> *Sincerely,*
> *Gloria S.*

The psychological changes that occur during the 28-Day Plan refocus the lens through which you view the world. The results are astonishing. You will naturally overcome your previously programmed food cravings and false beliefs. You will overcome your resistance to exercise. It will be natural for you not to want to eat junk. It will be natural that the very thought of red meat and cow's milk will almost nauseate you. You will naturally seek out fresh fruits, veggies, and other foods—with delight!

This plan is not about deprivation, either. Small amounts of butter are perfectly acceptable for cooking delicious recipes. Olive and canola oils are also fine in moderation. Olive oil, more physical activity, and a zest for life are why Mediterranean people are so healthy!

Some say Mediterranean people are healthier because of the red wine that abounds in their diet. This is questionable. We have already seen how nutritional science is severely tainted by economic agendas that have no place in good science. Recently, an article in the *Journal of the American Medical Association* purported that two alcoholic drinks a day increased longevity. Thanks to the wine industry, advertisements as to the benefits of wine suddenly appeared everywhere in the media, literally drenching the public with the "healthy news." I was appalled by this "news" because I have attended many autopsies in which the fatty changes of cirrhosis were present in the livers of individuals who regularly had just two drinks a day. Fortunately, another study in a different AMA journal appeared one month later, showing that two drinks a day were associated with a significant increase in breast cancer among women.

Wine is probably fine in moderation. But too much alcohol is not compatible with *Total Health Rejuvenation* and it makes losing weight virtually impossible because it changes the body's metabolism and ability to burn fat. It's best to limit your alcohol intake to about a drink (a glass of wine, a bottle of beer, or a cocktail) no more than two or three times a week; the less, the better.

Making Progress

No one is born fat. Therefore, no matter how overweight you or your family members are, you still have an inner healing force striving at all times to preserve a healthful energy balance in your body. Being overweight means that your energy is out of balance. It's an illness.

Despite the common misperception, it is common for people to successfully lose weight and keep it off. My patients have terrific rates of personal success. I personally lost 10 percent of my weight fifteen years ago. I went from 200 to 180 pounds. That's twenty pounds I can, *and will*, surely live without.

We simply eat too much dead food and are too sedentary. People sit in front of their computers all day at work and then go home and sit in front of their TVs until bedtime, while they are eating, drinking, and snacking.

The good news is that there is a little bit of hope in everyone, and it seems to be on the rise. A recent study conducted by the National Weight Control Registry and the University of Pittsburgh found nearly two thousand people who refused to stay fat. Instead, they lost an average of sixty pounds and kept if off for an average of six years. Most of the participants in this study were women. About half were between the ages of thirty-four and fifty-five. On average, they dropped from 220 to 154 pounds. Most went from being overweight to what they felt was a normal, healthy weight.

We can learn a great deal from these remarkable people. Remember: The goal promoted in this book is to lose a reasonable 10 percent of your weight. This is about ten to twenty-five pounds for most people. As you lose weight, *how you feel* is most important. Even without a scale, you will know you are losing weight. Your belt/dress size is a fine guide.

You may believe that if you have been overweight since childhood, you will really have to struggle to lose weight and keep it off now. This is a false perception! Almost 50 percent of the successful weight losers in the above study were overweight since they were ten years old, and another 25 percent were overweight from the time they were eighteen.

It is very likely that you also believe that losing weight is especially hard if being overweight runs in your family. Again, this is not so! Seventy percent of the successful weight losers in the above study had at least one obese parent. How did their beat their genes? By refusing to believe that they were destined to be overweight.

Almost all participants in this study reported that they had tried to lose weight before. In this case, 90 percent of them attributed their success to eating less food overall, and eating much less fatty food. They made these changes even while eating out an average of four times per week. They also engaged in very high levels of physical activity, about twice as much as the experts usually recommend. Most participants walked for exercise, while others bicycled, did aerobics, stair climbing, or weight lifting and running.

Surprisingly, 75 percent reported that a specific experience ignited their decision to lose weight. Men were more likely to report a medical event such as back pain, fatigue, high cholesterol, or varicose veins. Women were most likely to report an emotional event: "My husband left me and my lawyer told me it was because I was fat" or "I was going to my tenth reunion and I saw myself in the mirror." For many, the triggering event was someone just commenting on their weight.

Even more surprisingly, although most people believe that it is much harder to maintain weight loss than to lose weight, these successful weight losers said otherwise. About half said that keeping the weight off was actually easier than losing it in the first place. They were not miserable, nor did they spend their time dreaming about food. Ninety-five percent said that the overall quality of their lives improved, and 92 percent said they had greater energy.

Psychologist John Sklare studied thousands of overweight people who sought medical help to lose weight. He discovered that stress was the most common reason that people fail to lose weight permanently. His conclusion? Unless patients address the underlying issues that motivate them to overeat and make poor nutritional choices, they are sure to repeat their old habits and continue to struggle. In Sklare's words, "If you keep doing what you've always done, you'll keep getting what you've always got."

Most people have to try over and over again to overcome unhealthy habits. Overweight people often have to make New Year's resolutions for many years before they keep their promises. Understanding the mental processes that overweight people go through on their way to overcoming their harmful eating habits, however, will help you reach your goals *this year*, not many years from now.

The human psyche goes through a fairly predictable process before it prepares to surrender detrimental habits for better habits.

Psychologists James Prochaska, Carlo DiClemente, and John Norcross identified some of these stages as "precontemplation," "contemplation," "preparation," and "action."

Are you a precontemplator? Precontemplators are people who deny that a problem exists. If this describes you, then you really have no intention of changing your eating habits; you really don't even want to admit that your habits are detrimental to your health. We have all seen troublesome drinkers who deny they have a problem or hacking smokers who say they are just fine. Overweight precontemplators resist change, but all is not yet lost. You can still make progress if you are given the right tools at the right time. A nurturing relationship with a non-nagging spouse, or a friend who is unwilling to give up on you, can help. The 28-Day Plan is a sure strategy to propel you out of the precontemplator's trap.

Contemplators are people who recognize that they have a problem and begin to make plans to change their behavior. But their plans are more or less indefinite. Contemplators will eagerly talk about being overweight, and they will also make promises to change their behavior *someday*. Contemplators are chronic procrastinators. If you're a contemplator, you probably hope for some "magic moment" when you'll know that it's right for you to change your eating habits forever. Or perhaps you're engaged in some wishful thinking, such as hoping that an effective diet pill will be developed. As a contemplator, you may even have taken action prematurely in the past, long before you were really ready to change. Then you could say to yourself, "I just knew I couldn't do it."

Contemplators truly want to change but face a subconscious resistance that causes anxiety and fear and prolongs the procrastination. Contemplators get anxious about sacrificing something comfortable and familiar in their life for something unfamiliar. Additionally, contemplators fear failure once they really do make a commitment to change. If you are a contemplator, your internal fear can be paralyzing. For some people, according to psychologist James Bugental, fear of change is "a fate worse than death."

If you are an overweight contemplator, getting your adrenaline flowing is the best way to ascend from procrastination to preparation to action. In other words, you need some serious emotional and physical arousal to kick-start your final decision to change. The best way for you to get such a boost is to start eating lots of fresh fruit, particularly in the morning. Fruit is particularly full of the life-energy you need to stoke up your mental and physical furnace. It's important to get your endorphins flowing with more physical activity, especially long, brisk walks. Finally, it's necessary to enlist the power of your imagination. Take time to imagine what you might look like and how you might feel if you were happier, healthier, more energetic, and leaner. Just for a moment, imagine how you want look in the future. Imagination is a powerful force, the root of all creativity. We need imagination to plan a meal, build a bridge, write a poem, compose a song, make a friend, build a family. Imagination, along with emotional and physical energy, is your key to move from procrastination to preparation to action for a leaner life.

We have discussed the "thinking, planning, but not accomplishing" phase of weight loss. If that describes you, then it is time for you to cross the bridge to the "proactive and committed" phase of weight loss. Soon you will learn about a *Personal Wellness Retreat* that is designed to help you cross that bridge. Because you are where you are, you probably are familiar with some of the following statements:

"I want to lose weight."
"I know I should lose weight."
"I sure hope I can lose weight."
"I'm not totally sure I can handle the cravings."
"It's going to be very difficult to get some exercise every day."
"I'll never be as thin as the people on TV or in the magazines."
"I wonder whether I can keep the weight off once I lose it."
"How will I manage without hamburgers, french fries, milkshakes, potato chips, and ice cream sundaes?"

As you cross the bridge, you will be saying instead:

"I will lose weight."
"I will be able to handle the cravings."
"I will do some exercise every day that gets me at least a little bit sweaty and breathing faster."
"I'm not supposed to be as lean as the fashion models."

The 28-Day Plan introduced later in this book will help you to establish a lifetime of healthy eating habits, to cross the bridge from procrastination to proactive living once and for all. No matter how old you are, if you want to lose weight permanently, you must create a new frontier in your mind and *build a new path of least resistance* to get you over that bridge. *Balance Your Body, Balance Your Life* is all about creating that new result.

The four crucial elements in creating that new result are the following:

1. **self-respect**
2. **connectedness to others**
3. **accurate nutritional information**
4. **willingness to exercise**

My patient Mary L. provides an outstanding example of the above. She was enrolled in a hospital-sponsored 28-Day Plan I conducted ten years ago:

Dear Dr. Taub:

I saw you on TV last evening and just had to write to let you know how well I am doing. I completed your 28-day stress and weight loss class ten years ago, and I am happy to report to you that because of your teachings on meditation, yoga, exercise, and eating live-energy foods, not dead foods, I am maintaining a very reasonable weight and am very happy with myself.

I just thought of how many of your teachings I do without thinking. I eat low-fat foods, lots of fruit, and exercise regularly. I am sixty years old and have more energy than ever. I can control my stress by using the relaxation techniques I learned in our 28-day class. I have high self-esteem and self-confidence because I am now in control of what gets put into my body. I had dieted all my life, but since completing your 28-day plan ten years ago, I no longer diet, I eat healthy, exercise (even though I do not want to), and practice the relaxation techniques that come out of your classes. I no longer go on yo-yo diets; I simply go back to watching what I put in my mouth.

Most of my friends are overweight and have let themselves go. Of course, as we grow older we slow down and have a tendency to give up on some things. But I refuse to do this. I want to remain young in spirit and healthy enough to keep up with my two-year-old granddaughter. I want her to be proud of her grandmother.

I am so glad that I took your 28-day course because I work eight hours a day, take care of my granddaughter four hours every week-

day, and have an eighty-six-year-old mother who lives with me, so I need to be healthy. I take very few medications and I am never sick. I make sure my eighty-six-year-old mom follows your teachings, too, and she is never sick. She climbs stairs to my apartment every day, walks on a daily basis, does my housework, bakes (healthy foods), crochets, and is super independent. I thank you for this. I thank you for teaching me how to take control of my body and respect what I put into it. Giving myself permission to relax and take time for my-self has also helped a lot. Everything I learned from you has bene-fited my mom as well as myself over the past ten years and we are both thankful for your 28-day plan. We can attest to the fact that eating wise and living well pays off!

I am using your teachings about food with Sara, my granddaugh-ter. If she can learn good habits now, she will be able to control what goes into her mouth and how she acts in years to come. Self-respect, self-discipline, self-esteem, and knowing you are in control can help anyone. Thank you for helping me to gain control of my life.

Sincerely,
Mary L.

Change Is in the Air

Change is in the air and it is time to make your move. A journey of a thousand miles starts with the first step. But to address the fact that, deep down, most people fear making changes when their familiar habits are at stake, let's reconsider science and some more natural laws.

Modern science was launched when Isaac Newton (1642–1727) imagined that the universe was like a giant clock, the motion of its slowly moving external hands caused by the motion of its smaller internal gears. In much the same way, all natural phenomena in the world around us are the result of natural laws working below the surface of what's immediately evident. Newton described the natural laws that apply to motion as follows:

Anything that moves does so in response to the action of one or more forces. This is why blood cells travel through our veins (the heart pumps it), a baseball hurtles through the air (a bat applies a force), and water cascades downward off a cliff (the force of gravity). *Can you see any parallels in human behavior?*

There are two types of motion in nature: uniform motion and changing motion. Uniform motion means that something is either standing still or moving in a straight line at a constant speed. Therefore, both a book that is standing on a book shelf and a rocket that is traveling to the moon at a thousand miles per hour can be said to be in uniform motion. Changing motion means that an object either speeds up, slows down, or changes direction. Thus, a rolling ball that is slowing down or rolling down a hill faster and faster, or veering off in another direction, is said to be in changing motion.

An object at rest will continue to stay at rest unless it is compelled to change by a sufficient force applied to it. Likewise, an object that is moving in a straight line at a constant speed will keep doing so unless it is compelled to change by a force applied to it. When such a force is applied, the object will either slow down, speed up, or change its direction. *Now can you see any parallels in human behavior?*

The tendency of an object to resist a change in motion is called *inertia*. Inertia explains why objects continue doing exactly what they are doing. A book keeps sitting on a table and a rolling ball keeps rolling until a sufficient force is applied. The book moves if it is pushed and the ball eventually slows down because of friction. If the book is pushed far enough, it might also fall from the table, impelled by gravity to follow a new path of least resistance. Likewise, the ball might take a new direction down a steeper slope and also follow a new path of least resistance.

Human behavior is exactly like this! We live by inertia. We resist change. We tend to value what's most comfortable and familiar to us. We follow the most comfortable and familiar path that is available to us. It's all a system of natural laws.

If you habitually eat too much food, or too much junk food, your eating habits, food urges, and cravings naturally direct you toward the comfortable and familiar path of least resistance—appetite and taste bud pleasuring. The curative power of *Balance Your Body, Balance Your Life* is based on creating a **new** path that allows you to neutralize and overcome your food urges and cravings.

Perhaps at this very moment you are still feeling discomfort and apprehension over the very notion of real change. When stressed, people are especially likely to choose the familiar and comfortable path over even temporary psychological discomfort. It's easier to give in to your senses. With detrimental eating habits, the involved senses are always taste, smell, and what we call appetite. Unfortunately, being overweight also inflames your appetite. You mistake your mental appetite for physical hunger and eat more and more food.

This is why you will often eat beyond what is comfortable, even to feeling unpleasantly full. You will also mistake good smells for what people sniff at with delight on television—fat-laden dishes like pepperoni pizza and fried chicken. Finally, you will mistake good taste for lots of sugar, salt, artificial flavors, and fat. Fortunately, taste buds can be reprogrammed to appreciate the taste of fresh fruits and fresh vegetables, especially if you begin subconsciously to reason in a brand-new way: *This carrot is supplying life-energy for my body to stay well, avoid constipation, and burn off its excess fat. It also really does taste good.*

By taking advantage of a system of natural laws, you can begin to consistently override your food urges and cravings. It all depends on creating a new way of living marked by feelings of satisfaction rather than deprivation, and it must lead in the direction of good physical health rather than overweight and fatigue.

Here is a vital new mindset that makes you feel energized and invigorated. It will guide you toward happiness, healthiness, and permanent weight loss. Your food choices will naturally drift toward and travel down this new path.

Picture a woman in a canoe atop a swiftly flowing stream. If she doesn't paddle hard against the current, the canoe just proceeds downstream; it's the natural path of least resistance. Of course, the woman could paddle hard upstream if that is her destination, but when she stops, the canoe will stop and once again float downstream. In much the same way, people who go on a diet discover it's only a temporary fix. When they stop, the river carries them back. *An object in motion will head toward the path of least resistance, and efforts to overcome such a natural system are eventually futile.*

Perhaps there is nothing in life more discouraging than futile and hopeless effort. Sisyphus was a character in Greek mythology. For certain sins, he was condemned by the gods to spend all of his days and nights rolling a huge stone to the top of a mountain. Then, upon reaching the summit, the rock would tumble back down the mountain, and Sisyphus would begin his task once again. Nobel laureate Albert Camus portrayed the torment of Sisyphus straining to push the huge stone up the slope, his face contorted, his cheek against the stone, his shoulder bracing the boulder, his foot wedging it, his arms outstretched and his battered hands covered with earth. Then, at the end of his long effort, Sisyphus watches the stone rushing back down the mountain from whence he will have to push it up again. His face that toiled so close to the stone looks like the stone itself as he goes back down the mountain with heavy steps. But we are left with the feeling that Sisyphus is superior to his fate. He is stronger than his rock. He never gives up. His descent down the mountain is mixed with scorn and joy. Sisyphus believes that all will be well and the struggle toward the heights is enough to fill his heart.

What if Sisyphus found a way to succeed in his task and be reborn? What if he sought a more gentle slope around the mountain? What if he greased the ground in front of the boulder? Or put the boulder on a platform with wheels? Or crushed the boulder into smaller pieces? Sometimes in life you have to travel the path of most resistance to reach the path of least resistance. Perhaps Sisyphus realized that the night is darkest just before the dawn—and so can you. For you can't solve the problem of food cravings and urges that you have accumulated over so many decades just by wanting to. But you can begin there, and you can begin now.

You can build your own new path of least resistance by developing a strong personal vision. Losing weight and growing thinner, however, is not enough. You must develop a personal vision of being healthier, happier, more energetic, more loving, less stressed, and more lean. Then you will break free from the mental inertia that sustains you, yes, but at too great a cost! Your new personal vision will spark a paradigm shift!

By first creating in your mind the person you want to be, as well as the body you want to have, you take advantage of a natural system that Goethe described this way:

> *What you can do, or*
> *Dream you can do, begin it.*
> *Boldness has genius, power and magic in it.*
> *Only engage, and then*
> *The mind grows heartened.*
> *Begin it, and the work will be completed.*

Paradigm Shift

What if the woman paddling her canoe toward the direction of her dreams suddenly determines that she no longer wants to travel in the familiar, comfortable stream driven by currents beyond her control? What if, instead, she determines to reposition her canoe, pointing it in the direction of her greatest dreams, using the natural currents to aid her? With a change in current, a paradigm shift occurs. Her canoe begins to glide effortlessly toward her dreamed-of destination.

A crystal-clear vision and a thorough understanding of your present reality will help you get to where you want to be. No more traveling upstream with fad diets, unused health club memberships, and diet pills. Before we go further, let's look at the paddler's adventure again to ascertain what made the difference. First, she had to realize that the stream was taking her in a direction in which she didn't want to go. Then she had to clarify her desired destination and create a vision to help her determine her destiny.

How open are you to change? Are there some things you won't

budge on: your religion, the hand with which you write, even the side of your head on which you part your hair? Like the canoer, we mostly find ourselves adrift in currents that are too comfortable and familiar to change. There are thousands of books on the subject of personal change, but unless you personally want to change, the books are of no help. Self-help books are only effective if you are motivated to help yourself.

If change seems difficult, what about *improvement*? Nearly everyone says he or she is interested in improving some aspect of his or her life—relationships, appearance, health, job, outlook. Like change, improvement takes people out of their comfort zone and into an arena of uncertainty that has the potential for discomfort or pain.

Why won't people make a persistent effort to even slightly improve their eating habits and lifestyle? Because improvement alone is not a sufficient force to move an object that is quite comfortable at rest. Nor is the force sufficient to change the direction of a life already in motion in another direction. *It's all about a system of natural laws.*

Why do people choose this path in their everyday lives? Often they don't know other paths exist. It's a little like driving a car at night; you can only see the road hit by your headlights. Why do people who have accurate information about other paths and other directions choose to remain where they are? Because it involves moving out of the "comfort zone." Inaccurate information and fear of letting go fuel human inertia. Fear of letting go is why people stay in abusive relationships or unsatisfying jobs. Fear of the unknown is why people resist changing abusive eating habits and lifestyles. It's human inertia!

But imagine this: *Years of inertia can be a powerful springboard for progress!* Progressing toward a healthier lifestyle and attitude about eating doesn't have to be uncomfortable. Rather than saying good-bye to your comfort zone, you simply broaden that comfort zone to embrace new and healthier tastes and habits. The tools I will give you will increase your happiness, comfort, and well-being. I will help you let go of fear and progress toward your vision. Making progress will give you more physical comfort and eating pleasure than you can imagine.

Banish Fear

"The wise man in the storm prays to God,
not for safety from danger, but for deliverance from fear.
It is the storm within that endangers him, not the storm without."
—RALPH WALDO EMERSON

Previously, we discussed the stage at which you contemplate changing your lifestyle. Contemplators can also procrastinate because they experience a subconscious resistance that causes them too much anxiety and fear. We usually grow anxious about giving up what's comfortable and familiar. It's true that change can seem frightening. If you contemplate only to procrastinate about losing weight permanently, however, your fear may paralyze you!

Remember: a human being is a complex energy system, and energy always moves along the path of least resistance. The reason your body is overweight is because this is the path of least resistance that you have followed. The flow of water from a mountain stream in the Adirondacks to a river in New York City, then to the Atlantic Ocean, follows the path of least resistance. The flow of wind over the Great Lakes and through the widest streets of Chicago follows the path of least resistance. The flow of electricity from a far-off generator to your home, then to your toaster, television, or computer, follows the path of least resistance.

Energy always moves along the path of least resistance, and that's why people tend to move in the direction in which it is easiest for them to go. The reason you are overweight is because, like a river, electricity, and the wind, you have followed the path of least resistance. In our society, the path of least resistance means eating more dead food and becoming increasingly inactive.

Unless you open up a new frontier by building a *new* path of least resistance to get you there, you will always be paddling against the current or pushing the boulder up a never-ending mountain. But you can create an even larger river flowing in the new direction in which you wish to go. Or you can move the boulder sideways around the mountain. Either way, the only thing truly stopping you from creating a *new* path of least resistance is fear of pain and discomfort.

To leave your current path, you must be brave enough to seek a new frontier by finding an alternative path that leads to your desired destination. If you can't direct your canoe to a current leading where you want to go from your present stream, then you may have to pick up your canoe and move it to a different body of water altogether. Instead of searching for a new way around the mountain, you may just have to move to a new mountain. The only thing getting in between you and your progress up that mountain is fear.

Fear is rampant because stress is the raging epidemic of our times. Once you have good nutritional information, fear and stress are the most common obstacles to your quest for permanent weight loss. Your mind tells you that the discomfort or suffering will make life too unpleasant. Your mind also tells you to fear failure and convinces you that success is impossible to attain.

It is important to realize that your fear is only an emotional illusion that has acquired a life of its own because of stress. Unfortunately, though fear exists in your mind, it creates a stranglehold that prevents you from living in peace. President Franklin Delano Roosevelt, himself crippled by polio, inspired the entire free world—faced by the most evil army ever known—with this one moving statement: *The only thing you have to fear is fear itself.*

Unfortunately, you cannot use fearful thoughts to diminish your fear. Just think: Trying to analyze or escape fear with a fearful mind is like fighting fire with fire. But just as your thoughts are able to create fear, they can also create peace. You can learn to replace a restless, worried, or troubled mind with a tranquil, calm, and peaceful mind. The 28-Day Plan described in this book is designed to overcome stress and release you from the bondage of your fear. Freedom from fear requires only that you lift the veil that now obscures your own truth.

Only a quiet mind can dispel fear. You can begin to calmly observe your fear and release it. As you learn to meditate, you will be living more in the here and now instead of mulling over past defeats or worrying about future hopes. If you live in the present, there can be no fear that represents the chains of the past or the pull of the future. The simple relaxation-meditation technique introduced in the first part of this book (see page 34) is powerful. Even the busiest person can set aside five or ten minutes a day to meditate.

Just read this letter I received from Melanie W., a forty-eight-year-old woman, who thought she was in relatively good health:

Dear Dr. Taub:

Just about three years ago, my doctor told me, after a routine checkup, that my cholesterol was mega-high and my EKG was abnormal. Then he warned me that I had better change the way I was eating—completely. I was really sorry that I went to see him in the first place because all I ever suffered with was low energy, headaches off and on, some constipation, and maybe some PMS. And, of course, I was considerably overweight.

I was thrown for a loop, so totally disappointed and upset that I couldn't speak with anyone for a few days. I was literally frightened. No more croissants with bacon and butter for breakfast? No more barbecued steaks with that nice fatty crust? No more ice cream and chocolate creamy cakes? No more mayonnaise slathered on my sandwiches? No more salami and knockwurst? I can never do that! Impossible!

I was totally resistant to change because I love to cook and love to eat. After all, I prided myself on being a gourmet cook, and I loved to create new recipes. How could I just stop all that when I wasn't even that much overweight—maybe twenty pounds or so, just like most of my friends? Actually, to tell you the truth, I was too scared to make a real commitment because it all felt so painful. I thought I'd rather die than change, and that made me scared. Then I thought I'd try but probably fail, and that made me even more scared.

Everything felt like a real catastrophe and I was really in the pits, when my doctor urged me to attend your 28-day weight loss class at the hospital because he had personally benefited so much from it. He told me that he and his wife attended your program, and as a result, never felt better. "Oh sure," I thought, "give me a break!"

I guess what finally convinced me was when my doctor told me he was so impressed by your strategy that he decided to create an entire physician's advisory board just to support your work. I really trust my doctor, after growing up with him caring for me and now having him care for my own kids; so, reluctantly, I tried your plan. Slowly, I began looking at some of your wife Anneli's recipes, while still making a big circle around them; honestly, they didn't make a lot of sense at first. But then, when you actually held a class right smack in the middle of a supermarket aisle, I was stunned to really see, for the first time, that the shelves, the coolers, and virtually all the display cases in there were filled with processed, refined, and fake foods—what you call "dead energy."

And then it finally dawned on me that the contents of my refrigerator were just as appalling! I began shopping and cooking differently and started meditating and wellness walking every day, briskly as you say, "not just loping along." I cooked Anneli's recipes and found them to be even more savory than my old favorites, which just provided a sugar or grease high for my taste buds. For example, when I just had to have some fried potatoes, I got out my Teflon pan and vegetable spray and made them nice and crunchy without the fat. During weekends, when I love to make dishes like spinach, champignons, and cheese sauce, I tried some lot-fat milk instead of heavy cream—I liked it just fine. Same with some low-fat yogurt instead of ice cream, although I still indulge in ice cream now and then, without feeling guilty, because I remember your motto: "Everything in moderation—including moderation."

What was really amazing was the fact that in just four weeks, I lost a bunch of pounds as a bonus, without really thinking about it. What I really just wanted to do was lower my cholesterol rather than take off my excess pounds, which I had given up on long ago. Surprise! It's now five years later and I'm twenty pounds lighter. But the best thing is that I am holding my weight at the present level and it's no problem, because the most wonderful part of my experience is the fact that my taste buds have changed. Everyone else in our class began experiencing the same transformation, too. It seems that our taste buds change after about two weeks and adjust to fewer sweets, less grease, and less fake food. Actually, the previous stuff I used to eat is now much too sweet and greasy. Eating the old way also makes me gassy and upsets my stomach. My taste buds now find concentrated sugar or pure fat disgusting. Steaks, hamburgers, and all the glasses of milk I used to drink revolt me, and I guard against eating them. It's obvious that we don't need a lot of flesh, fat, salt, and sugar to ensure the pleasure of eating. These healthy changes will naturally happen to everybody's common sense as well as to their nose and taste buds. I guarantee it!

From a grateful patient,
Melanie W.

Needless to say, letters of this nature, which I receive all the time, make my heart feel wonderful!

The journey of the human cycle of life is inward as well as upward, striving to attain what Plato called "The Ideal of the Good" and what Aristotle called "the divinity in everything." Every body—every unhealthy, stressed, and overweight body—has the potential to feel better and lose weight permanently.

To realize this potential requires some of the fearlessness of an infant learning to walk for the first time. Fostering this fearlessness requires only a challenge to think differently about your body and your beliefs. The Roman philosopher Seneca said, "It is not because things are difficult that we do not dare; it is because we do not dare that they are difficult."

You are about to move beyond the "contemplating" stage to the "do it" stage. Read on now, so that you will understand your Personal Wellness Retreat and the entire 28-Day Plan that follows it. But before you continue, make sure you have completed the Health Profile in Part Two of this book.

Your Personal Wellness Retreat

I consistently observe that many of my patients become aware of their inner healing strength much quicker than I imagine possible (almost in the space of a heartbeat). The awareness is a function of their heightened self-value and reverence for life. Their experiences led me to create a much simpler, more practical pathway to the wellness and weight loss paradigm. It begins with a One-Day Personal Wellness Retreat.

The key to the therapeutic effectiveness of this one day will be the short but intensive effort you make to set your paradigm shift in motion. Some overweight people may choose to ignore the new paradigm for a while, but it will remain in their consciousness like a seed ready to sprout.

More than ever before, people feel an urgent need for more free time to regain control of their lives. Overweight people are already so enslaved by their senses that it would be ridiculous for them to embark on a lifelong journey to a leaner body without first taking some precious free time for themselves. If you are seriously committed to losing weight, it is time for you to set aside just a day for your Personal Wellness Retreat.

This is a necessary time-out before you begin to regain control of your weight. It can be any day you choose. Even if you have to take some time off from work, it's well worth it. What's more important than your health? You'll be better at work when you return. Your Personal Wellness Retreat will allow you to begin building a new path of least resistance to a healthier and leaner body. You will experience benefits to last a lifetime.

During your Personal Wellness Retreat your main goal is clear: defining your future vision and taking stock of your current situation. After all, you wouldn't rush into redecorating your house or creating an important presentation for your boss without first taking time to clarify what you want to accomplish and how you plan to do it. We are most successful at accomplishing our goals when we have a clear vision.

Make no mistake, this will be a crucial time of reflection for you. The results of the reality check I ask you to take in a moment may disturb you. But don't be discouraged, because your past ended one moment ago and the power of your body to bring itself back into balance is enormous. After all, during the one day of your Personal Wellness Retreat, your heart will beat around 100,000 times and your body will give birth to about 100 billion new red blood cells.

In the same natural way, your mind will ready itself to give birth to a new reality over the twenty-eight days that follow. A healthier and leaner body awaits you, as long as you are ready to embark on a *new* path of least resistance.

The goal of your Personal Wellness Retreat is to create a new vision of a healthier, happier, more energized, and leaner you. During this one day, you will begin focusing in on that vision, making it so intense that it infuses your entire being. Instead of merely problem solving, which is almost always a temporary fix at best, you will be creating a new and permanent result.

Over the twenty-eight days that follow, your mindset and your notion of reality will change—your paradigm will shift. First, you will catch a clear glimpse of who you wish to become. You will be so drawn to the image that you will be able to visualize your future more powerfully than your past. You will experience a physical, emotional, and spiritual epiphany when doing so. Your biochemistry and metabolism will actually shift toward homeostasis, as *your body remembers wellness.* New feelings of self-confidence will cast out fear to allow you to make progress toward your goal. Rediscovering love for yourself, for others, and for nature will make you feel worthy once more of life's blessings.

During the special day of your Personal Wellness Retreat, you will learn simple and reasonable steps to begin determining your own health destiny. Just the smallest effort, when part of a larger and focused vision, can unleash a harvest of health for you. In the space of a day, you will start shattering the physical, mental, and emotional chains that have weakened your own natural healing forces.

The guidelines for your Personal Wellness Retreat are straightforward and allow plenty of room for individual creativity. Commit yourself to following the guidelines, because this day will only be as good as you vow to make it. Your effort begins by taking small steps that stimulate your powerful body-mind connection. It's important for you to realize how much your health depends on your own personal responsibility, self-value, and reverence for life. What is in your heart and on your mind affects your physical well-being, and vice versa.

Quiet time and solitude is essential. If you think there are too many distractions at home, consider asking your spouse or getting a baby-sitter to help with the kids. It would be even better if you could get more in touch with nature by driving or taking a train to somewhere in the countryside. If you have a friend or a mate, you might wish to retreat together. It's wonderful when couples commit to this time together, but it certainly is not necessary. If you are with another person, it is important to be supportive but to still be by yourself. In other words, be together but not too together, because your main goal is to experience peace and quiet.

Have your answering machine take phone messages for the day, or simply unplug the phone. If other members of your family will be around, ask them not to interrupt you unnecessarily. You might want to make an announcement to everyone old enough to understand that their support and understanding will be appreciated. In any case, plan ahead to work together with your family to have everything go as smoothly as possible.

Here are the basic ingredients of *your* special day: healthy food, fresh air, exercise, good reading, soft music, and quiet time for meditation, writing, and prayer. *No* TV, *no* phone calls, *no* movies, *no* newspapers, *no* magazines, *no* radio (except for relaxing music).

Your Personal Wellness Retreat provides you with a good opportunity to relax with an amusing, educational, or inspirational book. It's also a great time to revisit some of your favorite records, CDs, and cassettes. Soft, relaxing music might be nice during, as well as before and after, meals. Dim the lights sometime during the day and light a candle or two for a while, perhaps while eating, bathing, writing, or while just doing nothing. This day is to quiet the mind and focus on *you*.

Make sure to go to bed early the night before, after taking some extra time for personal care: a pedicure or manicure, a bubble bath, facial, or massage. Also, cleansing your inside is as important as cleaning your outside. Many people may benefit from a Fleets enema, a Dulcolax suppository or a mild herbal laxative.

NUTRITION

It's important that you personally shop for your food for this special day. Take your time to carefully select lots of fresh, colorful, ripe fruits, and plenty of fresh vegetables. Pay careful attention to the colors, shapes, and consistencies, and make sure to get what's especially in season. Avoid all types of junk food. Instead, eat fruits and vegetables for snacks. You'll need to drink at least six to eight glasses of fresh water during the day too. Also, begin taking a comprehensive multivitamin and mineral supplement.

The Food Energy Ladder is described in detail in Part Six of this book. Foods at the top of the ladder are high in life-energy and help your body burn its excess fat. Conversely, foods near the bottom steps of the ladder, especially foods that have been processed or refined, are low in life-energy. Foods at the bottom of the ladder cause your body to accumulate fat. The object of this day is to stay as high on the Food Energy Ladder as possible. *It's as simple as that!*

Do not drink any alcoholic beverages or soft drinks during this day, and limit your coffee or non-herbal tea to just a cup. Used excessively, alcohol, refined sugar, and caffeine disrupt the balance of life-energy in your body and lead to harmful effects. Don't smoke! If you must smoke cigarettes though, smoke only outside, and try cutting your usual amount in half.

During the morning, before noontime, consume only fresh fruit and fresh juice. Eat as much and as wide a variety of fruits as you wish, as long as they are fresh. Many people who are not used to so much fruit find that lots of bananas, cantaloupe, and honeydews are best.

Lunch should consist mostly of fresh vegetables, salad and good whole-grain bread. Dinner should consist mostly of rice, pasta, or potatoes, along with vegetables. If you prefer, you can make lunch the heartier meal of the day and have a lighter dinner.

Eliminate flesh food during this day unless you can find some very fresh fish or wish to make some good chicken soup. Drink 6 to 8 glasses of water. Eat only small amounts of eggs and dairy products, essentially, just as needed ingredients for recipes. The recipes in this book will show you that you don't have to give up flavor just because you are cutting back on flesh food, dairy, sugar, and fat. It is best that you not eat anything after 8:00 P.M. If hunger intrudes upon your comfort later in the evening, however, have an apple, a banana, or some other fresh fruit.

PHYSICAL ACTIVITY

One of the major aspects of your Personal Wellness Retreat is reacquainting yourself with nature. If you can arrange it, the benefits of relaxing in a country setting, or near the sea, are tremendous. Wherever you are during this day, get outside as much as you can—just bundle up if it's cold or wet.

Open the windows in your house, weather permitting. Visit a park, walk on the beach, or work in the garden—repotting and transplanting are as healing to our own lives as to plant lives. In the fall, raking leaves is great exercise. In the winter, you might practice such long-forgotten skills as making snow angels and snowmen. Exercise is a major key to permanent weight loss.

Make sure to wake up by 7:00 A.M. on this special morning. Do the simple "wellness yoga" stretches in the exercise part of this book for about ten to twenty minutes, then take a brisk "wellness walk" for at least twenty minutes. Be sure to get at least a little bit sweaty and short of breath. Pick up your legs a little more than usual, swivel your hips, and swing your arms so that you feel like you are dancing or gliding along. The sillier you look, the better you are probably doing it. If you are unable to walk for twenty minutes, then just do what you can. This type of exercise helps to balance your metabolism and burn your excess body fat. It also releases vital endorphins, which heighten your self-confidence and motivation.

My patients unanimously agree that exercise is the turning point on their journey to a leaner life. It is important to take another "wellness walk" in the afternoon, with a few minutes of stretching beforehand. Use your walks to become aware of all the living things around you. This is a time to enjoy nature. Can you imagine God's presence in every living thing? Be sure to listen for sounds of life around you: children's play, birds, pets, etc. Also, pay attention to the colors in your environment. Smell the flowers. Finally, take a leisurely after-dinner stroll to look at the moon and gaze at the stars.

MEDITATION, JOURNAL WRITING, AND PRAYER

Get a notebook to create a journal that is dedicated to your Personal Wellness Retreat and the 28-Day Plan. Twice during the day, take some quiet time for meditation and writing in your journal. Use the simple five- to ten-minute meditation technique described in the first part of this book.

After you meditate, begin writing in your journal as if you are talking to your most trusted friend. Take at least ten to twenty minutes to do this.

Write about your feelings, your purpose, and meaning in this life, and about all sorts of dreams and aspirations. Write steadily without reading over what you are writing until you feel you have finished. Be honest! Admit to your journal what you might not admit to anyone else. Challenge yourself with different modes of expression; you might want to write a poem or write a dialogue between yourself and another person. Always date your journal entries.

Meditate and write in a quiet place where you will not be disturbed. In meditation, you bring your thoughts to stillness. Most people are always thinking, planning, strategizing, worrying, reflecting, or remembering. When you still your thoughts, your body releases endorphins that help overcome stress, stimulate homeostasis, and decrease appetite. Without meditation, your resolve to lose weight may be as superficial as a Band-Aid that covers a wound while the source of the problem continues to fester. An eight-year-old patient once informed me that meditation was the very best way for her to say her bedtime prayers; when she asked God for help, her thoughts were quiet enough so she could hear the answer.

Speaking of prayer, use this special day as an opportunity to renew your soul. Let bedtime be a reminder of your childhood by saying a prayer that was special to you when you were a child. If you wish, kneel down at the side of your bed. This is a wonderful time to think about how your soul touches the souls of others, and how their souls touch yours. However you wish to pray, before you finish, perhaps you might wish to say these words slowly and softly to yourself, over and over: *God Loves Me . . . God Loves Me . . . God Loves Me.*

BEING LOVING

Love is your own inner physician, and its healing energy is more powerful than any medicine. Your Personal Wellness Retreat is meant to balance body, mind, and soul. Balance has many definitions, one of which is "to bring into harmony or proportion." Beneath all physical and emotional imbalance, including being overweight, lies a longing for love. Nothing influences your overall well-being more profoundly than love, not only the love that you receive, but also the love you give. When you feel loved, and when you are being loving, you experience a sense of wholeness that helps heal the feelings of isolation that fuel your detrimental eating habits. Indeed, in this age of incredible stress, I-L-L is equivalent to "*I Lack Love!*"

"*Love one another*" is a core belief of Judeo-Christianity. Yet most people spend their lives fluctuating somewhere between wholeness and isolation. A sense of wholeness helps to keep your energy in balance. Isolation has the opposite effect. Before you can truly lose weight permanently, you must address the emotional and spiritual aches of "feeling alone." The potential to lose weight is immeasurably increased when you are able to offer your unconditional love to someone.

You may say, "But I have enough love. What I need right now is to lose weight." Maybe you are loved *by* others, but your soul still longs to be more loving *toward* others. When you are more loving, the music of your soul reverberates throughout your body and mind, helping to bring them into healthful balance. When you make a vow to love someone in your life unconditionally, it literally means without conditions. It means that no matter what that person says or does, nothing diminishes your feelings of love. Whether you choose your child, spouse, parent, brother, sister, grandparent, or someone else, nothing the person says or does, no matter how infuriating or insensitive, affects your love for him or her. This type of love overpowers hurt and anger. Unconditional love is offered selflessly, without expectation of receiving anything in return. It is love for love's sake.

In the center of a blank page of your journal, write out the following vow. Make sure to fill in the name of someone special and then sign it and date it:

"*I vow to love [   ] unconditionally.*"

LIVING ETHICALLY

When we are overweight, we often dislike what we see in the mirror, and we dislike ourselves. Trapped in this vicious cycle, even though we know there is a remedy, we usually choose not to take advantage of it. When we dislike ourselves, we don't feel worthy of effort or attention.

You must begin doing whatever it takes to make you feel worthy of having the best in life. Otherwise, a low level of self-respect will eventually wear down even your most intense resolve to lose weight. Your appetite will conjure up a dozen reasons to succumb to your food urges and cravings. Irresistible impulses will become just that!

The single most important factor you must deal with is developing enough self-respect to feel worthy of making progress toward your envisioned goal. You must learn to care for yourself enough to create a vision for the future and to focus on it so intently that you will become that vision.

"God's primary demand of human beings is ethical behavior" is another core belief of Judeo-Christianity. Ethical behavior inspires powerful feelings of self-value and personal confidence. Thus, you must make a personal vow that you will be the very best person you can be. Commit to being a decent, kind, loving, and honest person. This vow will be the framework that makes you feel worthy of progressing toward your goal. Ethics can become a very tangled topic, so you can follow this very elemental principle for your behavior: If you even think that it might be wrong, just don't do it!

In the center of a blank page of your journal, write out the following vow. Make sure to sign it and date it.

"I vow to do nothing that I feel in my heart is wrong."

Personal Wellness Retreat Schedule

Your Personal Wellness Retreat requires only about four hours of your time to accomplish essential and enjoyable tasks.

During the morning:

- Twenty minutes for simple "wellness yoga stretches"
- Twenty minutes for a "wellness walk"
- Twenty minutes for meditation and journal writing
- Sixty minutes for "creating your vision"

During the afternoon:

- Twenty minutes for a "wellness walk"
- Sixty minutes for your "reality check"
- Twenty minutes for meditation and journal writing

During the evening:

- Twenty minutes for meditation and journal writing
- Twenty minutes for an after dinner stroll
- Time for a bedtime prayer

Creating Your Vision

When your mind is exceptionally clear and you are feeling in a peak state (after you've done your wellness yoga stretches, meditation and walk), set aside at least an hour of time to answer the following questions as completely and honestly as possible.

First, take some time to review your answers to the Health Profile in Part Two. This will give you many new insights and ideas. You will be building a new path of least resistance to the vision you are about to create, so be sure to come back to your journal at any time to make any additions. After you read each question below, close your eyes and ponder your answer. This will help keep your thoughts focused. Write down your answers. Make sure no one will disturb your concentration as you identify the following:

"WHERE I WANT TO BE ONE YEAR FROM NOW"

- What will my health be like?
- In one year from now, about how much do I want to weigh?
- After achieving this weight, what three characteristics will best describe my life?

- What will I be doing for fun, and how much fun will I be having?
- What kind of exercise will I be doing?
- What will my body look like?
- How much will I respect myself?
- How much alcohol will I be drinking?
- How many cigarettes will I be smoking?
- How loved will I feel?
- How loving will I be?

Reality Check

The second part of creating a new path of least resistance is to gain a clear idea of where you are right now, and how you will be five years from now if you do not make any progress toward fulfilling a new vision of yourself. In other words, if your plan is to continue living and eating the same way that you do now, then what will you look like five years from now? To avoid the pain that results from resisting progress now, it is crucial to spend some serious time contemplating this type of future.

The reality check may be an emotional jolt, and perhaps somewhat painful, but it is critical in progressing toward becoming leaner. This is meant to be a wake-up call.

After taking an afternoon walk, take some time to once again review your Health Profile from Part Two of the book, then spend at least five minutes standing in front of a mirror with all or most of your clothes off. Treat what you see with honesty but kindness. Look especially at your face, arms, chest, abdomen, hips, thighs, buttocks, and legs. Also look at your skin and hair. Notice your natural curves. After you have observed your body, write down your thoughts in your journal.

Now answer the following questions as thoughtfully and completely as possible (write down your answers):

"WHERE I AM RIGHT NOW"

- What is my health like?
- About how much do I weigh right now?
- What three characteristics most describe my life?
- What am I doing for fun, and how much fun am I having?
- What kind of exercise do I do?
- What kinds of physical pain am I experiencing?
- How sedentary ("couch potato") am I?
- What does my body look like?
- How much do I respect myself?
- How much alcohol do I drink?
- How many cigarettes do I smoke?
- How stressed am I?
- How loved do I feel?
- How loving am I?

Now imagine how you will be five years from now if you continue to live and eat as you currently do. Answer the following questions as honestly and completely as possible as you identify the following *(write down your answers):*

"THIS DESCRIBES ME FIVE YEARS FROM NOW, IF I CONTINUE TO FOLLOW MY PRESENT LIFESTYLE AND EATING HABITS"

- What will my health be like?
- About how much will I weigh?
- What three characteristics will most describe my life?
- What will I be doing for fun, and how much fun will I be having?
- What kind of exercise will I be doing?
- What kinds of physical pain will I be experiencing?
- How sedentary will I be?
- What will my body look like?
- How much alcohol will I be drinking?
- How many cigarettes will I be smoking?
- How stressed will I be?

- How loved will I feel?
- How loving will I be?
- How much will I respect myself?

Now that you have clarified where you want to be (*created your vision*) and where you currently are, or will be if you don't change (*your reality check*), consider the following:

We all resist change. Even promises of better health, more money, or increased happiness don't cause lasting change. Yet, our brain readily embraces making progress toward a clearly envisioned goal. Once your new mindset is established, it will take on a life of its own.

The object of your One Day Personal Wellness Retreat is to define the result that you want to live for the rest of your life. The 28-Day Plan builds on this empowering day and spurs your progress toward your vision. This is much more powerful than problem-solving. It's about creating a new result. Enjoy!

Part Six

FOOD IS ENERGY:

A New Mindset and Plan for Permanent Weight Loss and Balanced Energy Throughout the Cycle of Life . . . The Blueprint

The Hardest Work Is Behind You

Before we get into Part Six, I would like to make a strong suggestion. As soon as you finish reading the entire book, please set your date for your Personal Wellness Retreat. Give yourself some planning time, but not too much. Don't put it off. Just do it!

You have begun to dust away the cobwebs in your mind that have tangled you up in unhealthful eating habits. Through what you've read so far, you have learned about the nutritional needs of your body throughout the cycle of life. You now can recognize how your attitudes toward food have been shaped by Madison Avenue and the multibillion-dollar foot and diet industries. Following the questionnaires you've already taken, you should take stock of your present state of wellness and weigh the strengths and weaknesses of your Health Profile. Set your sights on reasonable, attainable weight goals. You are almost ready for your *personal action plan*. A plan so simple, it will keep you motivated, feeling energetic and alive—a plan that will take *diet* (that four-letter word!) out of your vocabulary forever.

Most of the hard work is already done. Identifying the sources of your misperceptions about food by determining your current Health Profile required great courage, honesty, and self-value. By this process, you have begun to ignite your will to *eat wise and live well*. You should feel empowered and motivated by what you've read so far!

The knowledge of where you have been, and where you are presently, will motivate you as you embark on a twenty-eight-day journey toward greater health and energy. But the journey doesn't end after twenty-eight days; that is just the beginning. If you follow the action plan described in this part of the book for *just 28 days*, you and your family will be firmly on the path toward your naturally desired weight and energy for the rest of your life.

Permanent weight loss comes from within, not from without. It doesn't come in a bottle, a jar, or even a book. Throughout this book, I aim to give you the resources, knowledge, and tools that will help strengthen the source of wellness within you. This *natural source* is your key to permanent weight loss and radiant energy. I will teach you simple guidelines to follow for twenty-eight days—guidelines that will allow you to tap into this natural healing source and stimulate its power to keep you physically and emotionally well.

As you prepare to begin your twenty-eight-day journey toward wellness, keep in mind that short-term weight loss is *not* your goal. You are reaching for much more, and it is all within your reach! During these twenty-eight days, you will establish the eating habits and tastes that will bring you and your family a lifetime of improved health and balanced weight. Your journey to wellness doesn't end after just four weeks—you are establishing a *blueprint* for wellness and a healthier weight *for life*.

Put Your Mind on the Meal

Now that you've cleaned out your mental refrigerator and tossed away all your harmful thoughts, feelings, and emotions about food, you have begun to create a new mindset toward food and nutrition. This mindset will guide you toward healthful choices about the foods that you eat and feed your family—*naturally*. This mindset will also free you from calorie-counting, restrictive diets, and the favorite weight-loss fad of the moment.

At this point, you may be saying to yourself, "Dr. Taub, quit worrying about what I think and get to the point: *What should I eat?*"

Dear reader, remember that *you eat only as well as you think*. You will not change the way you eat (at least not in a lasting way) until you change your mind. And that is exactly what you have been doing. What is in your mind directly guides what you choose to put in your mouth. What is in your mind affects *every single cell* of your body. Why? Because your body is more than the sum of its parts. It is a magnificent system of energy, and your mind is the motor. What you think, along with what you eat, either helps keep your energy in perfect balance, which is your *natural state of health*, or disrupts your energy, which is the *unnatural state of illness*.

The essential key to losing weight is to change the way you think about food. From reading earlier parts of this book, you are already beginning to break out of your old mindset and rebuild a new, healthful one. It is important that I work on your mindset for just a bit longer, so hang in there!

One of the leading reasons so many of us are overweight to begin with is that *we don't think about what we eat*. How can we? Most of us eat while engaged in some other activity. We eat breakfast in the car on the way to work; in fact, a whole range of breakfast foods has been created to accommodate the needs of the commuting eater! We grab lunch and take it back to our desk to eat while finishing that report that was supposed to be finished yesterday. When we do have dinner at home, it's often while reading the newspaper or watching television. Simply swallowing our food is commonplace, and chewing our food properly is rare!

Think about the last meal you ate. Was it really a meal? What did you eat? Where were you when you ate it? Were you sitting down? These may sound like peculiar questions, but so many people eat in a rush on their way to somewhere else. Where was your mind during that meal? On the newspaper? On the phone call you made while eating? On the meeting in the next hour? On what you have to do when you're done eating?

Perhaps your eating habits are not unlike Barbara's. Barbara is a young professional, works long hours, and seems to be always "on the go." When I met Barbara, she was on the first vacation she had taken since graduating college. She was on a cruise ship sailing through Mexico, and on her first day aboard she happened to walk into my seminar on wellness, a program I created for cruise ships around the globe to transform a regular vacation into a Voyage to Wellness. For Barbara, it was a long overdue week of restoring some control to her otherwise chaotic life.

Barbara had perfected the skill of eating on the run. On her morning commute to work, she'd munch a bagel and cream cheese and down her first of many cups of coffee for the day, paying more attention to the traffic than her food. For lunch, which really just meant any fifteen minutes she could sneak away from the office in the afternoon, she frequented fast-food places downtown near work, then inhaled her food during her quick walk back to the office. Dinner wasn't much better. She alternated between five restaurants on her path home from work, ordering the same takeout dinners week after week. Barbara ate her takeout in front of the television, watching the evening news, since she never had time to read a newspaper.

Barbara stayed to hear what the Voyage to Wellness was all about, and decided to stay with the course for the week. When we began to talk about mindful eating, eating with awareness, she was one of the first to resist. "I'm sorry, Dr. Taub, but I just don't have the time to sit down and linger over an enjoyable meal."

Then I asked Barbara, "When was the last time you really enjoyed what you ate?" She said it was that very morning. She was sitting on the deck, enjoying the early morning sun, eating a plate of fresh pineapple, mango, and kiwi. She said she'd forgotten how delicious fresh fruit was. I asked her how she was feeling then, at midmorning. "I feel wonderful, energetic, ready to go explore when we pull into port." She went on to say that in fact she could not remember the last time she felt so good. "Really, I usually feel like I'm dragging after a meal, or my stomach gets upset."

As Barbara evaluated her current health profile, it became apparent that the illnesses she experienced, the daily discomforts she endured, were all related to her eating habits. She complained of indigestion, constipation alternating with diarrhea, and fatigue. She was at least ten to fifteen pounds heavier than she should be and her cholesterol was much too high.

During the seven-day cruise, I asked Barbara to eat every meal mindfully. This can be difficult on a cruise ship, where a banquet of rich, decadent food is available around the clock. But Barbara did it! She ate her fruit breakfasts on the deck every morning. She enjoyed more fruit and vegetables for lunch. She dined each night with fellow passengers enrolled in the Voyage to Wellness. Here is a letter I received from Barbara a month after the cruise:

Dear Dr. Taub:

Thank you for taking me on a Voyage to Wellness. I had really forgotten what a true pleasure eating is. I took food for granted, and I took my health for granted. But after seven days of thinking about what I ate, taking the time to enjoy my meals and savoring all of the flavors, my eating habits have changed forever. I realized that in the time it took me to park, jump out of my car, then wait in line for a bagel and coffee, I could have sat peacefully at home enjoying my fresh fruit. And I can't eat watching the news at night anymore—it just upsets my stomach! Since I've been eating mindfully and staying on the top five steps of your Food Energy Ladder, I have not had one bout of indigestion, constipation, or diarrhea. And I have more energy than ever. Thank you!

Many of us are just like Barbara. We rarely have our minds on the meal, the food, the taste. When we're eating, we're seldom thinking about the food we put in our mouth; so many other things are going on. Other activities are distracting us. That isn't eating at all! It's ingesting, inhaling, consuming—our minds are elsewhere.

When your mind is elsewhere, you are likely to make poor food choices. And you're also much more likely to overeat. On the other hand, when you eat with awareness, as Barbara learned, you are likely to choose foods that are healthy and recognize when your body is telling you that your stomach is full. Not only do you appreciate the taste of food more, but you also eat less. This is a much better feeling than the impulse to loosen your belt buckle, swallow a few antacids, and lie down after a meal.

Think about what you eat. Awareness is so important. And when you eat with awareness, rather than on autopilot, you will enjoy the foods you are eating much more. When you eat with awareness, every mouthful becomes more pleasurable and satisfying. Every mouthful counts. Eating this way, you are less likely to overeat.

You Need a "Blueprint" for Action

Empowered with knowledge and understanding, you are ready to move forward. In Part Six of this book you will learn how to put your new mental blueprint into action for permanent weight loss and radiant energy. This blueprint is the foundation for achieving your naturally ideal weight and energy *for the rest of your life*. It will guide you to make the small changes in your eating habits and activities that your body is begging you to make, changes that will boost your energy, balance your weight, and enhance your body's innate ability to stay well.

I will not ask you to embark on any changes that seem unreasonable to you. Diets fail because they require changes that are impossible to sustain over the long haul. I will ask you to learn *a new way of eating for life.* The steps you will take during this month are so much simpler than the strict dietary regimens with which you are probably all too familiar and disillusioned. Yet the effect of these steps is profound and everlasting.

I urge you to follow the steps described for twenty-eight days. After that, you will be lighter, more energetic, and healthier. At the end of four weeks, your feelings of wellness and energy will motivate you to continue to eat this way for the rest of your life. It will seem like the most natural thing to do.

Think of an architect's blueprint for a house. It's the master plan, the foundation. Would you even consider building a new house with a temporary blueprint? Of course not. A blueprint has to be the foundation for a long-lasting, solid, sound structure. Think of your body and health in the same way. After all, you may move from house to house in your lifetime, but you only live in one body. Be the architect of your own health. Put into action a sound and solid blueprint that will ensure healthy weight and well-being.

During the twenty-eight days it will take to establish a solid blueprint for lifelong health and ideal weight, you will begin to feel more enthusiastic and more focused. Your body's own natural healing forces will thrive and you will experience a greater sense of well-being, self-esteem, and happiness. It will be exciting for you to experience firsthand how small improvements in your diet can reap such big benefits throughout your cycle of life.

You have read about the dynamic relationship between nutrition and health in previous parts of this book. Don't take lightly what dramatic improvements you can make in your health through the foods you eat. Weight loss is only one of the many significant health benefits you will experience through proper nutrition.

A nutritional strategy high in fruits and vegetables and low in animal fat and fake foods has the proven power to help prevent and even reverse heart disease, lower the risk of many types of cancer, control diabetes, and increase longevity.

In this 28-Day Plan, you will learn how to harness the power of food for weight loss and improved health. Why does it take twenty-eight days to put your new blueprint into action? You may think that sounds like a long time—actually twice as long as a two-week starvation diet. Let's put this into perspective. It took you a lifetime to develop the unhealthful eating habits you have now. If it takes you only twenty-eight days to dissolve these habits forever, isn't that a good return on your investment? Twenty-eight days in the span of a lifetime is just a drop in the bucket, but it is going to make an enormous splash for the rest of your life.

You might as well choose a two-week starvation diet regimen if all you want to do is lose a few pounds quickly and don't mind gaining them back within the next few months. However, if lifelong health and achieving your ideal weight is your goal, it takes only twenty-eight days to put the process permanently in motion. During that time, you will be teaching your body new tastes and learning new ways of preparing your foods. You are creating new, healthful eating habits. They are lessons in eating your body will respond to immediately. After twenty-eight days, you will be feeling so good, so energetic, and so much lighter that you will continue on your path to wellness for life.

Unlike a strict diet of two weeks of feeling deprived, hungry, and dissatisfied, these twenty-eight days are filled with delicious, appetizing, and filling foods. Why punish yourself for a few weeks when you can pamper yourself for four weeks and beyond? You will discover how simple it is to eat well. No diet foods. No diet pills. No diet drinks. No confusing formulas to remember. Just a sensible, natural approach to eating that will help you gain energy and health while losing weight. It doesn't get any better than that!

Food Is Energy . . . Or It's Not

Food is energy. This is the basic scientific principle underlying the way of eating that I advocate. Remember what you learned in the previous parts of this book: Your body is an energy system; every single process in your body requires energy to work. Circulation, metabolism, respiration, digestion—everything needs energy! Every muscle, every organ, every cell needs energy to function healthily. When your energy is low, your body doesn't have the resources it needs to function healthily, and that is when illness results. When your energy is high, health and ideal weight are in your hands. And, as you also learned earlier, food is the source of energy your body needs most.

Food either gives you energy or it takes energy away from you. Food is nature's medicine for nourishing your energy. What you eat either nourishes and helps balance your energy system or it eats away at that balance. In the pages that follow, you will learn a very simple, instinctive way of distinguishing high-energy foods from low-energy foods so that you can feed your body with the proper fuel to lose weight and be well.

If you feel sluggish throughout the day, if you have to drag yourself out of bed and to work, if you rely on coffee to keep you semialert, your energy supply is running dangerously low. If you feel down, unmotivated, as if you are just getting by, your energy is nearly drained. Rather than focus on losing weight, turn your pursuits toward increasing your energy and bringing it back into balance through the foods you eat. Good health, ideal weight, an optimistic outlook, and a peaceful mind will follow.

Nourish Your Body's Natural Capacity to Lose Weight

Yes, I've said it over and over and I will say it again: the best way to lose excess weight and burn fat is to eat foods bursting with nature's life-energy. When you feed your body foods that are high in energy, your body will naturally begin to burn excess fat and lose weight. Your body has more wisdom than all of the diet gurus and the nutritional scientists combined! You just need to eat foods that feed your body's innate wisdom and allow it to do its work.

Most of us don't eat enough "live" energy foods and eat too much food with "dead" energy. If you fill up on dead foods, you are actually starving your body of the energy it requires to be well. Dead food depletes your energy. When you feel sluggish or sleepy after a heavy meal, it's because your body must work overtime, using its life-energy to digest too many dead foods. You feel energy-less because you are.

Specialty diet foods do not give your body proper energy. You may feel as if you are eating something that is low in fat, but foods that are empty of live energy will not help you lose weight. When you lose energy, your body cannot lose weight over the long term in a healthy manner. Diets that restrict you from eating tend to restrict your energy. Your body can only do its natural work of burning your excess fat when it has abundant live energy to do so.

When you emphasize live, high-energy foods in your meals, eating will become an entirely different and more pleasurable experience. The pleasure extends beyond the meal, because after you eat a meal abundant in live foods, your body will thrive from the food's energy. Live food helps your body burn fat, stave off illness and disease, and makes homeostasis soar!

When we understand food as energy, we understand "convenience foods" in an entirely different way. Convenience doesn't come in a can or ready-made microwavable meal. Dead foods are a terrible inconvenience to your body. They give your body less than it needs, and they use up bodily energy to digest them. Digestion requires more energy than any other function your body performs, and digesting dead foods places an incredible burden on your digestive system. If you frequently eat foods marketed as "convenient," ask yourself, "How convenient is it to eat something that robs my body of energy, vitality, and health?"

If you are trying to lose weight, feel healthier, and more fit, the most convenient foods you can eat are alive with energy. Live foods give your body the energy it needs to burn its excess fat efficiently.

Your body certainly recognizes the difference between live and dead food. But remember that when it comes to food, your natural instincts have been suppressed; our culture has trapped your taste buds. You know this as well, even if it's hard to admit. There are no fields of flowing white bread, no potato chips sprouting under the soil, no rivers of soda pop. When was the last time you saw jelly doughnuts growing on trees?

The Food Energy Ladder

Here we are—you are ready! Thank you for your patience and let's go on. You need a ladder to help climb up and out of the traps our culture has set for your taste buds. Thus, I have created the Food Energy Ladder to help you climb back up to foods that are alive and filled with energy and avoid foods that weaken your energy. The Food Energy Ladder is an easy, common-sense tool to help you visualize foods that are alive and filled with energy, as well as foods that are dead and energy depleting. When you care for your body with high-level fuel, you have the highest potential for achieving *Total Health Rejuvenation* and natural weight loss permanently.

Look at the Food Energy Ladder. The food at the top of the ladder is high in energy. The food at the bottom is virtually *energy-less*. Foods at the top of the ladder are natural, while foods at the bottom of the ladder tend to be artificial, processed, and chemically engineered. Your goal for the next twenty-eight days is to stay on the top five steps of the ladder, eating foods that are highest in energy. The 28-Day Plan is as simple as that!

It doesn't mean that the foods at the bottom steps are forbidden.

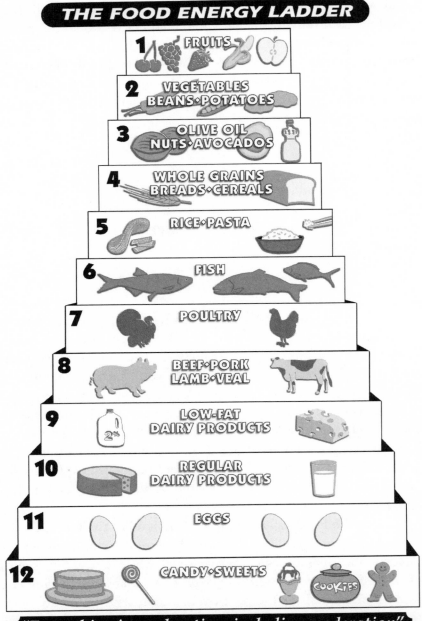

THE FOOD ENERGY LADDER

1 FRUITS

2 VEGETABLES BEANS·POTATOES

3 OLIVE OIL NUTS·AVOCADOS

4 WHOLE GRAINS BREADS·CEREALS

5 RICE·PASTA

6 FISH

7 POULTRY

8 BEEF·PORK LAMB·VEAL

9 LOW-FAT DAIRY PRODUCTS

10 REGULAR DAIRY PRODUCTS

11 EGGS

12 CANDY·SWEETS

"Everything in moderation, including moderation"

Indeed, some of the recipes that follow use small amounts of dairy or eggs. Remember, this is not about deprivation! If you feel deprived of something you want, you will only hunger for it more. That is why it is important to eat primarily foods at the top of the ladder, then *only occasionally* and *moderately* from the foods at the bottom of the ladder. If you slide down the ladder, all you have to do is climb right back up to where you were.

These twenty-eight days, along with your Personal Wellness Retreat, are going to jump-start your energy gain and weight loss. The twenty-eight days of eating high on the Food Energy Ladder will engrain these healthful habits within you and activate your will to continue to *eat wise and live well* beyond the twenty-eight days. **For maximum momentum, stay on the top five steps of the ladder as much as possible.** For most people, weekends are the most likely time for eating lower on the ladder. Allow yourself those moments, but in moderation. An occasional ice cream is not going to sabotage your energy. Where you need to be most diligent, however, is with flesh foods. Poultry and fish are fine, but not more than once every three days. There is even room in this nutritional strategy for a hamburger or steak, but *not* more than once a week. Any more than that and you will not gain the momentum and motivation you need to activate this blueprint for life.

Once you begin to eat the energy way, you will naturally be inclined to stay within the top five steps of the ladder because you will know and feel that these foods enhance your energy, while you will know and feel that the foods at the bottom sap your energy. You will know this by the end of twenty-eight days. When you climb to the top half of the Food Energy Ladder, you will leave your weight worries behind. When you eat at that level, enjoying all of those naturally energy-enhancing foods, your struggles with weight will come to an end—naturally. If you slip down the ladder from time to time, don't punish yourself or feel that you've failed. There is no pit of fire at the bottom of the ladder! If you find yourself at the bottom of the ladder, just climb right back up with your next meal.

To follow the Food Energy Ladder, the basic principles are simple and straightforward:

◆

> Eat foods from the top five steps
> in abundance and variety.
>
> ◆
>
> Before noon, eat mostly
> fresh fruits and juices,
> with whole grain breads and cereals.
>
> ◆
>
> Eat flesh food in moderation:
> Eat fish or poultry no more than once every three days;
> limit red meat to no more than once a week.
>
> ◆
>
> Eat with awareness
> and remember this motto:
>
> *"Everything in moderation . . .*
> *including moderation!"*

Let's climb up the ladder together, step-by-step, so that you understand why the foods are categorized as they are. Remember that the higher on the ladder you eat, the higher the food's energy. And the greater the energy, the more fat you will lose.

At the bottom step of the ladder, *Step 12*, are refined sweets, including chocolate and sugar. The surge of energy you may feel after eating a candy bar is temporary. After the surge subsides, your energy is lower than it was before you ate the sweet. These foods provide a quick jolt but then make your energy dive. The sugar low that follows quickly after the sugar high earns these foods their place at the bottom rung of the Food Energy Ladder. To satisfy your sweet tooth, turn to nature. Nature's fruit is both sweet and sweet on energy.

Eggs have taken a real beating in the last few years. You should eat eggs in moderation, not only because they are *the leading source of high cholesterol* in the American diet, but also because they are dead energy. That is why they are at *Step 11*.

Eggs are only energy when they grow into chickens. Whether you boil, fry, scramble, or poach them, eggs stay low on the ladder. Especially avoid eggs for breakfast—they do not provide the energy you need to begin your day. If you must eat eggs, most grocery stores carry fresh eggs from free-range chickens. And whenever possible, remove the yolks.

Dairy foods are at *Steps 9* and *10*. Nearly every dairy food is now available in a low- or nonfat variety that is generally healthier for you. Cheddar, jack, mozzarella, cottage, and cream cheeses are available in reduced-fat versions. Yogurt from skim milk is almost entirely fat-free. These are more healthful than regular dairy products, not only because they contain less fat, but also because they are easier to digest and don't burden your mucous membranes as much. Still, these foods are difficult to digest, and impossible to digest for some. Remember, cow's milk is wonderful nourishment, if you're a baby cow.

You will find some dairy products in the recipes in this book because most of us are simply not ready to give dairy up completely; remember the motto, *Everything in moderation . . . including moderation*. It is important for you though to stop drinking all the glasses of milk you've been taught are so healthy. My favorite cartoon character, the witty but perennially misunderstood young Calvin of Bill Waterson's *"Calvin and Hobbes,"* showed that wonderful intelligence only children possess when he pondered the question of cow's milk. Calvin asked his animated, stuffed tiger Hobbes, "Who was the guy who first looked at a cow and said, 'I think I'll drink whatever comes out of these things when I squeeze 'em?' " Only humans believe they need the milk of another species to be healthy!

You may protest here, since you know dairy is a source of calcium which is necessary for healthy bones and body. Consider the following foods not only as alternative sources of calcium, but as full of life-energy: broccoli, spinach, brussel sprouts, celery, carrots, artichokes, lima beans, and swiss chard.

Energy eating doesn't mean you have to become a vegetarian, but flesh foods, especially red meat, have low energy. The foods on *Step 8* of the ladder should be downplayed in your diet. Because red meat takes so much energy to digest, it is a burden on your system. If you must eat red meat, then limit yourself to no more than once a week. This will at least give your body the ample time it usually requires to fully digest and eliminate red meat before challenging your system with more of it. The more you burden your body, the less energy you will have for burning fat and protecting yourself from illness.

The average American eats about 175 pounds of meat every year. Red meat is one of the leading sources of fat in the American diet. Remember what you've learned so far about all the health consequences of a diet heavy in meat: *Even just cutting down on how much red meat you eat, and choosing leaner cuts, will lower your animal fat intake and benefit your energy, weight and overall health.* Also keep in mind that when you eat red meat, you are being subjected to the hormones and antibiotics regularly injected into the animals we eat, and these substances are foreign energy to your body.

Poultry, on *Step 7*, is a better alternative than red meat, and many people are already substituting poultry for red meat at the dinner table. Of course, chicken deep-fried with the skin on is just as fatty as red meat. White, skinless chicken breast, grilled or broiled, is the healthier alternative. You can go a step further by eating chicken in smaller amounts, in a sauté of vegetables or with lots of rice. But remember, the concern here is not just about fat. While it is important for you to reduce fat in your diet, the emphasis in this plan is on *increasing your energy*. Poultry, as with other animal foods, is low in efficient live energy. When you do eat poultry, accompany it with lots of fresh vegetables.

Fish, *Step 6*, is the healthiest of flesh foods, higher in energy than red meat or poultry. But it is important to know where the fish comes from. In many parts of the United States, contaminated waters can lower the nutritional value of fish and, in some cases, pose dangerous health risks. If there are toxins in the fish, then that is toxic foreign energy to your body. Fresh fish, from healthy waters, are an excellent, low-fat source of protein. Enjoy fish in moderation, with generous amounts of vegetables!

In fact, whenever you eat red meat, poultry or fish, follow this same energy-wise guideline: Instead of serving vegetables on the side, make the vegetables as prominent as the flesh food part of your meal. You can even try serving vegetables, pasta, and rice as the main dish, with smaller amounts of flesh food on the side. This is the best way to "have your meat and eat it, too."

Remember: The foods between *Steps 6* and *12* should be eaten only on occasion. Flesh foods, such as poultry and fish, should not be eaten more often than once every three days during the next twenty-eight days. Fresh fish is best. Red meat, such as beef and pork, should not be eaten more often than once a week during the next twenty-eight days. Adding it up, that's about two or three meals of flesh food each week.

As for other foods on the lower steps of the ladder, it's okay to have a little cheese grated over your pasta, some slivers of chicken in your vegetable soup, some hard-boiled egg on your chef's salad, some cream in your coffee or milk in your cereal. Again, some of the recipes in this book use dairy products and eggs. These small amounts on occasion are inconsequential, as long as 90 percent of your meal consists of foods from the top five steps.

Pasta and rice, the complex carbohydrates on *Step 5*, are a healthful source of energy. These foods are slow-burning, so they provide sustained energy. Build your dinners around these high-energy foods, accompanying them with fresh vegetables. Like bread, brown rice is higher in energy and fiber than processed white rice. Likewise, seek out higher quality, less processed pasta.

The whole grain foods on *Step 4* are satisfying, filling, healthful, and loaded with energy. Breads and cereals made from whole or unrefined grains such as corn, wheat, rye oats, and rice are a wonderful source of healthy, complex carbohydrates. These are also much higher in fiber than refined, processed white breads or junk cereals. Fiber is an essential ingredient in a healthy diet. Recent studies show that for every ten grams of fiber you add to your diet, your risk of heart attack declines by 20 percent. Whole grain breads, rice, oat products, and cereals are optimal sources of fiber.

As you come to *Step 3* on the ladder—nuts, avocados, and olive oil—you may think you've climbed your way right to high-fat heaven! True, these foods are rich and high in fat, but they are also valuable sources of natural energy. They come from the earth, grow in the sun, and contain no cholesterol. The energy of the fat in an olive, a nut, or an avocado is not the same as the energy of the fat in a strip of bacon! Mediterranean cuisine is laden with olive oil, but people living in that region have some of the lowest rates of heart disease on earth. Also a handful of walnuts every other day seems to reduce, not increase, the risk of heart attack among Americans. But how can this be if fatty foods are supposedly in the danger zone? While these foods are high in plant-based fat, they are abundant in life-energy—and thus have a place high upon the Food Energy Ladder. Eat them in moderation and enjoy!

If you want to eat for energy and to lose weight, there is simply no better source than an abundant daily supply of fresh vegetables and fruits from *Step 1* and *Step 2*. Vegetables and fruits should be the leading foods in your diet. Every day you should eat more of these foods than any other. Plant foods are full of life-energy from the sun that nourishes them. Eating plenty of plant foods nourishes your body naturally and stimulates your body's innate healing abilities.

Eat generously from the top two steps of the ladder, making fruits and vegetables the centerpiece at every meal. These plant foods are filled with fiber, and four or five servings of fruits and vegetables a day will give you the 25–40 grams of fiber your body needs each day. As you have already learned, fiber is absolutely essential for proper elimination, which is vital to weight loss and overall health. Most Americans don't eat nearly the amounts of fruits and vegetables they need. In fact, most Americans don't even eat a single piece of fruit a day; not even their apple a day to keep the doctor away! No wonder Americans are so low in energy and stressed out. Eat more fruits and vegetables!

You've climbed the Food Energy Ladder. For the next twenty-eight days, your ultimate goal is to eat from the variety of foods on the top five steps. When you eat on those top five steps, eating an abundance of fresh fruits and vegetables, your weight will gradually return to its *natural ideal*. That's how homeostasis works. Your body remembers wellness and strives toward balance. If you feed your body naturally, it will naturally achieve its balance. *And then you will not have to worry about excess weight*.

Remember, this is a ladder, not a law. If you eat something on the lower steps, you have not broken any law. We all know too well that restricting foods makes them more appealing, which is why diets drive us crazy. *The goal here is to reduce, not restrict*.

Let's Take the Confusion Out of Food Combining

More than a decade ago, I wrote the foreword to the #1 best-selling nutritional book, *Fit For Life*, a book that revolutionized the way millions of people around the world think about nutrition. The book proposed that, to obtain the most energy from the foods you eat, certain foods should be combined in certain ways. Many people swear by the combinations offered in *Fit For Life*. But others lost their way in the complicated guidelines of what food combinations to emphasize and what to avoid.

Nutritional science has progressed in the last ten years, and we now know that some of the combinations cautioned against in *Fit For Life* can be ignored. So, in a streamlined, scientific update of the principles set forward in that book, the following simple guidelines will help maximize your energy as you eat among the top five steps of the Food Energy Ladder. These guidelines take the confusion and complexities out of food combining.

BREAKFAST AND BEFORE LUNCH

Skipping breakfast is a sure path to sagging energy by lunch time. Your body needs energy to get started in the morning. For breakfast, the following foods will give you an abundant supply of long-lasting energy:

- *Fresh fruit and fruit juice—as much as you want*
- *Whole grain, low-fat cereals without added sugar*
- *Use nonfat, 2% milk, rice or soy milk*
- *Whole grain breads, muffins or bagels with little, if any, butter*
- *Limit coffee to two cups*

This breakfast menu departs from the strict principles of *Fit For Life*, which recommended that fruit be eaten alone, never in combination with other foods. The reasoning behind this rule is that fruit requires very little energy to digest, but when combined with other foods, fruit requires more energy to digest.

Some fruits, however, may actually assist in the process of digesting other foods. Also, combining fruit with other nutritious foods is much better for you than the typical American breakfast combination of eggs, bacon, and toast. If you want to eat fruit and whole grain toast or a bagel for breakfast, go right ahead. You can even enjoy a nutritious whole grain waffle with sliced strawberries (hold the whipped cream, and if you must have syrup, make sure it's real maple!). Eat as much fruit as you want before noon, but don't stuff yourself.

This breakfast may be different from what you now eat in the morning. Some of my patients have given up a thirty-year habit of eggs, toast, and bacon, and swear by a breakfast full of fresh fruit, fruit juice, and some whole grain cereals and breads. Just give it a try—the proof is in the experience! You'll love all the energy this breakfast gives you, and at about eleven o'clock at the office, when you'd typically be reaching for that third cup of coffee, you'll appreciate it even more.

LUNCHTIME TO DINNER

From lunch to dinner, emphasize vegetables, whole grains, and more fruit. If you are likely to have flesh food at dinner, be absolutely sure to avoid flesh at lunch. A lunch of soup, salad, and good bread will fill you with energy during the day and, unlike a heavy lunch, won't make you feel sluggish or in need of nap. The ideal lunch is loaded with raw, fresh vegetables. Eat a generous salad with low-fat dressing and a bowl of vegetable soup, or try layering fresh vegetables in a whole wheat pita or between two layers of fresh, crusty Italian bread. There are endless healthful possibilities, many of which you will find in the recipe section of this book.

DINNER AND BEYOND

For dinner, emphasize complex carbohydrates such as potatoes, rice, and pasta. Eat more vegetables and avoid animal foods. When you eat poultry or fish (not more than once every three days), eat it in smaller amounts, in a sauté of vegetables or accompanied by pasta or rice.

If you do eat red meat (not more than once a week), then on the following day try to eat only fruits and vegetables. This is because red meat is a shock to your energy system, and eating only fruits and vegetables the next day will help your body retain its energy balance.

It's important not to get fanatical about the above guidelines. Remember the Food Energy Ladder motto: *Everything in moderation—including moderation!* Fanaticism fuels failure. Just remember that fruits and vegetables should be in greatest abundance with most of your meals. If the only green you are seeing on your plate is the parsley being used for garnish, then you aren't eating enough vegetables!

Avoid eating after eight o'clock in the evening. By this time, you're gearing up for the rest and rejuvenation your body requires to begin its elimination cycle. Eating after 8:00 P.M., can divert the energy necessary for eliminating wastes from your body to ongoing digestion. You will also miss those vital hours of complete, internal rest so necessary for you to replenish your body with. People who eat late in the evening frequently complain of restless sleep. In great part, such restlessness comes from the new digestive work you've asked your body to perform when it should be doing otherwise: eliminating the unused food you've eaten during the day.

If you absolutely must eat later at night, then it's best to limit your food to a piece of fruit or some raw vegetables. Be assured that if you don't eat after eight at night, you will sleep much more soundly and feel more refreshed and energetic when you awake in the morning.

If you work the night or graveyard shift, the eight o'clock guideline will not work for you. That's okay. Just don't eat at least three hours before going to bed. Your body will adjust very soon and you will never feel dead on the graveyard shift again.

Let's review what and how you should be eating for the next twenty-eight days. First, keep your mind on your meal. When you eat with awareness, every mouthful is more satisfying, and you are much less likely to overeat. Then just follow the guidelines of the

Food Energy Ladder. Stay mainly on the top five steps. If you slide down, climb back up at your next meal. Eat an abundance of fresh fruit in the morning. Eat an abundance of vegetables, especially in soups and salads, along with good whole grain bread and fresh fruit for lunch. Emphasize green leafy vegetables, potatoes and beans, along with complex carbohydrates (rice or pasta) at dinner. Keep in mind that soybean products may be very beneficial in protecting against breast cancer and prostate cancer. Limit poultry and fish to not more often than once every three days. Eat fresh fish if it is available. Don't eat red meat more than once a week. And don't eat after eight o'clock (or three hours before going to bed).

During these twenty-eight days, you are putting into action your new blueprint for a lifetime of nutritional wellness, ideal weight, and balanced energy. In twenty-eight days, you will have imprinted this blueprint into every cell of your body. Remember, your goal isn't fast, temporary weight loss. Your goal is to increase your energy so that your body will burn more fat and your immune system will be stimulated to prevent illness and disease—weight loss will come naturally.

In Part Seven, you'll find a variety of recipes for delicious, satisfying meals that nourish your body with energy and nutrients without burdening your digestive system. Eating naturally for optimal energy doesn't mean you have to go out of your way to shop at a health-food store. Eating naturally actually streamlines your kitchen requirements. Your main ingredients are fresh fruits, fresh vegetables, potatoes, whole grains, pasta, and rice. All these foods should be readily available in your neighborhood supermarket. If not, it is worthwhile to go a little farther. Because the produce is fresh and locally grown, a trip to the local farmer's market is ideal in this regard. As you'll find out in Part Seven, if there is one rule to the recipes, it is this: they are made of easily acquired foods. There are no obstacles to eating well the natural way!

Behind Every Healthy Body Is a Strong Mind: Don't Let Stress Sidetrack Your Will to Eat Wise and Live Well!

Stress is a major obstacle to eating well. Stress affects what you eat. From time to time, as you reach for the top five steps of the ladder, the negative thoughts caused by stress may tug at your heels. You can shake off these thoughts and break free from stress, however, if you possess effective tools to strengthen your resilience. You can learn to surmount stress so that it doesn't sabotage your will to eat well.

Everyone has a certain amount of normal stress in his or her life. Managing this stress by disarming its power to divert you from your goals is especially important when making positive changes in your life, particularly in your attitude toward food and your eating patterns. Stress is the major trigger for overeating and for eating poorly. Because diets play on feelings of guilt, anxiety, and deprivation—all stressful emotions—they undermine your self-value and will to be well. Diets put you under so much mental and emotional stress, they have a built-in mechanism for failure!

Stress begins in your mind. That doesn't mean there aren't people and circumstances that ignite stress; it's your mental and emotional response to them that does the damage. Yes, our culture and environment trigger stress. But in response, you can cultivate a strong mind that will help protect you. That is why your new mental blueprint is such a vital foundation for the changes in nutrition you are making! The blueprint puts *you* in control, so that stress doesn't control you and what you eat.

Healthful, high-energy food can help you in dealing with stress. But if food is one of the ways you typically respond to stress, then understand why dead, low-energy food really is no escape. If a bag of fudge cookies is your common weapon against stress, you are losing the battle. On the other hand, if you nourish your body with live, high-energy foods during stressful times, you will remain in control and help give your body and mind the strength you need to resolve the stress you face.

When you are stressed out, your energy burns up. Most people greet a stressful situation with worry, anger, fear, and anxiety. As a result, you pour so much energy into the source of your stress that you feel drained. In fact, you *are* drained—drained of the vital energy that you need to keep body and mind well.

Stress, in fact, is a national epidemic. It is the leading factor that makes us susceptible to illness and disease. Stress diminishes your body's amazing ability to keep you well. Nonetheless, you have a tremendous healing force within you, a healing force with the wisdom to keep well and close to your naturally ideal weight. Stress burdens that healing force within you. At the same time, stress weakens your body's immune system, and if stress persists you may not be able to defend against infection and disease.

Stress is largely the result of feeling you have no options left, are at the end of your rope and ready to give in. It's easy to feel this way if you have little or no energy. But when you supercharge your energy, as you will when you eat high on the Food Energy Ladder, you will feel empowered instead of hopeless, bold instead of broken, and determined instead of depressed. That is why the nutritional ladder you are learning to climb is such a powerful tool for stress management. When you climb up the Food Energy Ladder, you boost your energy and your will to be well. You feel healthier, more vital, more energetic, and positive. These feelings of self-value protect you from the harmful effects of stress. *Feelings of self-esteem take the steam out of stress!*

You can vaccinate yourself against stress as you would against viruses. Yet it doesn't require a needle and it is perfectly painless. And the only side effects are wonderfully positive. Your protection against stress comes from inside of you. Balanced energy inoculates you against stress. Eating high on the Food Energy Ladder naturally bolsters your energy and stops your stress in its tracks, before it stops you in yours!

Eating high on the Food Energy Ladder will also help you stay out of the vicious stress/food cycle. People commonly react to stress by overeating, eating junk food, or both. Stress triggers eating, and eating triggers more stress. When stress causes you to be upset, depressed, sad, anxious, or worried, it leads you to indulge in poor eating habits. When under emotional distress, you are more likely to fall back down the ladder and indulge in the very eating habits you are currently trying to change.

The power of emotional distress to plunge you back into behaviors you are trying to inhibit is called the "stress disinhibition effect." I've seen this effect in many of my patients, who drink, smoke, and eat too much. Allen, a thirtysomething stockbroker, came to me with his blood pressure skyhigh. He was headed straight for a heart attack before he turned forty: He was fifty pounds overweight and his only exercise was waving his arms wildly on the stockmarket floor. If he was going to ward off the heart attack that was just around the corner, Allen knew lifestyle changes were absolutely necessary, and we both knew that the first place to begin was with his eating habits. He began to eat according to the principles of the Food Energy Ladder, and in just two months he looked remarkably healthier, felt better, and his blood pressure fell dramatically.

Allen's climb up the Food Energy Ladder was temporarily stymied when the stress of a sudden stockmarket decline crashed down upon him. He was terrified of losing everything: his clients, his job, his savings, his home. His emotional distress over the situation triggered his slide back into the very eating habits he was working so hard to overcome. Allen returned to my office again with his blood pressure dangerously high.

First I asked Allen to take several deep breaths. As he began to relax, I asked him to tell me about the sources of his stress. Like many people, he identified work as the main culprit. Worry over finances, time pressure, job security, and future prospects all heightened his stress. Once Allen identified his sources of stress, which also triggered his overeating, we were ready to discuss how to cope with it all. Overeating wasn't solving his stress. In fact, overeating caused him more stress in regard to his health.

In the questionnaire answered earlier, you identified what causes stress in your life. You, too, can now begin to control your response to the people, events, and circumstances you associate with stress. That doesn't mean you can lead a stress-free life just like that! But you can devise an action plan that will strengthen your energy to surmount stress and prevent you from overeating or eating poorly in response to your stress.

Extreme stress overwhelms the human body's energy system. It's a bit like turning on every light and appliance in your house at the same time. The fuse box or circuit breaker overloads and blows out. Stress robs your energy and leaves you out of balance and without the mental resources to make healthy eating choices. This is why it is so crucial to take stock of the stressful situations in your life and work to either change those that you can or change your reaction and response to those that you can't. Everyone has some level of stress in their life that cannot be avoided, and it's in those situations that you need positive, effective methods for conquering stress, so that it doesn't conquer you.

The good news is that you are already taking momentous steps to build up your resistance to stress! Climbing the Food Energy Ladder cultivates your inner strength and energy and your will to eat wise and live well. The higher you climb, the lower your chances of experiencing the negative impact of stress. During stressful times, it is especially important to stay among the top five steps of the ladder and especially to avoid sweets (the "sugar blues" is a poor state to be in under stress). Eating well is one of the best forms of stress prevention. The investment you make in your energy now will save you from stress in the future.

In all of my years working with patients one thing has become especially clear: If you are trying to make lifestyle changes involving food, alcohol, or nicotine, the key to your success is an effective way to manage stress. Your climb up the Food Energy Ladder will be permanently successful once you learn how to effectively deal with stressful situations that can cause you to give in to temptation.

Stress sidetracks your resolve. So much of your body's energy is mobilized to fight the harmful physical effects of stress that you are left with little energy to help maintain your will to eat wise and live well. Excessive stress consumes your energy, leaving you with a weakened ability to cope. But this 28-Day *Action* Plan will help you keep your mindset right on track.

Unless you have the resources and tools, psychological and emotional stress can create a downward spiral all too difficult to avoid.

Under stress, people turn to food for comfort. But indulging in the very behaviors you're trying to control just makes you feel more stressed out. You feel bad for eating poorly, for falling back on the old habits from which you are trying to free yourself. And when your self-value drops, your stress rises. One of the greatest benefits of climbing the Food Energy Ladder is that the longer you stay among the top five steps, the more powerful your resolve becomes, and the better able you are to fight the stress disinhibition effect.

According to the diet industry, failure to lose weight is a personal fault. How many times have we heard these "ifs": *If she only tried harder . . . If he only had more willpower . . . If she just had more determination . . .* These negative messages probably do more harm than the diets themselves—they are part of your mental blueprint and it's time to erase them. It is time for you to show yourself deep compassion and realize that it is not your lack of personal strength that has undermined your past efforts to lose weight. The underlying cause of a dieter's relapse is almost always the lack of effective skills for coping with stressful situations and demands. Without such skills, even a person with the strongest inner resolve is likely to lapse back into poor eating behaviors.

It is crucial to remember that if, during the twenty-eight days, you occasionally eat foods from the bottom of the Food Energy Ladder, *you have not failed*. This is *not* an all-or-nothing diet. This is not about deprivation. Moderation is your motto. Don't judge yourself if you have an occasional bowl of ice cream. You are not doomed to failure if you do. Don't beat yourself up for lacking willpower. Instead, ask yourself: Why do I want to eat ice cream? Is it a response to a stressful situation? Or do I simply want a little bit of something sweet? If stress is causing you to crave ice cream, remind yourself that it won't make the stress go away. And if the stress remains, you are likely to feel tempted again. If you just want a little ice cream, remind yourself of your long-term goals and try a low-fat variety or nonfat frozen yogurt. Or just have a *little bit* of ice cream. That's part of moderation.

For many people, food is a habitual escape from stress. Eating through a pint quart of ice cream, a chocolate cake, or a bag of fast-food hamburgers and fries may seem to offer a temporary escape from worries and troubles. For the moment, the act of eating takes your mind off your worries; it indulges your senses, giving you feelings of pleasure. But the effect is fleeting. Once the act of indulgence is over—the ice cream is gone, not a crumb of cake remains, the bag of fast food is empty—the feelings of stress return, and most people feel worse than they did before binging.

Should you find yourself in the above scenario, don't attribute your lapse to personal inadequacy or failure. Just recognize that you are learning how to develop the tools for effectively managing stress in the future. Don't berate yourself or judge yourself harshly. Feelings of low self-esteem just add fuel to the fire of stress. Show yourself some compassion and climb right back up the Food Energy Ladder at your next meal.

During the first twenty-eight days of eating high on the Food Energy Ladder, you are reprogramming your thoughts and your taste buds. Remember, you are putting a new blueprint into action. And, as you learn how to eat well, and continue to eat well over time, you will *unlearn* the negative habit of overeating in response to stress.

Regularly renewing your body's energy supply with fresh, live foods is one major step in combatting stress. Renewing your mental energy is equally important; reducing negative thoughts reduces your harmful responses to stress. Mental relaxation provides nourishment for your mind. You previously read about the mental relaxation exercises that bolster your will to eat wise and live well. Regularly practicing these exercises is a wonderful form of stress insurance. Unlike physical exercise, it's impossible to overdo it! (Just don't practice mental relaxation while driving!) The more timeouts you give your mind, the more opportunity you take for moments of peace and calm, the greater your ability to respond to stress effectively. Remember, regular mental relaxation builds a strong and healthy mind. And a strong and healthy mind won't be rattled by stress.

Keep practicing the mental relaxation exercises. Increase your practice when you feel stressed out. This is especially important when a stressful situation triggers emotional hungers for foods low on the Food Energy Ladder. Now that you have identified the situations that trigger stress in your life, prepare yourself for those moments with mental relaxation. If family visits are high on your list of stressors, be sure that during the visit you take your own personal timeout, ten minutes to practice your mental relaxation. I assure you, you will be able to cope with even the most tense family situations afterwards.

Shortly, in Parts Eight, Nine and Ten, respectively, you will learn how physical activity helps inoculate you against stress and about nutritional supplements that enhance your energy, which is especially important during stressful times. For now, understand that the new mindset you have created and are putting into action empowers you with knowledge that is essential to being well, losing weight, and beating stress. Twenty-eight days may seem like a lot right now, but what you do during those days will establish your blueprint for the rest of your life. Climbing the Food Energy Ladder will strengthen your ability to achieve your ideal weight and lead a healthy, stress-free life.

During these twenty-eight days, *don't* obsess about weight loss. *Don't* hop on the scale every morning after you shower. *Don't* be in a rush to see if your size eight jeans from five years ago fit again. Just relax and enjoy the process of taking good care of yourself. Think about the process itself, not the desired result. If you enjoy the process, and stay with it long enough so it becomes a natural habit to eat and mentally relax, the desired weight loss will naturally result. Keep your mind in the present and don't worry about the future. Feel good about yourself for taking such good care of your body. Put your best foot forward and climb up the ladder. Remember, this is not just about losing weight; it is about improving your health and energy forever! It is about enhancing homeostasis—the basis of *Total Health Rejuvenation*. Nature will take care of the rest.

The Power of the Written Word

In the twenty-eight days that it takes to turn energy eating into a natural habit, your progress will be visible in many ways. Your weight loss will show, your increased energy will shine through, your eyes will light up with radiant health, and your uplifted outlook will be clear to all. Your feelings about yourself, your body, and your health should be soaring right now! You have already done the hardest work of all. That hard work of introspection, self-reflection, and personal evaluation has put you firmly on the path to natural weight loss and radiant energy. You are on the ladder toward *Total Health Rejuvenation*, upward bound!

Keep in mind that your eyes have been trained to see yourself in a certain way—probably much more critically than others actually see you. Many people who experience weight loss have a difficult time adjusting their self-image to their new, more slender, healthier self. Many of us look at ourselves as if through a funhouse mirror: Our self-image is distorted and out of perspective.

A positive self-image is vital to your motivation to continue to climb up the Food Energy Ladder. It is especially important to change your feelings about your body. Remember, as you have learned, your body image influences how well you care for your body. A poor body image encourages poor care in eating.

I don't want you to lose sight of all that you have already accomplished. Remember, changing your mindset is the most important step—it is the *key* to changing your diet. Believe it or not, you have already made tremendous efforts to establish a new mindset to support your new eating habits. Just by reading this book, you've proven that you are interested in change. What your eyes may not see in the mirror can be seen on paper, if you write it down. The best way to see all the progress you are making, all the important ways you are caring for your health, is to keep a daily journal.

Think of keeping your journal as if it was a love letter to yourself. Praise yourself for all the good you are doing. Congratulate yourself for eating high on the Food Energy Ladder. Every day, write down at least one thing you are proud of. For example, if you had a wonderful garden salad for lunch instead of a hamburger, write it down so that you can remember how good that made you feel. If you conquered a craving for chocolate by eating a naturally sweet piece of fruit instead, write that down!

Your journal is also a great place to note your responses to your daily meditations. Take some time after you finish your meditation and write down how you are feeling. Write down anything interesting or inspiring that came up during the meditation, an image or a feeling. Make notes about how you feel before and after meditating. What are the differences? Keeping a journal of these experiences leaves you with proof positive that you can see and touch, a record to remind you of the revolutionary steps you are personally taking to increase your energy, and achieve your naturally ideal weight. Total health rejuvenation!

Emphasize the positive in your journal, but don't ignore any hurdles you find yourself leaping. Writing down the difficulties is not to remind you of a weakness or to make you feel guilty if, for example, you fall down the ladder now and then. But it can help you overcome those hurdles the next time you face them. You will be infinitely more appreciative of the progress you are making when you see how far you have come.

Keeping a journal is a powerful strategy for stress management. When you feel stressed out, taking a moment just to write down how you feel, especially about whatever is making you stressed, has the same effect as a tea kettle that reaches the boiling point and then lets off steam. Writing it down helps relieve the pressure of stress before it reaches the boiling point—before *you* boil over. When stress triggers an emotional hunger to eat poorly or to overeat, sit down and begin writing. The process of writing it down may be just the pressure valve you need. Remember that food is only a fleeting escape from stress. Let your journal be a comforting and constructive source for blowing off stress.

♦

Your journal is so important to your journey that I have included space for a "model therapeutic journal" and inspirational quotes for each of the days. Make sure to purchase a special journal or notebook that you will carry with you. Just follow the model provided. It is especially important that every day you note whether you stayed on the top five steps of the Food Energy Ladder. *You don't have to count the cream in your coffee, milk in your cereal or the small amounts of dairy and eggs in this book's recipes.*

In the upper righthand corner of the page of your journal, make a ✓ if all of your meals for that day came from the top five steps. If you ate below Step 5, mark the box with an ✗. At the end of the twenty-eight days, count up all of the ✗s. Hopefully, there are no more than ten because you need to stay among the top five steps for the majority of the twenty-eight days to jump-start the process of permanent weight loss. If you have more than twelve ✗s, begin the twenty-eight days again. Don't punish yourself. You are making big improvements. *Just begin again . . . and know that this time you will do it! Total Health Rejuvenation* is worth it!

At the end of the twenty-eight-day period, I want you to make a special entry in your journal. Give yourself tremendous praise for taking twenty-eight days to improve your weight and wellness for the rest of your life. Take a look back at the journey. It wasn't so difficult, was it? Don't you feel ready to continue eating this way for the rest of your life? *Pledge to yourself that you will continue to climb up—and stay on top of—the Food Energy Ladder.*

With your new mindset about food, your feet firmly on the Food Energy Ladder, and a journal in hand to track your progress, you are ready for action. You are in control. You have a blueprint and a ladder! That's all you need to climb up to new personal health and energy peaks. You will be amazed by how good you look and feel after just twenty-eight days. People will comment on how rested, radiant, light and energized you appear. *They will want to know what you are doing to look so great.*

Total Health Rejuvenation requires you to treat your body as a temple for your soul during the 28-Day Plan—meditating, exercising, staying high on the Food Energy Ladder, and keeping a therapeutic journal . . . *not a lot to ask of yourself!*

MODEL THERAPEUTIC JOURNAL

1. Every day, after you finish your meditation, write down how you are feeling.

2. Every day, write down at least one thing you are proud of for that day.

3. Stay among the top 5 steps of the Food Energy Ladder for most of the next 28 days. Mark a ☑ in the box if you do. Mark an ☒ in the box if you don't.

4. Be sure to do your wellness yoga stretching and your wellness walking five days a week. Also, be sure to do the simple strength training exercises two or three days a week, especially if you are over 50. (see Parts Eight and Nine)

Please get a notebook. Just use the "Model Therapeutic Journal" on the following pages as a guide to what you should be writing down in your own notebook each day. Please take the time to reflect on each day's very special inspirational quote, which I have chosen to be part of your daily dose of self-administered TLC—*Tender Loving Care.*

DAY 1

I had an incredible meditation experience. I always pray a lot and ask God a lot of questions. But with my mind becoming so quiet, I felt that I could finally hear God's answers. They made me cry because I could see how much strength I really have and I could truly feel how much God loves me.

Before noon, I had a glass of fresh orange juice and I ate half of a cantaloupe as well as a banana, which made me feel great all day! I had a big salad and some good whole wheat bread for lunch. My family loved the vegetable lasagna I made for our Sunday dinner. No meat at all, today. That's amazing for me—for my kids and husband too.

Let's see . . . I did my yoga stretches and my wellness walk and I actually enjoyed it, which is no small matter for a couch potato like me. Where did I get all this energy? What a great start!

DAY 2

A wonderful meditation again! I felt like I did when I was a little girl and I used to lie on the grass during summer evenings and watch the stars. I must have drifted really deeply because when I opened my eyes, I felt like a child again!

Last night I slept great—maybe because I didn't eat after 8 PM. Also, I set the alarm for an hour earlier so I could meditate, exercise, and still have time to get to work.

I know I'll really sleep like a baby tonight because I did the entire set of strength training exercises— with 5 pound weights! Now I'm really proud of myself! Starting the day with so much fruit seems to be giving me an incredible amount of energy. I just love it.

❧ DAY 1 ❑

Look at a day when you are supremely
satisfied at the end. It's not a day when
you lounge around doing nothing, it's
when you've had everything to do, and
you've done it.
—MARGARET THATCHER

❧ DAY 2 ❑

Look after yourself every day and put
forth your best effort to love yourself
enough to do what's best.
—OPRAH WINFREY

❧ DAY 3 ❑

The world cares very little about what
a man or woman knows; it is what a
man or woman is able to do that
counts.
—BOOKER T. WASHINGTON

❧ DAY 4 ❑

It's okay to make mistakes. Mistakes
are our teachers—they help us to learn.
—JOHN BRADSHAW

❧ DAY 5 ❑

If you want your dreams to come true,
don't sleep, act!
—YIDDISH PROVERB

❧ DAY 6 ❑

The only place where your dream
becomes impossible is in your own
thinking.
—ROBERT H. SCHULLER

❧ DAY 7 ❑

There is hunger for ordinary bread but
there is also hunger for love, for
kindness and for thoughtfulness. This
is the great poverty that makes people
suffer so much.
—MOTHER TERESA

❧ DAY 8 ❑

If opportunity doesn't knock, build a
door.
—MILTON BERLE

DAY 9 ❑

Our greatest glory is not in never
falling, but in rising every time we fall.
—CONFUCIUS

DAY 10 ❑

You must do the very thing you think
you cannot do.
—ELEANOR ROOSEVELT

DAY 11 ❑

We all have ability. The difference is
how we use it.
—STEVIE WONDER

DAY 12 ❑

They can conquer who believe they
can. He has not learned the first lesson
of life who does not every day
surmount a fear.
—RALPH WALDO EMERSON

❧ DAY 13 ❑

We can do anything we want if we stick to it long enough.
—HELEN KELLER

❧ DAY 14 ❑

If I'd known I was gonna live this long, I'd have taken better care of myself.
—EUBIE BLAKE AT AGE 100

❧ DAY 15 ❑

Dining is, after all, a spiritual experience.
—NICOS KAZANTAKIS

❧ DAY 16 ❑

Strength does not come from physical capacity. It comes from an indomitable will.
—MAHATMA GANDHI

DAY 17 ❏

When you win . . . you won't
remember the pain.
—JOE NAMATH

DAY 18 ❏

The ultimate measure of a man is not
where he stands in moments of
comfort and convenience, but where he
stands in times of challenge.
—MARTIN LUTHER KING

DAY 19 ❏

We write our own destiny. We become
what we do.
—MADAME CHIANG KAI-SHEK

DAY 20 ❏

Never wait for trouble. Be prepared
for it.
—CHUCK YAEGER

DAY 21 ❑

The doctor of the future will give no
medicine, but will interest his patients
in the care of the human frame, in diet,
and in the cause of disease.
—THOMAS EDISON

DAY 22 ❑

Every blade of grass has its Angel that
bends over it and whispers, *"Grow . . .
Grow."*
—THE TALMUD

DAY 23 ❑

Resolve, and you are free!
—HENRY WADSWORTH LONGFELLOW

DAY 24 ❑

Never let the fear of striking out get in
your way.
—BABE RUTH

DAY 25 ❏

The journey of a thousand miles begins
with one step.
—LAO-TSZE

DAY 26 ❏

The whole of science is nothing more
than a refinement of everyday
thinking.
—ALBERT EINSTEIN

DAY 27 ❏

Everyone's life is a fairy tale written by
God's fingers.
—HANS CHRISTIAN ANDERSON

DAY 28 ❏

Start the day with love. Fill the day
with love. End the day with love.
—SATHYA SAI BABA

DAY 28

I'm really proud of myself . . . I feel like I've been living my life as a prayer for the past 28 days. I've meditated every day, exercised almost every day, eaten foods high on the Food Energy Ladder, and kept writing in my journal.

The exercise was truly fun but very surprising. As a former devoted couch potato, I still can't believe how well I'm doing with wellness yoga stretching, wellness walking and lifting weights.

I know that I'll never be able to look at food in the same way again. No milk for me means no gas. I love it! Also, when I add up my (checks) and my (x's) in the journal, I see that I've eaten turkey or chicken 4 times and fish 4 times. And no beef or pork . . . not bad for having spent my childhood growing up in Kansas City!

Also, I'm no longer so fearful and worried so much of the time—it's like my stress level is lower than it's been in years because now I know just how I can cope. After all, I have strength and God loves me!

One last thing. It has felt completely natural for me to continue living the way that I did during my one day Personal Wellness Retreat . . . in other words, no doing anything wrong and also being more loving. I feel great, I know I look good . . . and I'm really proud of myself!

Part Seven

THE COOKBOOK

Recipes for Radiant Energy and Weight Loss That Lasts

A WORD FROM ANNELI TAUB

Many people have asked me how I cook for a wellnesss medical doctor. I reply in words attributed to Zorba the Greek that I once saw written on the ceiling of an old country inn in Corsica: "I have decided, after all, that dining is a spiritual experience."

I grew up in Europe with a mother who made everything from scratch. So it would never cross my mind to use a so-called ready-made meal from the supermarket freezer. I never hesitate to drive the extra miles to a farmer's market where I can pick through the freshest produce available, produce still clinging to vines, still dusted with soil. I'll splurge on a good olive oil and balsamic vine-gar to accent and bring out the flavors of these delicious foods. A good bakery is a must for the best bread. When I shop at the local supermarket, I especially look for fruits and vegetables that are in season and locally grown because I want foods that are ripened naturally by the sun. My extra efforts are rewarded with the joy of my husband (and our guests) eating foods full of energy that taste as if they originated from my own garden.

I used to be a big meat eater. But once I moved away from fatty, fleshy foods to cleaner, fresher, live-energy foods, I had very little need to go back to my old ways. Do the same and your body will thank you for it.

I'm happy to share with you some of our favorite recipes for delicious meals. I've also included a few recipes from *Seven Steps To Self-Healing* by Edward A. Taub, M.D., *The Low Fat Jewish Vegetarian Cookbook* by Debra Wasserman and *Great Tastes—Healthy Cooking From Canyon Ranch*. I believe you'll find all the recipes to be healthy, savory, and easy to prepare. Simplicity and common sense are the most important aspects of my cooking. I don't count calories or fat grams. I just try to stay among the top five steps of the Food Energy Ladder. Taste is subjective, so a recipe shouldn't be measured exactly by one teaspoon of this and two teaspoons of that. I encourage you to improvise—I'd much rather inspire you than direct you.

Here, then, is what and how we eat in our home. Hopefully, as it is for us, eating will become a spiritual experience for you. *L'Chaim—To Life.*

SALADS

Antipasto di Anneli

MAKES 4 SERVINGS

Serve this antipasto on a spring or summer evening, with your favorite red wine and fresh bread.

12 *stalks asparagus, steamed until tender, and halved*
1 *12-ounce jar artichoke hearts in water, drained*
1 *red bell pepper, sliced in thin strips*
1 *red onion, thinly sliced*
1 *cup sundried tomatoes (softened in a bowl of hot water, drained and chopped)*
1 *8-ounce can Kalamata olives in water, drained*
8 *leaves fresh basil, chopped coarsely*
2 *tablespoons olive oil*
2 *tablespoons balsamic vinegar*
2 *tablespoons lemon juice*
1/2 *cup shaved asagio cheese*
Salt and pepper to taste

NOTE: To soften sundried tomatoes: place sun dried tomatoes in a bowl of scalding water and set aside for 15–20 minutes. Drain and chop.

1. On a large platter or serving plate, arrange asparagus, artichoke hearts, bell pepper, and onion.

2. Top with sundried tomatoes, olives, and basil.

3. Mix together olive oil, balsamic vinegar, and lemon juice. Drizzle over vegetables.

4. Top antipasto with asagio cheese and season to taste with salt and pepper.

◆

Traditional Italian antipasto salads are so high in fat and calories. The vegetables are drenched in oil and soggy, with layers of processed meats.

◆

This low-fat, vegetarian variety brings out the best flavors of an antipasto. It's filled with Italian delicacies, such as artichoke hearts and sumptuous olives, but goes light on the high-fat cheeses and unhealthy oils.

Caesar Salad

MAKES 2 SERVINGS

Our family and friends agree that this recipe has all of the goodness of a traditional Caesar salad without the unhealthy traditional raw egg.

½ cup Parmesan cheese, grated
1 tablespoon low-fat plain yogurt
4 garlic cloves, minced
Juice of half a lemon
1 tablespoon Worcestershire sauce
½ tablespoon Dijon mustard
Black pepper to taste
8 leaves romaine lettuce, washed and torn

1. To prepare the dressing, combine the first 6 ingredients in a medium-size mixing bowl and whisk well. Season dressing to taste with pepper.

2. Pour dressing over lettuce and toss to coat leaves thoroughly.

There are endless "healthful" variations on this timeless classic. Unfortunately, most lack the flavor of a true Caesar salad. Here's a variation that tastes just like a Caesar salad is supposed to taste!

Quick Noodle Salad

MAKES 2 SERVINGS

This cool salad is perfect for a warm summer day or evening. It's light and refreshing—the perfect salad for a picnic.

> 2 *tablespoons lime juice*
> 1 *tablespoon soy sauce*
> 1 *tablespoon canola oil*
> 2 *cucumbers, peeled, halved, seeded, and sliced*
> ½ *red bell pepper, seeded and thinly sliced*
> 6 *ounces plain ramen, soba, or vermicelli noodles*
> 2 *cups water*
> 2 *tablespoons cilantro, chopped*

1. Mix the lime juice, soy sauce, and oil. Add the cucumbers and bell peppers and toss well.

2. Put the ramen in a bowl and cover with boiling water. Let the noodles stand until al dente—about ten minutes—then strain. Let ramen cool, then combine with the vegetable mixture.

3. Garnish with cilantro and serve.

NOTE: If using soba or vermicelli noodles, follow cooking instructions on package.

For a delicious variation with added protein, top noodles with ½ cup of toasted peanuts or cashews, chopped coarsely.

Be creative about adding more grains to your diet. Along with traditional pastas, other varieties of noodles are high in complex carbohydrates, fiber, and vitamins.

Ramen or soba noodles are available in most supermarkets and natural food stores. If your store does not carry them, vermicelli pasta is a fine substitute.

Most ramen noodles come in a package with a seasoning pack. Keep the noodles, but throw away the seasoning pack—most are loaded with high-fat tropical oils and animal products.

◆

Tomato Mozzarella Salad

MAKES 2 SERVINGS

On warm evenings, we dine on this salad for dinner alone. With fresh bread for soaking up the zesty vinaigrette, it is a substantial and healthy meal.

> 2 tablespoons pine nuts, toasted (walnuts are suitable, too)
> 2 cloves garlic, mashed
> 1/2 tablespoon olive oil
> 1/2 cup Arugula, washed and torn in bite-size pieces
> 5 leaves Romaine lettuce, washed and torn in bite-size pieces
> 1/2 tablespoon balsamic vinegar
> Salt and pepper to taste
> 1 tablespoon raisins, soaked in water for 10 minutes
> 2 large tomatoes, cut in wedges
> 8 ounces low-fat mozzarella cheese, cut in 1/4 inch slices

1. Combine nuts with garlic and olive oil. Spread on a foil-covered baking sheet and toast in 350° oven for 5 minutes, until golden brown. (Keep a close eye on this because it browns quickly).

2. In a large bowl, toss greens with vinegar and season to taste with salt and pepper. Stir in raisins and toasted nuts.

3. On a platter, arrange tomato wedges and cheese slices around the tossed greens.

4. Serve with crunchy Italian bread or fresh baguettes.

The fresh and tangy tastes of this salad make a delicious meal in itself. Wonderfully light and crisp, and easy to prepare, this salad is full of energy and protein.

◆

Pine nuts come from the cones of the stone pine and have a deep, rich flavor. Combined with low-fat mozzarella, this light salad packs a protein punch.

◆

For a lively variation, substitute small bits of apple for the raisins.

◆

Anneli's Tomato Salad

MAKES 4 SERVINGS

This is a simple yet sensational salad. The freshest vine-ripened tomatoes will create the most flavorful salad.

8 medium tomatoes, cut in small wedges
1 tablespoon rice vinegar, (seasoned)
½ small onion, minced
1 tablespoon parsley, finely chopped
½ teaspoon salt
1 teaspoon sugar
Black pepper to taste

1. Place tomato wedges in a medium bowl. Set aside.

2. In another bowl, mix together vinegar, onion, parsley, salt, sugar, and pepper, beating well with a fork.

3. Pour mixture over tomatoes and toss lightly.

4. Try serving with Veggie Burgers and fresh corn.

Tomatoes are a versatile vegetable, high in vitamin C. To keep tomatoes fresh and flavorful, do not refrigerate them. This may seem counterintuitive, but it's true. The cold refrigerator not only destroys a fresh tomato's flavor, it may destroy its vitamins.

◆

When buying tomatoes, buy only as much as you can use in the next three or four days. The extra trip to the store or farmer's market will be well worth it.

◆

Rice vinegar gives this salad loads of flavor without loading it with the fat of traditional salad dressings. This salad is virtually fat free.

◆

For variety, use cucumbers instead of tomatoes, or try a combination of both.

Swabian Potato Salad

MAKES 4 SERVINGS

This salad originates from the southwestern region of Germany. When I was growing up, no Sunday meal was complete at my house without this salad (which we called Grossmutter's Kartoffel Salat). It's much more flavorful (and healthful!) than the traditional potato salad made with mayonnaise.

> 6 medium potatoes (Yukon Gold is best), peeled and
>   boiled until just soft, thinly sliced
> ½ small onion, finely grated
> 2 tablespoons white vinegar
> 2 tablespoons canola oil
> 1 tablespoon chopped chives
> ½ teaspoon salt
> ½ teaspoon pepper
> 1 teaspoon sugar
> 1 teaspoon Dijon mustard

1. Place sliced potatoes in a large bowl. Set aside.

2. Mix all remaining ingredients together in a small bowl, stirring vigorously till creamy.

3. Add mixture to potatoes. Stir gently. If too dry, add some hot water.

NOTE: If time allows, cook the potatoes a few hours before, so they are easier to slice very thin.

Potatoes are loaded with healthful complex carbohydrates and are a wonderful source of vitamin C, iron, and fiber. It's only how we prepare them that sometimes makes them high in fat and unhealthy. Unlike traditional potato salads doused in mayonnaise, this one gets its creamy texture from vinegar and Dijon mustard.

◆

When it comes to satisfying foods that fill you up without all the calories and fat, potatoes cannot be beat.

◆

◆

Accompany this dish with Swabian Cucumber Salad for a memorable summer picnic. You can even combine the two salads into one. Because it's free of mayonnaise, this potato salad will not spoil.

◆

For dinner, this salad marries wonderfully with Chicken Goulash or Turkey Patties.

Fast Green Bean Salad

MAKES 2 SERVINGS

Savory, tasty and tangy, this salad is a treat for the tastebuds and so easy to prepare. Use fresh green beans if they are in season.

1 14-ounce can French-cut green beans, drained
1 tablespoon onion, finely grated
1 tablespoon parsley, finely chopped
1 tablespoon white vinegar
¼ teaspoon salt
½ teaspoon Maggi
Dash each of pepper and sugar
1 tablespoon canola oil

1. Drain the water from the beans and empty them into a bowl. Add the remaining ingredients and mix well, so that all the beans are coated with dressing.

Green beans are a high-fiber vegetable. A great, tasty way to get most of the nutritional fiber you need in a day is to enjoy this salad.

◆

This is quick and simple but has a distinct flavor, thanks to the blend of Maggi, pepper and sugar. Maggi is a condiment which has a nutty, round taste and is widely used in Germany. It's also great for soups, instead of salt. Look for Maggi in the gourmet foods or condiment section at your market.

Mango Dressing

MAKES 2 CUPS

This delicious, aromatic dressing complements a fresh salad of spinach leaves or other greens. It's tropical flavors are perfect any time as long as mangos are available.

> 1 *small mango, peeled and cored*
> 1 *garlic clove, mashed*
> 2 *tablespoons nonfat yogurt or silken tofu*
> 1 *tablespoon cilantro*
> $1/2$ *teaspoon pepper*
> 2 *teaspoons lemon juice*
> *Salt to taste*

1. Put all ingredients in a blender or food processor and blend until creamy.

2. Chill well and serve over your favorite salad, or for something different, over rice.

Mangos are freshest and most flavorful in late spring and summer, when they are in season.

◆

This sweet-smelling and succulent fruit is a wonderful source of vitamin A and potassium.

◆

Be sure to pick mangos that are not overripe or bruised.

◆

Tahini Dip or Dressing

MAKES APPROXIMATELY 1 CUP

Tahini and garlic are a tangy combination that liven up any sandwich or salad. For dip, follow the directions below. To thin dip for a salad dressing, add water until desired consistency.

> 1/4 cup tahini (sesame seed paste)
> 1 tablespoon lemon juice
> 1 tablespoon soy sauce
> 1 tablespoon white vinegar
> 1 garlic clove, mashed
> 2 tablespoons water (more for a thinner dressing)

1. In a bowl, whisk together all ingredients. For a creamier texture, use a blender.

2. Add more water for dressing. If you add too much water and dressing is too runny, just add more tahini.

Tahini is a traditional middle-eastern ingredient used in dips and dressings. Tahini comes from sesame seeds and is a rich source of protein.

◆

Thick, this makes a wonderful sandwich spread or dip for fresh vegetables and pita bread. Thinned with additional water, this is the perfect dressing for a fresh spinach salad.

SAUCES

Simply Fresh Tomato Sauce

MAKES 2 SERVINGS

The best tomato sauce comes from the freshest ingredients—tomatoes and basil soaked with the energy of the sun. On the coast of the Italian Riviera, we asked the chef of our favorite restaurant what the secret to his great sauce was, and he exclaimed, *"Il sole! The sun!"*

½ tablespoon olive oil
1 small onion, finely diced
3 cloves garlic, crushed
1 small carrot, peeled and shredded
6 ripe tomatoes, diced
2 tablespoons fresh basil, chopped
Salt and pepper to taste
Dash of sugar

1. Heat oil in a medium-size pan and add onion, garlic, and carrot. Sauté over medium heat for about 8 minutes, until onion is soft but not brown.

2. Add the tomatoes and basil and simmer on low heat for 15 minutes, stirring often. Season to taste with salt, pepper, and sugar.

This sauce is so low in fat, and its ingredients come mainly from the very top of the Food Energy Ladder. Served with a plate of steaming pasta, this makes a low-fat, high-energy meal.

◆

Select fresh tomatoes carefully. Look for bruises or soft spots. Choose vine-ripened tomatoes if available.

When basil is not in season, or for variation, use fresh parsley in the recipe.

A little sugar helps bring out the taste in tomatoes.

For a pure, healthy and easy to prepare tomato sauce, this recipe can't be beat.

♦

Lycopene gives tomatoes their red color and it is probably the substance that decreases prostate cancer significantly in men who eat lots of tomato sauce.

◆

Best Basic Tomato Sauce

MAKES 2 SERVINGS

This simple, tasty sauce is better than any jar tomato sauce you'll find in the store—I assure you. And if you are in a hurry, this sauce will be ready in almost as little time as it takes your pasta to boil.

> 28-ounce can whole tomatoes with juice
> 1 tablespoon olive oil
> 5 garlic cloves, crushed
> 1/2 small yellow onion, finely diced
> 1/2 carrot peeled and sliced very thin
> 1 tablespoon Italian herbs (i.e., basil, parsley, oregano)
> Juice of 1 medium orange
> 1 teaspoon sugar
> 3/4 teaspoon salt
> Pepper to taste

1. Tear or cut tomatoes into small pieces, removing any hard stems. Set aside.

2. Heat oil in a medium pot and add garlic, onion, carrot, and Italian herbs. Sauté until garlic is golden, stirring well.

3. Add tomatoes, orange juice, sugar, salt, and pepper. Simmer on low heat for 20 minutes and serve over hot pasta.

When fresh tomatoes are unavailable, or you are short on time, terrific tomato sauce can start from canned tomatoes.

◆

Orange juice revitalizes canned tomatoes and brings out their flavor.

◆

Select whole canned tomatoes in juice. Some varieties contain added salt and other spices. Plain, simple whole tomatoes are all you need.

◆

Canning fresh tomatoes yourself is a wonderful summer activity and will guarantee you delicious tomato sauce throughout the year.

Mushroom Spinach Sauce for Baked Potatoes

MAKES ABOUT 2 CUPS

Turn a plain baked potato into a delicious low-fat meal. One taste and you will forget the high-fat butter and sour cream commonly served over baked potatoes.

4 baked potatoes
1 tablespoon canola oil
2 cups onions, minced
2 tablespoons all purpose flour
1 1/2 cups water
2 cups mushrooms, chopped
1 cup frozen chopped spinach, thawed and drained, or 1
   cup fresh spinach, washed and chopped
Juice of 1/2 lemon
Salt and pepper to taste

1. Bake potatoes in a 450° oven for approximately 1 hour, or until soft.

2. In a large skillet, heat oil and add onion. Sauté until translucent, stirring frequently. Add mushrooms and sauté 3–5 minutes (pan will become dry). Add flour and water and stir well until creamy.

3. Add spinach and lemon juice and stir well. Season to taste with salt and pepper.

4. Turn heat to low and simmer for 8 minutes, stirring frequently.

5. Slice open potatoes down the center and top with sauce.

Americans love potatoes, and one of the most popular ways to eat them is baked.

◆

Fresh baked potatoes are typically turned into a nutrition nightmare by smothering them with high-fat toppings. Two tablespoons of butter adds 24 grams of fat!

◆

Potatoes are super sources of potassium, vitamin C, and fiber. Their skins are especially nutritious—loaded with more fiber, iron, calcium, zinc, and B vitamins.

Here is a delicious topping to enjoy over baked potatoes without adding fat and calories. The mushrooms are an excellent source of potassium and phosphorous.

For variety, substitute swiss chard for spinach and add a few chopped walnuts.

This sauce was created to top baked potatoes but it can also be enjoyed over steamed cauliflower.

Serve with a fresh baguette.

SOUPS

Cold Tsatziki Soup

MAKES 4 SERVINGS

Smooth and cool, this authentic Greek soup comes together in hardly any time. It's perfect for a light lunch, and tastes even better on the second day.

> 2 cucumbers, peeled and coarsely grated
> Salt and pepper to taste
> 1 pint low-fat plain yogurt
> Juice of ½ lemon
> 1 garlic clove, mashed
> 2 cups water
> 2 tablespoons fresh mint, finely chopped

1. Place cucumbers in a medium bowl and season to taste with salt and pepper. Set aside.

2. In another bowl, mix yogurt with lemon juice, garlic, and water.

3. Combine the cucumbers and yogurt mixture, add mint leaves, and stir well.

This soup is perfect for a hot summer day. The cool and crisp flavors of cucumber and mint are delicious and refreshing.

◆

Fresh mint gives this soup its distinct taste. Mint is easy to grow. If you don't have a garden, even a small container on the windowsill will produce amazing results.

◆

If mint is too strong for your tastes, substitute fresh parsley for a more subtle soup.

◆

Savory Green Bean Soup

MAKES 4 SERVINGS

This soup is hearty and healthful, the perfect meal in itself.

5 cups water
1 teaspoon summer savory herb
3 cups green beans
2½ tablespoons canola oil (½ tablespoon for browning
    onions, 2 tablespoons for browning flour)
2 medium onions, finely diced
3 tablespoons all purpose flour
1 tablespoon vinegar
2 teaspoons salt
2 teaspoons sugar
1 pound wide egg noodles

1. Bring water to a boil with summer savory. Add beans to boiling water and cook for 20 minutes.

2. While beans cook, heat ½ tablespoon canola oil in a small skillet and sauté onions until brown. Transfer onions to a small bowl and set aside. In the same skillet, heat 2 tablespoons canola oil and add flour, stirring constantly to avoid clumping. Cook flour until golden brown and barely smoking. Watch carefully, flour turns from brown to burned very quickly!

3. Add onions and flour to the beans and water and stir. Add vinegar, salt, and sugar, and let simmer for 15 minutes.

4. While soup simmers, boil water for noodles. Cook noodles until al dente. Serve soup hot, over noodles.

Garden-fresh green beans are the key to this flavorful soup. Green beans picked from the garden are loaded with life-energy. Look for a local farmer's market for the freshest beans available. If fresh beans are not possible, frozen or canned beans are a good alternative.

◆

If you have children, involve them in the preparations. Children love the popping sound that beans make when they break off the ends!

◆

Carrot and Orange Soup

MAKES 4 SERVINGS

This is a refreshing, light soup. Ginger, coriander, turmeric, chili powder, and cumin create a delightful palette of spices and herbs.

    2 teaspoons olive oil
    1 small onion, minced
    1-inch slice of fresh ginger, peeled and minced (optional)
    1 garlic clove, minced
    1/2 teaspoon ground coriander
    1/2 teaspoon ground cumin
    1/2 teaspoon ground chili powder
    1/4 teaspoon turmeric
    1/4 pound carrots, thinly sliced (About 5 large carrots)
    Grated zest and juice of 1 large orange
    1 large orange, peeled and chopped
    3 cups fresh vegetable broth or bouillion
    1–2 teaspoons fresh lemon juice
    Salt and pepper to taste
    Cilantro leaves or twists of orange zest for garnish
        (optional)

1. Heat oil in a saucepan. Add onion, ginger, garlic, and spices. Sauté gently for 3–5 minutes. Add carrots and cook 8 more minutes, stirring frequently.

2. Add orange zest, chopped orange flesh, and broth to the pan. Bring to a boil, then reduce heat, cover, and simmer gently for 20 minutes.

3. Purée soup in a blender or food processor. Reheat gently, then stir in the orange and lemon juices and season to taste.

4. Serve garnished with cilantro leaves or twists of orange zest, if desired.

"Soup up" your energy and immune system with this delicious soup!

Carrots are an outstanding source of beta-carotene, which boosts the immune system and helps to prevent cataracts, cancer and heart disease.

It's common knowledge that the vitamin C found in oranges boosts the immune system and helps relieve colds, but research also suggests that it may help guard against cancers of the breast, cervix, and gastrointestinal system.

Fresh Vegetable Broth

MAKES ABOUT 5 CUPS

The perfect way to use up vegetables in the fridge. This broth gives Vegetable Risotto a wonderful flavor.

2 *large carrots, sliced*
1 *large onion, sliced*
2 *celery stalks, outer, sliced*
A few celery leaves
A few parsley stems
2 *sprigs each of fresh thyme and marjoram*
2 *bay leaves*
3 *garlic cloves, crushed with the side of a knife*
A strip of lemon peel
10 *black peppercorns*
6 *cups water*

1. Put all ingredients in a large saucepan. Bring to a boil, then reduce the heat, cover the pan, and simmer until vegetables are just soft but not mushy, about 45 minutes. Let cool.

2. Strain broth through a sieve into a large container, pressing the solids to extract as much liquid as possible. Keep covered in the refrigerator. Use broth within four days.

Vegetable broth is simple and satisfying to make. Homemade is much healthier, and lower in sodium, than store-bought broth. You will taste the difference!

Broccoli Soup with Walnuts

MAKES 4 SERVINGS

This is a favorite autumn or winter soup, the perfect overture to a good meal, or a perfect meal, in itself. Serve with a loaf of crusty bread for dipping in this savory soup.

> 1 medium onion, chopped
> 4–5 cups fresh broccoli, stems sliced and florets separated
> 1 tablespoon butter
> 1 cup vegetable bouillion or water
> 1 cup milk or plain soy or rice milk
> 1/4 cup half-and-half
> Salt and pepper to taste
> 3 tablespoons walnuts, chopped and toasted

1. In a large pot sauté onion and broccoli in butter for 5 minutes.

2. Add bouillion (or water) and milk and simmer gently for 30 minutes, or until broccoli is tender.

3. Transfer to food processor or blender, purée until smooth, and return to pot.

4. Add half-and-half and walnuts. Season to taste with salt and pepper.

This soup provides plentiful amounts of fiber to your diet. Broccoli and nuts are both high in fiber. Fiber helps remove excess cholesterol from the blood, and thus helps keep your heart healthy.

♦

Broccoli may be the most maligned vegetable, but it is also one of the most healthful vegetables you can eat. Broccoli is loaded with compounds that help protect against cancer, as well as vitamin C and beta-carotene.

♦

Nuts are wonderful for your health when eaten regularly and in moderation. The monounsaturated fat and vitamin E in nuts helps protect against heart disease.

Wonderful Mushroom Soup

MAKES 2 SERVINGS

This soup is so simple to prepare and so flavorful. The complex tastes of fennel and anise liqueur will linger on your tongue long after the last spoonful has been eaten.

1 tablespoon canola oil
1 small onion, diced
1 clove garlic, minced
1 stalk celery, diced
2 tablespoons fennel, diced
3 cups vegetable bouillion or water
8 ounces mushrooms (a brown variety), sliced
2 tablespoons parsley, chopped very thin
1 teaspoon butter
2 tablespoons cream
1 tablespoon anise liqueur or Pernod (optional)
Salt and pepper to taste

1. Heat oil in a medium pot and add onion, garlic, celery, and fennel. Sauté on medium heat for 10 minutes, stirring often. Add mushrooms and sauté for 5 minutes, stirring often.

2. Add bouillion or water and simmer on low heat for 30 minutes.

3. Let cool and transfer to blender. Purée soup until smooth.

4. Return to pot and add butter, cream, parsley, and liqueur.

5. Serve with a fresh baguette and boiled or mashed potatoes.

Mushrooms are a staple of fall and winter cooking, especially for hearty soups and stews.

◆

This soup is best prepared with a good brown mushroom that has a deep flavor, such as cremini or porcini.

◆

Fennel is at its freshest in fall, and its delightfully sweet licorice flavor mingles well with strong mushrooms.

Swabian Lentil Soup

MAKES 4 SERVINGS

When I was a child in Germany, many snowy, bitter-cold after-noons were warmed by the fragrance of a big pot of lentil soup simmering on the stove. This soup is especially flavorful the next day.

6 cups water
1 cup brown lentils
1 cup celery, peeled and cut into $^1/_2$ inch slices
1 carrot, peeled and cut into $^1/_2$ inch slices
2 tablespoons canola oil
1 medium onion, diced
1 tablespoon all purpose flour
Salt and pepper to taste
1 tablespoon white vinegar
1 teaspoon sugar
4 cups wide noodles

1. Rinse lentils with fresh water through a fine strainer.

2. Boil water, add lentils, celery, and carrots, and cook over low heat, simmering for 45 minutes.

3. Meanwhile, heat oil and sauté onions until just light brown. Add flour and stir constantly until golden brown and just starting to smoke. Watch carefully to avoid burning.

4. After the lentils and vegetables have simmered for 45 minutes, add the flour-onion mixture and stir well. Simmer for 10 minutes.

5. Add vinegar, sugar and season to taste with salt and pepper.

6. While soup simmers, cook noodles following directions on package.

7. Pour soup over noodles in soup bowls.

The nutty flavor of lentils combined with noodles makes a hearty winter soup.

The combination of lentils and noodles create a satisfying soup filled with fiber and loaded with energy.

The nutty flavor of lentils combined with noodles makes a hearty winter soup.

Lentils were one of the very first crops to be cultured and they are now grown all over the planet. India produces more than fifty varieties of different colors and sizes to help provide adequate protein and Vitamin B_1 (thiamin) to its population in the traditional dish called "dahl."

All of us would do well to eat more energy-rich lentils, and this delicious, savory soup is a wonderful way to do so because it is truly a meal in itself.

Chicken Soup with Savoy Cabbage

MAKES 4 SERVINGS

The scent of this soup cooking will fill your kitchen with a warm aroma in winter. When anyone in our family is feeling under the weather, this soup will boost his or her energy and help ward off a cold. This recipe combines my mother's favorite cabbage soup with Ed's mother's famous chicken soup. We think it's a perfect marriage of flavors and traditions.

> 6 cups water
> 4 skinless chicken breast fillets, sliced
> 1 small leek, cut in 1/2 inch chunks
> 2 carrots, peeled and cut in 2-inch chunks
> 1 celery root, peeled and cut in 1/2 inch chunks
> 1 bay leaf
> 1 small Savoy cabbage, cut in small pieces
> 1/4 cup chives, cut very thin (optional)
> 1/4 cup parsley, chopped
> Salt and pepper to taste

1. Bring water to a boil, and add chicken and leek. Cover and cook on medium heat for about 30 minutes.

2. Add carrots, celery root, bay leaf, and cabbage. Cover and cook for another 30 minutes on low heat.

3. Just before serving, add parsley or chives, and season to taste with salt and pepper.

4. Serve over rice, or just with some crusty fresh bread.

5. Remember to remove the bay leaf prior to eating the soup.

Wintertime is for soups, and this one is filled with hearty vegetables and chicken. Leftovers make a more flavorful soup the following day, and the broth can be used in many other recipes.

◆

Making a soup stock is a terrific way to use up the vegetables in your refrigerator. The vegetables fill the broth with a healthy supply of vitamins.

◆

This soup cooks fairly fast, in just an hour. The vegetables will be cooked but not soggy and flavorless. Overcooking vegetables in water or broth destroys their vitamins.

◆

Savoy cabbage, loaded with vitamin A and calcium, is dark and green with a tight and curly head and crinkly leaves.

◆

Celery root gives a delectable flavor to this hearty dish.

Potato Parsley Soup

MAKES 2 SERVINGS

Whenever I cook this soup, I am transported by its aroma to my mother's kitchen in Germany. At home in California, it reminds me of all the warmth and comfort I felt watching my mother cook.

> 5 cups cold water, lightly salted
> 4 medium potatoes, such as Idaho baking potatoes,
>   peeled and cut in 2-inch pieces
> 6 cloves garlic, peeled and left whole
> 1 medium onion, quartered
> ½ cup low-fat milk
> 1½ cups parsley, chopped fine
> Salt and pepper to taste

1. In a large pot, boil water and add potatoes, garlic, and onion. Cook until vegetables are very soft, about 30 minutes. Do not drain water.

2. Using a masher, mash potatoes, garlic and onion until smooth, creating a creamy soup. Add milk slowly, until desired consistency. Add parsley and stir well.

3. Simmer over low heat for 10 minutes. Add salt and pepper to taste and serve hot.

A creamy potato soup without the high-fat cream. This soup is actually almost entirely fat-free.

◆

Parsley comes off the sidelines in this recipes and plays a starring role. This soup proves that parsley has flavor worthy of more than just a garnish. For additional flavor, add chopped carrots or celery.

◆

Mexican Chicken Soup

MAKES 4 SERVINGS

On our visits to Zhijuatenejo, Mexico, we encountered this tangy, satisfying soup. Each time I sit down to enjoy it now, I have the memory of the festive mariachi players singing and dancing to colorful music.

1 tablespoon canola oil
1 medium onion, finely diced
2 limes, juiced
4 skinless chicken breast filets, cut in 1/2 inch pieces
5 cups chicken broth
4 tomatoes, diced
1/2 bell pepper, diced
6 corn tortillas
2 tablespoons canola oil
1/2 cup cilantro, chopped
Salt and pepper to taste

1. Heat 1 tablespoon oil in a large pot and sauté onions until translucent. Squeeze in juice of both limes, reduce heat, add chicken and sauté 3–5 minutes.

2. Add broth, tomatoes, and bell pepper. Cook about 45 minutes, until chicken is tender. Season to taste with salt and pepper.

3. In the meantime, cut 2 tortillas into small pieces. Heat 2 tablespoons oil and fry tortilla pieces until crisp and golden. Drain well on paper towels to remove excess oil.

4. Put chicken pieces in soup bowls, add tortilla pieces, and cover with broth. Sprinkle each bowl generously with cilantro.

5. Serve with steaming hot tortillas on the side and a dish of fresh salsa.

♦

This Mexican soup sparkles with the tangy flavors of lime and cilantro. This is the perfect soup for a refreshing meal on a summer evening. Leftovers are even more delicious the second day, after the flavors have mingled overnight.

♦

Tomatoes, bell pepper, and cilantro give this soup wonderful color, a real celebration of summertime. This soup is simple to prepare but dazzling to the eyes and stomach.

APPETIZERS

Portobello Appetizer

MAKES 4 SERVINGS

This is a wonderful party appetizer. For a side dish, the rich flavors complement a crisp Caesar salad. And what a great sandwich it makes with a little lettuce and tomato!

2 tablespoons olive oil
2 large portobello mushrooms, stems removed, sliced thin
2 tablespoons balsamic vinegar
Salt and pepper to taste
$\frac{1}{2}$ tablespoon fresh thyme, chopped
1 teaspoon fresh rosemary, chopped
(Substitute 3 teaspoons dried Italian herbs, if fresh herbs
    unavailable)
2 garlic cloves, peeled
$\frac{1}{2}$ cup parmesan cheese, grated

1. In a medium skillet, heat 1 tablespoon oil and sauté portobellos until deep brown. Drain on paper towel.

2. Arrange mushrooms on a plate, sprinkle with balsamic vinegar, salt and pepper.

3. In the same skillet, combine chopped herbs and garlic together and add 1 tablespoon olive oil. Mix well. Cook for 5 minutes on low heat.

4. Drizzle herb mixture over mushrooms.

5. Sprinkle mushrooms with parmesan.

6. Serve mushrooms alone or on a baguette with sprigs of arugula and sliced tomatoes.

Rich, plump portobellos are our favorite variety of mushrooms. Once found only in specialty food stores, they are now common in most supermarket produce sections.

◆

This is a pleasing appetizer. For variation, serve the sautéed mushrooms over a bed of rice or pasta for a main dish.

◆

Portobello mushrooms are as meaty and satisfying as a great piece of beef!

Mock Chopped Liver

MAKES 6 SERVINGS

Chopped liver fans will rave about this healthy, low-fat variation of a traditional paté. Deborah Wasserman's recipe captures all the strong flavors of the original classic but is much lower in fat and completely vegetarian.

½ pound green beans, chopped in bite-size pieces
¾ pounds mushrooms, chopped
1 small onion, peeled and finely chopped
1 teaspoon canola oil
¼ cup walnuts, chopped
Salt and pepper to taste
¼ cup water

1. Sauté green beans, mushrooms, and onion in oil over medium-high heat for 10 minutes.

2. Pour mixture into food processor bowl, add remaining ingredients, and blend until creamy.

3. Chill and serve on a bed of lettuce with pita bread or raw vegetables.

Thanks to Deborah Wasserman's creative cooking, snacking before dinner doesn't have to throw you off the top of the Food Energy Ladder.

◆

Giving a dinner party? Going to a potluck? This is an excellent, easy-to-prepare, low-fat appetizer that will please vegetarians and non-vegetarians alike.

◆

For variation, this can be spread on bread for a delicious vegetarian sandwich.

Curry Zucchini Dip

MAKES APPROXIMATELY 1 CUP

Guests always love this appetizer. The refreshing flavors of yogurt and curry make this a perfect pre-dinner treat.

1 teaspoon canola oil
1 medium onion, cut in quarters
2 zucchini, cut in 2-inch cubes
3 tablespoons low-fat plain yogurt
1 teaspoon lemon juice
1 ½ teaspoons curry powder
Dash sugar
Salt and pepper to taste

1. Heat oil and sauté onion and zucchini for 5 minutes.

2. Purée the mixture in a food processor or blender with yogurt, lemon juice, curry, and a dash of sugar. Add salt and pepper to taste.

Curry adds intense flavor to vegetables. This smooth, creamy dip makes a memorable appetizer served with crackers, warmed pita bread, or fresh carrot and celery sticks. Unlike most dips, it is low in fat and calories.

◆

You can also use this dip to enliven any sandwich.

French Salmon Spread

MAKES 4 SERVINGS

Many fans of French cuisine, like myself, have had to give up their favorite French dishes because they do not accommodate a low-fat lifestyle. Over the years, I have learned to transform traditionally rich French recipes into low-fat, high-energy variations that still maintain their distinct French flavors. This one is derived from an appetizer served in our favorite Parisian bistro. Bón appetit!

1 tablespoon mustard (preferably Dijon)
1 tablespoon olive oil
3 ounces smoked salmon, finely chopped
1 tablespoon onion, minced (optional)
1 tablespoon greens of spring onion, finely chopped (chives
    can be substituted)
Salt and pepper to taste

1. Mix mustard with oil until creamy.

2. Add salmon, onion, greens of spring onion or chives, season to taste with salt and pepper and mix well. Refrigerate for several hours before serving.

3. Simply tear off hunks of baguette and enjoy, or toast slices and top with spread.

Americans love appetizers. Unfortunately, most appetizers are high in fat and filled with meat. This dish is borrowed from the French and transformed into an intensely appetizing but not sinfully fattening spread.

◆

Traditional rillette is served throughout France, made of pork or rabbit. In this dish, salmon is substituted for a lighter, healthier spread, with terrific taste. If smoked salmon is unavailable, substitute another variety of smoked fish.

Rolled Salmon with Carrots

MAKES 4 SERVINGS

This is a favorite party appetizer. Splurge on a high-quality, very fresh smoked salmon—the added flavor is worth the extra cost!

8 slices smoked salmon
1 teaspoon horseradish or mustard
1 teaspoon honey
1 tablespoon fresh dill, chopped fine
Pepper
4 lettuce leaves, cut in thin strips
1 carrot, peeled and shredded with a potato peeler
½ lemon

1. Arrange slices of salmon next to each other on a plate.

2. Mix horseradish or mustard with honey, dill, and a dash of pepper. Spread evenly on each salmon slice. Top with lettuce strips and roll up.

3. Arrange carrot shavings on 4 plates and lay salmon rolls on top. Sprinkle lemon juice on top of each roll.

Seafood and vegetables combine to create a healthy meal rich in flavor, vitamins, and minerals.

◆

Smoked salmon is a wonderful source of omega-3 fatty acids, shown in research to reduce the risk of cardiac disease.

◆

Carrots add healthful beta-carotene and vitamin C to this dish.

◆

As a variation, substitute peeled cucumber slices for lettuce.

◆

Black Olive Tapenade

Our visit to Nice was memorable in part because of this delicious appetizer. Each time I make it I am transported back to that fine little restaurant by the market where we enjoyed this tapenade on a fresh baguette with a glass of Beaujolais. C'est magnifique!

2 *cups pitted black olives*
2 *tablespoons capers*
2 *anchovy fillets*
2 *garlic cloves, peeled*
2 *tablespoons fresh thyme (or 1 teaspoon dried thyme)*
1 *tablespoon Dijon mustard*
1 *teaspoon ground pepper*
1 *teaspoon Cognac (optional)*

1. Mix all ingredients in a food processor until smooth.

2. Serve with crusty sourdough bread or a French baguette.

The intense flavors of olives, capers, and anchovies create a heavenly appetizer. Their strong flavor is perfect for a tapenade spread lightly on a French baguette.

True, olives are high in fat, but of the mono-unsaturated type that is good for your heart!

This is a wonderful appetizer to make ahead of time. Covered tightly, it will stay fresh in the refrigerator for days.

◆

Any strong olive will do, but I like Kalamata or Black Nicoise best. These are no longer just gourmet store delicacies, but can be found in cans in most supermarkets. You can easily pit olives yourself by pressing the olive with the bottom of a cup.

◆

Hearty Garlic Spread

MAKES 1 ¹/₂ CUPS

This delicious spread earns its name because garlic truly is good for your heart. This is staple fare in the French countryside and Mediterranean. Combined with their zest for life, no wonder people from both areas have such low rates of heart disease! Traditionally, the spread is served to flavor crusty bread, fish soup, and seafood.

> I cup silken tofu, firm
> 6 cloves garlic, peeled
> I tablespoon lemon juice
> I tablespoon olive oil
> Salt and pepper to taste

1. Combine all ingredients in a food processor and blend until smooth. Season to taste with salt and pepper.

2. Refrigerate until serving in an airtight container; freshness lasts up to a week.

Peeling garlic can be frustrating if you don't know this simple trick: place single cloves on a cutting board or counter. With the flat side of a large wooden spoon or a wide chef's knife, smash them. The peels just fall away.

◆

Garlic is wonderful for your health. Scientific studies have shown its preventive value in warding off bacteria viruses, fungi, and other organisms that cause human disease. Chemicals in garlic also protect the heart. Researchers have shown that garlic has a cholesterol-lowering effect, reduces blood pressure, and can help prevent blood clots.

◆

Enjoy this as a dip for raw or steamed vegetables, or as a zesty sandwich spread.

Lentil Paté

MAKES 6 SERVINGS

This vegetarian paté is an excellent alternative to liver paté. It transforms the humble lentil into an elegant appetizer.

1 cup lentils
2¼ cups water
1 onion, peeled and minced
4 cloves garlic, peeled and minced
2 teaspoons canola oil
1 teaspoon pepper
½ teaspoon white vinegar

1. Cook lentils in water over medium heat for 45 minutes. Meanwhile, sauté onion and garlic in oil for 2 minutes.

2. When lentils are cooked, drain and pour them into food processor bowl. Add sautéed onion and garlic, pepper, and vinegar.

3. Blend in food processor until creamy, adding a little water if necessary. Season to taste with salt and pepper.

4. Chill and serve with pita bread, crackers, or raw vegetables.

Lentils are an inexpensive and low-fat source of carbohydrates, fiber and protein.

♦

Unlike other legumes, lentils can be prepared in less than an hour. They can be cooked without pre-soaking but remember to rinse and drain them several times before cooking.

♦

Many thanks to Deborah Wasserman for this creative vegetarian appetizer.

SIDE DISHES

Stuffed Cucumbers Nany

MAKES 4 SERVINGS

Swiss friends introduced us to this savory dish. It's light but surprisingly filling, topped with the Best Basic Tomato Sauce.

> 1 cup brown rice
> 2 cups water
> 1 8-ounce package low-fat cream cheese
> 2 tablespoons raisins
> Salt and pepper to taste
> 5 medium cucumbers, peeled, halved lengthwise and
>   seeded
> Best Basic or Simply Fresh Tomato Sauce (Recipe pages
>   228 and 230)

1. Cook brown rice according to directions on package, but 10 minutes less than required cooking time.

2. Drain rice and mix with cream cheese and raisins. Add salt and pepper to taste.

3. Fill half of the cucumbers with the rice mixture. Top each stuffed cucumber with another half and secure with toothpick.

4. Place stuffed cucumbers in a casserole dish.

5. Make one recipe of Best Basic Tomato Sauce and pour over stuffed cucumbers. Cover and bake for 45 minutes at 300 degrees

---

We love vegetables in their natural, raw, fresh state. When we cook them, we favor recipes that draw out the naturally delicious flavors. It's easy to overcook vegetables and destroy not only their flavor but their nutritional value.

◆

This delicious dish combines the cool taste of cucumbers with the sweetness of raisins and nutty taste of brown rice.

◆

Yes, this recipe uses cream cheese (low fat), but remember our motto for healthy eating: "Everything in moderation . . . including moderation!"

◆

For variation, substitute turkey for brown rice.

Mashed Potatoes and Vegetables Italiano

MAKES 2 SERVINGS

This dish turns plain old mashed potatoes into something truly wonderful! a traditional American favorite combined with some Italian culinary pizzazz . . . *buon appetito!*

3 medium potatoes
½ tablespoon olive oil
1 small onion, minced
4 cloves garlic, mashed
¼ cup skim, soy, or rice milk, scalded
½ cup pine nuts, toasted
½ cup red bell pepper, diced
1 cup mushrooms (any variety), cut in half
½ tablespoon lemon juice
1 cup tomato sauce (Recipe page 230)
½ teaspoon fennel seeds
1 teaspoon Italian herbs (i.e. basil, oregano, parsley page 230)
Salt, pepper, and sugar to taste
Pat butter (optional)
Shredded Parmesan cheese (optional)

1. Peel potatoes, cut in quarters, and boil in salted water until soft, approximately 20–25 minutes.

2. While potatoes boil, heat ½ tablespoon olive oil in large pot and sauté onion until translucent and add garlic. Stir frequently to avoid burning.

3. Add to pot all vegetables, lemon juice, tomato sauce, fennel seeds, and Italian herbs. Season with salt, pepper, and sugar to taste. Simmer on low heat for about 20 minutes.

4. When potatoes are done, drain them well, add hot milk, and mash well. Add a pat of butter if you like. Stir in pine nuts and season with salt and pepper to taste.

5. Transfer mashed potatoes to plates and top with the vegetables.
   Sprinkle with shredded parmesan if desired.

It's easy to find vegetarian inspiration in many of our favorite American dishes, including the humble mashed potato! Potatoes are a super high-energy food. This complex carbohydrate provides long-lasting energy, as well as abundant amounts of fiber, vitamin C, potassium, and other minerals.

◆

Yukon Gold potatoes are great for this dish because of their natural buttery taste and creamy consistency.

◆

Feel free to vary the vegetables according to your tastes and what is in season: eggplant, cauliflower, and green peas are a delicious variation.

Cooked Green Beans and Carrots

MAKES 2 SERVINGS

Want to create a quick vegetarian dish with just a few on-hand ingredients? This makes a great side dish.

2 *cups vegetable bouillion or water*
6 *small carrots, peeled and sliced lengthwise in quarters*
2 *cups green beans, trimmed*
1 *teaspoon olive oil*
1 *small onion, diced*
1 *small orange, washed, zest and juice*
Salt and pepper to taste
2 *tablespoons parsley, finely chopped*

1. Boil bouillion or water and cook carrots for 8 minutes. Remove carrots, leaving liquid in pot.

2. Add beans to liquid and cook for about 12 minutes, until crisp tender. Remove from liquid.

3. Keep beans and carrots warm.

4. Heat oil in a small skillet and sauté onions until translucent. While onions cook, grate orange peel, then add peel and juice of orange to onions. Add salt and pepper and sauté 5 more minutes.

5. Pour orange juice mixture over carrots and beans and toss well. Transfer to plates and sprinkle with parsley before serving.

6. This is delicious with a plate of rice.

Green beans are a terrific source of fiber and vitamin C. We use green beans in a variety of dishes because they are available year-round.

◆

Vegetables are most nutritious raw. To preserve their vitamins and minerals, vegetables should be cooked gently, until crispy tender, not wilted.

◆

For variety, in place of beans use another high-fiber vegetable, such as broccoli or cauliflower.

◆

Stewed Tomatoes and Cucumbers

MAKES 2 SERVINGS

Simplicity makes this combination of tomatoes and cucumbers work so well. The secret is in the sweetness of the tomatoes—fresh and vine-ripened are best.

  1 teaspoon canola oil
  2 medium cucumbers, peeled and sliced into 1/4-inch
     pieces
  2 large tomatoes, diced
  Salt and pepper to taste
  1/4 teaspoon sugar
  2 tablespoons parsley, chopped
  1 tablespoon Parmesan cheese, grated

1. Heat oil. Add cucumber and tomatoes and sauté on low heat for 15 minutes.

2. Add salt, pepper, and sugar to taste.

3. Sprinkle with parsley and parmesan cheese.

4. This is delicious served over brown rice or a light pasta, such as angel hair or cappellini.

Gently stewing tomatoes and cucumbers brings out the sweet flavors of these summer vegetables.

◆

This is an unusually tasty variation on a cool, crisp tomato-and-cucumber salad. This is a wonderfully light dish, perfect for a warm spring or summer evening.

◆

For variety, use this dish as a layer in a vegetarian lasagna.

Savory Red Cabbage

MAKES 4 SERVINGS

The beautiful color of red cabbage makes this a festive side dish for a special Thanksgiving meal. But it's wonderful anytime, served with potatoes for a strictly vegetarian meal, or with turkey or chicken.

> 2 *tablespoons canola oil*
> 1 *medium onion, diced*
> 1 *large red cabbage, cut in very thin slices (Discard thick*
>   *white stems)*
> 1 *large apple, peeled, cored, and cut in wedges*
> ½ *cup raisins*
> ½ *cup white vinegar*
> ¾ *cups water*
> *Salt and pepper to taste*

1. Heat oil in a large pot and sauté onions until translucent.

2. Add cabbage, apple, and raisins.

3. Immediately add vinegar and water.

4. Cover and cook for 45 minutes on low heat, stirring occasionally.

5. Add a little more water if cabbage gets too dry.

6. Add salt and pepper to taste.

Red cabbage is a super source of vitamin C. The most popular way of preparing cabbage is in a cole slaw, a typically high-fat, high-calorie dish.

Here is a flavorful, low-fat way to enjoy the goodness of cabbage. If you only ever eat cabbage in cole slaw, you are in for a delightful surprise!

Leeks in Vinaigrette

MAKES 2 SERVINGS

Aromatic balsamic vinegar adds dazzle to leeks. This recipe seems very gourmet but is so simple to prepare.

5 *cups water*
1 *teaspoon salt*
4 *medium leeks*
1 ½ *tablespoons canola oil*
1 *tablespoon balsamic vinegar*
1 *teaspoon Dijon mustard*
1 *tablespoon orange juice*
Salt and pepper to taste

1. Heat water in medium-size pot and add a teaspoon of salt for boiling.

2. Cut off roots and tops of leeks, clean well, and cut in 4-inch lengths. Drop into boiling water for about 15 minutes, or until just tender. Drain and set aside.

3. Mix oil, vinegar, mustard, orange juice, and season to taste with salt and pepper to a creamy consistency.

4. Arrange leeks on a plate and drizzle with dressing.

Leeks are commonly used to flavor broth but have wonderful flavor served on their own as a side dish.

◆

Not only are leeks an excellent source of dietary fiber, they also contain a chemical called allium, which is receiving a lot of attention for its cholesterol-lowering effect.

◆

Enjoy this as a side dish, or as a main dish accompanied with any potato recipe, or simply with peeled, soft boiled potato wedges.

Mashed Potatoes with Basil and Pine Nuts

MAKES 2 SERVINGS

Mashed potato fans will love this dish. The addition of fresh basil and toasted pine nuts make a classic meal even better!

> 6 potatoes (Yukon Gold if available), peeled and boiled in
>   3–4 cups of water until soft
> 1/2 cup hot milk (skim or soy)
> 1 packed cup fresh basil, very finely chopped (Reserve a
>   few whole leaves for garnish)
> 3 tablespoons pine nuts, toasted
> 1 tablespoon butter (optional)
> Salt and pepper to taste

1. Mash potatoes together with hot milk until creamy.

2. Add basil, pine nuts and butter (optional), and season to taste with salt and pepper, and mix until smooth.

3. Serve this dish alone, garnished with a few leaves of basil, or accompany it with a fresh tomato salad.

Once again, mashed potatoes provide the beginnings of a memorable, flavorful dish.

Puréed potatoes can be used as the basis for many variations on mashed potatoes that incorporate fresh vegetables and herbs.

There is no reason for people trying to lose weight to stay away from mashed potatoes. It's all in the way they are prepared. Traditional recipes are heavy on cream and butter, but potatoes mashed with just skim milk are surprisingly creamy and smooth.

◆

This recipe calls for pine nuts, but you can substitute chopped hazelnuts. To toast the nuts, place them in a nonstick skillet on very low heat. Stir frequently, because they burn easily.

Nouveau Kale

MAKES 4 SERVINGS

This winter dish was a staple in my mother's house. Although she made a traditional dish with lots of meat and sausage, this new version is tastier, lower in fat and higher in energy. The toasted nuts bring out the nutty flavor of this wonderful winter green.

1 tablespoon olive oil
1 small onion, diced
4 cloves garlic, minced
1½ pounds kale, cleaned and chopped
½ cup water
¼ cup raisins
¼ cup walnuts or pine nuts, toasted
Salt and pepper to taste

1. Heat olive oil in medium pot. Add onion and garlic and sauté until translucent.

2. Add remaining ingredients to pot and stir well.

3. Cook for approximately 10 minutes, until kale is soft.

4. Serve with rice or mashed potatoes.

Kale is a nutritious winter green. Like other leafy greens, it is a superb source of calcium, vitamin A, and iron.

◆

For readers who like to garden, kale is easy to grow when started from seed in spring or fall. The plants will be ready in time for late fall and winter meals.

◆

When choosing kale at the market, avoid the larger leaves (more than 10 inches), which are tough. Smaller leaves are tender.

Roasted Vegetables

MAKES 2 SERVINGS

While these vegetables roast in a balsamic marinade, your kitchen will become remarkably fragrant. The vinegar draws out the vegetables' subtle flavors. Vegetables never tasted so good!

1/2 tablespoon balsamic vinegar
1 1/2 tablespoons extra virgin olive oil
1 teaspoon salt
1 tablespoon rosemary
1 cup mushrooms, halved
1 cup green beans, broken in half
1 medium onion, sliced
1 medium sweet potato, peeled and cut in large chunks
1 large carrot, peeled and cut in large chunks
5 cloves garlic, peeled

1. Preheat oven to 450°.

2. Prepare marinade in a large bowl, combining vinegar, oil, salt, and rosemary.

3. Add vegetables (including garlic) to the marinade and coat evenly.

4. Spread vegetables out in a shallow baking pan and pour marinade on top.

5. Roast vegetables for 35–40 minutes (or until sweet potato is soft), stirring occasionally. Vegetables are done when they are a warm brown, caramel-like color.

There's nothing more delicious than the flavor of roasted fresh vegetables. Roasting vegetables brings out their naturally sweet juices.

♦

For variety, add other vegetables of your choice. Zucchini, red or green bell pepper, and Roma tomatoes roast very well.

♦

Enjoy roasted vegetables with fresh crusty bread, or spoon them over a plate of basmati rice.

Ciabatta Sandwich

MAKES 4 SERVINGS.

Radishes, oranges, and vinaigrette make this a spirited sandwich.

> 1 loaf Ciabatta or French bread
> 1 bunch watercress, stems removed
> 1 bunch radishes, thinly sliced
> 2 small oranges, peeled and thinly sliced
> 1 small cucumber, peeled and thinly sliced
> 1 tablespoon olive oil
> 1 tablespoon balsamic vinegar
> 1 teaspoon Dijon mustard
> 1 garlic clove, mashed

1. Cut bread lengthwise in half and divide into 4 pieces. Layer watercress, radishes, orange and cucumber slices on 4 halves.

2. Beat together olive oil, vinegar, mustard, and garlic with wire whisk until creamy.

3. Pour vinaigrette over vegetables and bread. Cover with remaining bread and serve.

Thin slices of radish give this sandwich punch. Radishes are high in vitamin C and are easily grown in a simple window box.

Topped with a tangy vinaigrette, this makes a delicious high-energy lunch.

Ciabatta, sometimes called "slipper bread" for its long flat shape, is our favorite Italian bread. It has a light and airy texture, sometimes we nibble on it so much there's very little left for a sandwich!

For variety, substitute watercress with spinach or arugula and add tomato slices.

Tomato Carrot Sandwich

MAKES 2 SERVINGS

This is the ultimate veggie sandwich. We always pack it when we take day hikes or spend the day at the beach.

Four slices whole wheat bread, toasted
1/2 cup Dijon mustard
3 tablespoons, honey
2 tablespoons, lemon juice
1/2 avocado, mashed
1/2 cup carrots, peeled and grated
1 tablespoon parsley, chopped
1 spring green onion, diced
1 medium tomato, sliced
2 pieces romaine lettuce

1. To prepare honey mustard see #1 on page 272.

2. Spread honey mustard on one slice of bread, avocado on the other slice.

3. Layer carrots, onion, tomato, lettuce, and parsley and top each sandwich with remaining slice of bread.

This sandwich is high in fiber and bursting with vitamin C. Carrots, onions, and avocado are good sources of fiber. You should eat at least two high-fiber foods each day—this sandwich helps meet your daily fiber needs.

◆

For variety, stuff sandwich ingredients in a whole-wheat pita bread or wrap them up in a fresh tortilla.

Sardine Sandwich

MAKES 2 SERVINGS

Simple to prepare but so delicious you will savor every bite. Pumpernickel and sardines are two strong flavors that complement each other well. This is a perfect high-energy lunch, especially when served with a fresh raw vegetable salad.

4 slices Pumpernickel bread
3³/₄-ounce can brisling sardines
4 scallions, thinly sliced
Fresh lemon juice

1. Break off tails of sardines.

2. Arrange a layer of sardines on one slice of bread, top with scallions, and drizzle with lemon juice. Top with second slice of bread and serve.

Canned brisling sardines are more than just a delicacy, they are healthy for you.

Sardines are one of the very best source of calcium to help prevent osteoporosis. They also provide special fatty acids (omega-3s) to help keep our arteries clean and prevent heart attacks and strokes. Sardines are also rich in selenium, zinc, chromium and iron.

◆

Sardines are obviously a wonderful addition to your regular diet and this tasty sardine sandwich will appeal even to those who have not been sardine lovers.

◆

Arugula, Lettuce, and Tomato Sandwich

MAKES 2 SERVINGS

This is a favorite lunch in spring or summer, when arugula is in abundance. Parmesan and tomato make this a surprisingly substantial sandwich, flavored with aromatic balsamic vinegar.

Baguette or any crusty bread
2 leafs lettuce
4 leafs arugula
1 medium tomato, sliced thin
1/2 teaspoon oil
1 teaspoon balsamic vinegar
Parmesan cheese, grated

1. Cut bread lengthwise in half and top with layers of vegetables, beginning with lettuce, arugula, and tomatoes.

2. Sprinkle vegetables with oil, vinegar, and Parmesan cheese. Top with another slice of bread or serve open-faced.

Fresh greens bring distinct and unusual flavors to any "garden-variety" salad. This salad is anything but ordinary—we serve it on bread!

◆

One of the keys to eating a more vegetarian-based diet is learning how to turn salads from simple into spectacular.

◆

For variety, and extra iron, use spinach instead of lettuce leaves.

Ecumenical Bagel

MAKES 2 SERVINGS

We love bagels, lox, and cream cheese for Sunday brunch, or lunch anytime, but sometimes we prefer this vegetarian version of the classic.

1 *medium green bell pepper, seeded and sliced*
2 *medium tomatoes, sliced ¼-inch thick*
1 *red onion, sliced ¼-inch thick*
2 *onion bagels, sliced in half*
Reduced fat cream cheese
Lemon pepper

1. Preheat oven to 400°.

2. Spread bell pepper, tomatoes, and onions on a sheet of aluminum foil (shiny side up).

3. Roast vegetables for about 15 minutes. Remove from oven and wrap foil around vegetables to keep them warm.

4. Toast bagels. Spread a thin layer of cream cheese on each half, top with roasted vegetables. Sprinkle with a dash of lemon pepper and serve open-faced.

This traditional Jewish sandwich doesn't have to be high in fat and calories. It can even be converted to suit a vegetarian's tastes.

◆

There are many reduced-fat cream cheeses, or you can use just a thin spread of regular cream cheese.

◆

We like to use onion bagels because they are so flavorful, but you can use any variety, such as sesame or poppy seed, egg or plain.

Roasted Vegetable Sandwich

MAKES 2 SERVINGS

Whenever we picnic with friends, we always include roasted vegetables. They make a delicious sandwich on a baguette.

2 *red bell peppers, sliced*
1 *large zucchini, sliced*
1 *large onion, thinly sliced*
2 *garlic cloves, peeled and thinly sliced*
1 *fresh baguette*
1/2 cup Parmesan cheese, grated

Marinade:
3 *tablespoons balsamic vinegar*
2 *tablespoons olive oil*
1 *tablespoon molasses*
1 *tablespoon fresh basil, chopped*
1 *tablespoon fresh thyme (or substitute 1 teaspoon Italian herbs, dried)*

1. Combine marinade ingredients in a large bowl. Add cut vegetables and let stand for 60 minutes, then drain. Arrange peppers, zucchini, onion and garlic on a baking sheet covered with foil (shiny side up) and bake at 400° for approximately 30 minutes, until vegetables are golden brown.

2. For sandwiches, slice baguette in half and layer vegetables on bread. Sprinkle with Parmesan cheese.

3. As a dinner suggestion, serve grilled vegetables over brown rice and complement with fresh green salad.

Vegetables are easy to roast in the oven. But if you have the time, vegetables turn a summertime barbecue into a healthy, low-fat delight.

◆

Summer is the perfect time for grilling, and the season offers a variety of flavorful vegetables.

◆

Whether you prepare these vegetables in the oven or over the coals, you'll enjoy their succulent, smoky sweet flavors.

Picnic Energy Sandwich

MAKES 2 SERVINGS

This sandwich has become legendary! We first encountered the original energy sandwich on St. John's Island, in The Caribbean, where we had the tangiest honey mustard ever! Back home, we tried infinite variations on this island favorite. Our friends and family say this one is the absolute best.

½ cup Dijon mustard
3 tablespoons honey
2 tablespoons lemon
2 small loaves of French bread
Garlic cheese spread (such as Rondele)
2 slices Norwegian smoked salmon (optional)
1 avocado, peeled and sliced
1 tomato, sliced
1 cup alfalfa sprouts

1. To prepare honey mustard: Combine the Dijon mustard, honey, and lemon juice. Whisk well.

2. Cut bread lengthwise and spread honey mustard on two halves.

3. On top of honey mustard, spread a thin layer of garlic cheese spread. Top with smoked salmon if desired. Then begin adding layers of vegetables in this order: avocado, tomato, sprouts.

4. Serve with plenty of napkins!

Be creative with sandwiches. They can be a great high-energy lunch in the middle of your working day or on a weekend picnic.

◆

We love to use avocado in sandwiches. We know it is high in fat, but the fat in an avocado is not the same as the fat in a strip of bacon or slice of pastrami! Avocados are a wonderful source of vitamins.

Very Veggie Burgers

MAKES 10 PATTIES

These burgers are delicious on fresh sourdough bread or a whole-wheat bun. Kids love them as much as adults.

1 tablespoon canola oil
½ pound mushrooms, quartered
1 small onion, diced
2 tablespoons walnuts or sunflower seeds
1 large carrot, coarsely grated
1 tablespoon apple peeled and grated
1 teaspoon marjoram
Salt and pepper to taste
1 cup green beans, cooked to crisp tender
1 cup Garbanzo beans, drained
1 tablespoon tahini or peanut butter
1 tablespoon Worcestershire sauce
3 tablespoons bread crumbs
1 egg white

1. Heat oil in a large skillet. Add mushrooms, onions, nuts, carrot, apple, and marjoram. Sauté until mushrooms appear golden brown. Add salt and pepper to taste.

2. Transfer vegetables to medium-size bowl and add green beans, garbanzos, tahini or peanut butter, Worcestershire sauce, and bread crumbs.

3. Combine everything well and put in a food processor. Pulse 3 or 4 times. Mixture should be a coarse consistency. Mix in egg white.

4. Form mixture into palm-sized patties.

5. Bake on a nonstick baking sheet in oven at 450° for 15 minutes; turn over patties and cook another 15 minutes. Alternatively, fry patties in a skillet with light coating of canola oil until golden brown.

We've searched all over the world for the best veggie burger. Some taste too much like soy, some have a gummy texture, some simply fall apart!

◆

Veggie burgers are a healthy alternative to hamburgers, but unless they are pleasurable to eat and tasty, why would anyone switch?

◆

Some veggie burgers try too hard to resemble hamburgers. That's not our goal with this recipe. We've created a healthy and delicious, low-fat burger that is sure to win over even the toughest skeptics!

◆

For variety, use this recipe to make a veggie loaf.

ENTREES

White Cabbage and Potatoes

MAKES 4 SERVINGS

This dish is sure to warm hearts and bellies on a late autumn or cold winter's night. Cabbage and potatoes are a soothing and filling combination.

> 1 tablespoon canola oil
> 1 medium onion, diced
> ½ teaspoon sugar
> 1 small white cabbage, shredded finely
> ½ cup water
> 1 teaspoon caraway seeds
> 5 medium-size potatoes (Yukon Gold if available), peeled
>   and cut in quarters
> Salt and pepper to taste

1. Heat oil in large pot, add onion, and sauté until golden. Sprinkle with sugar.

2. Add cabbage and cook on high heat until cabbage is slightly browned (about 10 minutes), stirring often to prevent burning.

3. Add water and caraway seeds, cover, and cook on low heat for 40 minutes. Season to taste with salt and pepper, and add more water if too dry.

4. While cabbage cooks, in a separate kettle boil potatoes until soft.

5. Drain potatoes and combine with cabbage. Serve warm.

Potatoes are a superior source of complex carbohydrates, vitamins, and minerals. Eating more of this type of carbohydrate is a wonderful way to cut down on fat in your diet without feeling starved. Potatoes are one of the most filling foods, and are so good for you.

◆

Potatoes only become high-fat when topped with butter and sour cream, or whipped with milk and butter.

◆

Here is a delicious way to enjoy potatoes, mixed with the goodness of cabbage. The presence of caraway seeds in this recipe is a wonderful remedy for the gassiness some people experience from cabbage.

Mushroom-Stuffed Pasta Shells

MAKES 4 SERVINGS

Every shell is stuffed with a delightful surprise of mushrooms and cheese. This is a perfect substantial dinner that is delicious any time of the year.

2 teaspoons olive or canola oil
1 small onion, minced (½ cup)
1 garlic clove, minced
1¼ pounds mushrooms, chopped
2 tablespoons chopped fresh rosemary
1 tablespoon chopped fresh parsley
1 cup crumbled feta cheese
½ cup pine nuts
¼ cup raisins
Salt and freshly ground black pepper
20 jumbo pasta shells
4 cups Simply Fresh or Best Basic Tomato Sauce (pages
   228 and 230)
Chopped parsley for garnish

1. Preheat oven to 350°.

2. Heat oil in a nonstick skillet, add the onion, and sauté 2–3 minutes. Add the garlic and mushrooms and sauté a few minutes more, stirring from time to time. Stir in the rosemary and parsley and continue to cook until the liquid from the mushrooms has evaporated. Remove from heat. Stir in half the cheese, the pine nuts, and the raisins, and season lightly. Let cool.

3. Cook the pasta shells in a large saucepan of boiling water until barely al dente. Drain well and dry on paper towels before filling.

4. Fill the pasta shells with the mushroom mixture. Arrange the filled shells in a large baking dish, pour the tomato sauce over and around them, and then sprinkle with the remaining cheese. Cover dish with foil and bake in the preheated oven for 30–40 minutes.

5. Sprinkle with chopped parsley.

Pasta shells can be stuffed with virtually any ingredients. Fresh mushrooms and herbs are the tastiest filling we've tried. This recipe is always a hit, even with meat-and-potato types!

◆

The addition of fresh rosemary makes this dish especially flavorful and fragrant.

◆

This dish is unbelievably good the next day—even cold!

Farfalle with Beans and Tuna

MAKES 4 SERVINGS

This is a perfect dish to prepare when you have unexpected guests.
It's simple but delicious and can be enjoyed year-round.

   1 *tablespoon olive oil*
   1 *large onion, finely diced*
   4 *cloves garlic, mashed*
   2 *tablespoons Vermouth Rosso (optional)*
   8 *fresh tomatoes, peeled and diced, or 1 28-ounce can*
       crushed tomatoes
   1 *10-ounce package frozen lima beans, defrosted*
   1 *teaspoon sugar*
Salt and pepper to taste
   1 *tablespoon oregano*
   1 *can tuna in water, drained and cut into small chunks*
   1 *pound farfalle (bowtie pasta)*

1. Heat olive oil in large pot. Add onion and garlic and sauté until
   translucent. Add vermouth.

2. Add tomatoes, beans, sugar, and oregano. Season to taste with
   salt and pepper. Cook on medium-low heat for 15 minutes.

3. Mix tuna into sauce and simmer for about 3 minutes, until tuna
   is just warm.

4. While sauce is simmering, cook pasta to al dente and, mix together with sauce, and serve.

This dish proves there are delicious ways to eat high-protein meals without rely-
ing on high-fat red meat.

◆

Pasta, beans, and tuna combine to create a dish packed with energy but low in
fat. This is a classic italian combination, where beans play a prominent role in
cooking.

◆

Not only are beans a super source of protein, they are also high in fiber, iron
and other minerals.

Spaghetti with Tomatoes and Arugula

MAKES 4 SERVINGS

The freshness of spring or summertime comes alive in this light but satisfying dish. It takes less than a half hour to prepare—perfect if you'd rather sit down and enjoy a beautiful sunset instead of toiling over a hot stove.

1 *pound spaghetti*
2 *tablespoons balsamic vinegar*
2 *tablespoons orange juice*
1/2 *teaspoon Dijon mustard*
1 *tablespoon olive oil*
Salt and pepper to taste
8 *medium tomatoes, diced*
1 *bunch arugula, chopped*

1. Cook spaghetti in boiling water until al dente.

2. While spaghetti cooks, mix vinegar, orange juice, and mustard in a medium bowl. Whisk together well.

3. Slowly add oil, and season with salt, and pepper. Add tomatoes and arugula and mix well.

4. Pour tomato mixture over spaghetti and gently toss.

Arugu-what? *Arugula . . . This flavorful leafy green has only recently made it into mainstream cooking. It is now a staple in California cuisine, and because it is rich in calcium and vitamins, we think it deserves its place in all healthy cooking.*

◆

If you garden, arugula is simple to grow. With a little care, one plant will thrive throughout the summer.

◆

Vegetable Risotto

MAKES 2 SERVINGS

This risotto is rich and creamy but very low in fat. Asparagus and asagio cheese are a memorable combination. Look for the freshest, most tender stalks of asparagus available.

2 cups trimmed asparagus tips
3 cups water
1 tablespoon olive or canola oil
2 shallots, chopped (about ¼ cup)
1 garlic clove, minced
1½ cups short-grain or Arborio rice
Vegetable broth recipe (page 237)
Pinch of saffron threads (optional)
Strip of lemon peel
1 tablespoon lemon juice
2 cups sliced button mushrooms
8 sundried tomatoes packed in oil, well drained and
    chopped
½ cup chopped walnuts or cashew nuts, toasted
Salt and freshly ground black pepper
Roughly chopped flat-leaf parsley and large shavings of
    Asagio cheese (optional) for garnish

1. Put asparagus in a small saucepan of boiling water and cook until barely tender, 2–3 minutes. Drain, reserving cooking liquid. Refresh the asparagus in ice water and set aside.

2. Heat oil in a heavy saucepan. Add shallots and garlic and sauté 2–3 minutes. Stir in rice and cook 3 minutes, stirring occasionally.

3. Add enough vegetable broth to the reserved asparagus cooking liquid to make 3 cups. Add to the pan the saffron threads, if using, and lemon peel and juice. Bring to a boil, then reduce heat, cover, and simmer 10 minutes.

4. Add mushrooms and sundried tomatoes and cook, covered, until rice is tender—another 10 minutes. Stir in asparagus and nuts for the last few minutes of cooking.

5. Remove lemon peel, season to taste, and transfer to a warm dish. Sprinkle with chopped parsley and large shavings of Asagio cheese, if using. Serve risotto at once.

Risotto is a wonderfully creamy Italian rice. It has a texture and flavor that is simply out of this world. This dish takes a little longer to prepare, but it is well worth the extra time.

◆

An endless variety of ingredients can be added to the basic risotto. Asparagus is a particularly delicious variation, but you can substitute radicchio, green peas, spring onions, mushrooms, or beans.

Rigatoni with Asparagus and Parsley

MAKES 4 SERVINGS

This is a delicious springtime pasta, when asparagus is abundant. We buy huge bunches of it at the farmer's market on Saturday mornings and enjoy it throughout the week. This is our favorite recipe, filled with the freshness and sweet flavors of spring.

½ pound asparagus, cut into 2-inch pieces
2 cups water
1 teaspoon salt
1 teaspoon olive oil
2 cloves garlic, mashed
2 tomatoes, peeled, cut in wedges
2 tablespoons parsley, finely chopped
Salt and pepper to taste
Shaved parmesan cheese
1 pound rigatoni

1. Put asparagus in medium-size pot. Add just enough water to cover asparagus. Add salt and cook for approximately 12 minutes (depending on size) until asparagus is crisp tender.

2. Heat oil and sauté garlic until just fragrant.

3. Add asparagus, tomatoes and parsley. Season to taste with salt, and pepper. Stir well. Cover and turn heat to lowest setting.

4. Cook pasta to al dente.

5. Drain pasta and combine with asparagus mixture. Divide onto four plates and top with shaved parmesan.

6. Serve with a fresh green salad.

Asparagus is our favorite spring vegetable, at its peak between April and July. Especially in California, where 70 percent of the country's asparagus is grown, we can even find it fresh in the stores between February and July.

◆

♦

When selecting asparagus, choose firm stalks with tightly closed tips.

♦

Asparagus is best served the day you buy it, but will keep in the refrigerator for four or five days. If fresh asparagus is not available, frozen stalks or canned asparagus will do.

♦

Asparagus is a wonderful source of vitamin A, which is beneficial for eyesight.

◆

Pasta with Bread Crumbs and Spinach

MAKES 4 SERVINGS

This Sicilian dish harmonizes the distinct flavors of garlic, lemon, and spinach with the sweetness of basil and raisins. Enjoy it with a glass of Chianti for a deeply pleasing meal.

1 tablespoon olive oil
1/2 yellow onion, diced
5 cloves garlic, minced
4 cups fresh spinach, stemmed and chopped; or one 10 ounce package frozen, chopped spinach, thawed and drained
2 tablespoons canola oil
1 cup plain bread crumbs
1/2 cup shredded parmesan cheese
1 cup fresh basil chopped, or 1 tablespoon dried basil
1 tablespoon grated lemon or orange zest
1/4 cup raisins
1 pound farfalle (bowtie pasta)
Salt and pepper to taste

1. In a large sauté pan or skillet heat 1 tablespoon olive oil and sauté onion and garlic until golden brown. Add spinach and cook until just wilted. Season to taste with salt and pepper. Transfer spinach to a bowl and set aside.

2. In the *same pan* heat 2 tablespoons canola oil and stir in bread crumbs.

3. Add breadcrumbs, parmesan cheese, basil, lemon or orange zest, and raisins. Sauté over *low* heat 3–5 minutes, stirring frequently. Remove from heat.

4. Cook pasta al dente, drain, and transfer to large serving bowl. Combine pasta with spinach and bread crumb mixture and serve immediately.

This dish has its origins in Sicily and fits perfectly with the new low-fat tastes of more and more Americans.

◆

Greens and grains make this a healthful dinner, high in fiber and vitamins and low in calories and animal fat.

◆

Enjoy variations on this dish by substituting any winter green, such as Swiss chard or kale. These winter greens are abundant sources of vitamins and iron.

◆

Healthy Lasagna or Roll-ups

MAKES 6 SERVINGS

This wonderful pasta dish inspired by our very good friend Debbie Oliphant is absolutely delicious. You'll fill up on a healthy dish and look forward to leftovers the next day.

> 2 pounds fresh spinach, blanched
> 1 cup pine nuts, toasted (or substitute chopped walnuts)
> 2 cloves garlic, mashed
> 1 cup low-fat mozzarella cheese, shredded
> ½ cup raisins
> 1 egg white
> Salt and pepper to taste
> 9–12 lasagna noodles, cooked al dente
> Tomato sauce (according to season, use Simply Fresh or
>   Best Basic recipes on pages 228 and 230)

1. Drain blanched spinach, let cool down, and squeeze out all liquid. Chop fine.

2. Add toasted nuts, garlic, mozzarella, raisins and egg white to the spinach. Season to taste with salt and pepper.

3. Cover bottom of 9-inch × 9-inch baking dish with a little tomato sauce.

4. Place one layer of lasagna noodles, then one layer of spinach mixture. Add another layer of sauce, then noodles, then spinach mixture and repeat using remaining noodles, spinach mixture and sauce, making 3–4 layers total. Top with tomato sauce.

5. Cover with foil and bake at 350° for 30 minutes. Remove foil and bake another 15 minutes.

6. To make roll-ups, lay lasagna noodles on a flat surface and spread about 2 tablespoons of spinach mixture on top of each noodle. Roll noodles up and place them seam-side down in the baking dish. Top with tomato sauce, cover with foil and bake.

7. Serve with Caesar salad.

One variation to try: make your mixture using half spinach and half kale, which packs a healthy punch of vitamins and anti-oxidants.

◆

A handful of nuts a few times a week, such as in this recipe, seems to make for a healthier heart, and this is a great way to have them. Along with the sauce of your choice, you can also add sliced mushrooms and red peppers.

◆

You will only need about 9 noodles, but in cooking some will break so be sure to cook more if you are making roll-ups.

Spaghetti with Lentil Tomato Sauce

MAKES 2 SERVINGS

Even spaghetti and meatball lovers will rave about this dish! Lentils give this recipe great flavor and texture.

> 2 teaspoons olive oil
> 1 medium carrot, thinly sliced
> 1 medium onion, diced
> 3 garlic cloves, minced
> 1 28-ounce can whole peeled tomatoes
> 1 teaspoon Italian herbs (i.e., basil, parsley, oregano)
> 3/4 cup dried brown or green lentils
> Salt, pepper, and sugar to taste
> 1 16-ounce package spaghetti

1. Heat oil in medium-size pot and sauté carrot, onion, and garlic over medium heat for about 5 minutes. Stir frequently so garlic doesn't burn.

2. Empty the canned tomatoes together with liquid into a medium-size bowl and mash with potato masher.

3. Add mashed tomatoes, Italian herbs, and lentils to sautéed vegetables and stir well. Simmer over low to medium heat for about 40 minutes, adding water if necessary to keep the sauce from becoming too thick. Sauce should be the consistency of a meat or bolognese sauce. Season to taste with salt and pepper.

4. Cook spaghetti in boiling water until al dente. Combine pasta with sauce and serve.

This creative combination of grains and lentils provides plenty of carbohydrates, fiber, and protein.

◆

This meal will give your body long-lasting energy and satisfy your taste buds and hunger.

◆

Lentils are easy to prepare. They are the only legume that does not have to be pre-soaked before cooking.

◆

This makes a wonderful filling for lasagna. It tastes even better than ground up meat!

◆

Pasta with Buckwheat

MAKES 2 SERVINGS AS A MAIN DISH,
4 AS A SIDE DISH

The simplicity of this dish is the key to its good taste. Pasta and buckwheat blend in a wonderful texture. Our family calls this traditional dish, Kasha Varnishkes.

> 2 cups water
> 2 cups farfalle pasta (bowtie pasta)
> 1 cup kasha (roasted buckwheat groats)
> 1 teaspoon butter
> 1 medium onion, minced
> Salt and pepper to taste

1. Boil 2 cups of water in medium saucepan. Add the kasha and return to a boil. Reduce heat, cover and simmer gently until tender, about 10–15 minutes.

2. Cook the pasta until al dente.

3. Melt butter in a small skillet, add the onion, and sauté until lightly browned, stirring frequently.

4. Add the onion to the cooked kasha. Drain the pasta and lightly toss with the kasha and onion mixture. Serve immediately. Tastes great with cucumber salad as a side dish.

Buckwheat, also known as kasha, is a high-fiber grain. It also provides good supplies of magnesium, vitamin B_6, zinc, copper, and iron.

◆

This is a simple dish, combining pasta and kasha, for a filling high-fiber, high-energy meal.

Eggplant Rollatini

MAKES 4 SERVINGS

Thanks to the magnificent chefs at Canyon Ranch, this delicious and healthy meal is low in calories and fat. For variety, we sometimes substitute fresh garden zucchini for eggplant.

⅔ cup bread crumbs
1 tablespoon parmesan cheese
¼ teaspoon dried ground basil
¼ teaspoon dried ground rosemary
¼ teaspoon dried ground parsley
¼ teaspoon dried ground thyme
¾ cup part-skim ricotta cheese
1 pound eggplant, cut into 12 slices about ¼-inch thick
1 cup tomato sauce
2 tablespoons gratred part-skim mozzarella cheese
4 ounces spaghetti or linguini

1. Preheat oven to 350°.

2. Combine bread crumbs, parmesan cheese, and half of herbs in a small bowl and set aside.

3. In small bowl, mix remaining half of herbs into ricotta cheese and set aside.

4. Steam eggplant slices until pliable, about 3 to 5 minutes.

5. Lay each eggplant slice in bread crumbs, patting to be assured the coating will stick.

6. Spoon 1 tablespoon of ricotta cheese mixture near edge of each slice of eggplant and roll to form a tube.

7. Arrange eggplant rolls in shallow 8-inch × 11-inch baking dish. Sprinkle extra crumbs over them and top evenly with tomato sauce and mozzarella cheese. Bake until heated through, about 30 minutes.

8. While rollatini are baking, cook pasta, drain, and divide evenly among 4 plates.

9. Place 3 eggplant rollatini over pasta and serve immediately.

Italian cooking makes the most of fresh seasonal vegetables. Italian home cooking entails a daily trip to the market, where fresh vegetables fill the stands. One of the most enjoyable pastimes on our Italian vacations is to sit at a sidewalk café and watch the animated conversations between grocers and customers as they compare the size and color of fresh bell peppers, smell the fragrance of freshly picked basil, and select the firmest, reddest vine-ripened Roma tomatoes.

◆

Eggplant is a staple of Italian cooking. In Italy, eggplant is rarely fried, as it is here in the states. In this low-fat recipe (only 8 grams of fat per serving), the unique flavor of eggplant is enhanced with Italian herbs and tomatoes.

Pasta with Tomatoes and Cheese

MAKES 4 SERVINGS

This is a delicious dish in late summer, when tomatoes are at their ripest. The delicate cottage cheese balances the flavors of tomatoes, fresh basil, and garlic.

> 4 large beefsteak tomatoes, diced
> ³/₄ cup low-fat cottage cheese, large curd
> ¹/₄ cup fresh basil chopped
> 1 large garlic clove, minced
> 2 tablespoons olive oil
> Salt and pepper to taste
> 1 pound penne or fusilli pasta
> Freshly grated Romano cheese for garnish (optional)

1. Combine tomatoes, cottage cheese, basil, garlic, oil, salt, and pepper in bowl. Mix together gently. Time permitting, let stand for about 15 minutes so the flavors mingle.

2. Cook pasta until al dente. Drain and return to saucepan. Add tomato mixture and fold together gently.

3. Taste and adjust seasoning. Sprinkle with Romano cheese, if desired, and serve immediately.

4. Makes a great lunch the next day, served cold.

You can enjoy a creamy pasta sauce without the high fat. Instead of cream and butter, this sauce uses low-fat cottage cheese, which gives this recipe great texture.

◆

Cottage cheese comes in both 1 percent and 2 percent low-fat varieties, with 1 and 2 grams of fat per 4 ounce serving, respectively. Either is a small fraction of the fat content from the heavy creams that are usually the basis for a creamy pasta sauce.

Orange Couscous with Vegetables

MAKES 2 SERVINGS

As the couscous cooks, it soaks up the orange juice and garlic and becomes intensely aromatic and tasty. This meal is a delight for all your senses.

> 1 tablespoon canola oil
> Medium onion, finely diced
> 2 cloves garlic, minced
> 1/2 red pepper, cut into 1/2" slices
> 2 tablespoons raisins
> 1 cup orange juice
> 1/2 cup frozen lima beans, defrosted and blanched (fresh
>   lima beans, blanched if available)
> 1 cup water
> 3/4 cup couscous, uncooked
> Salt and pepper to taste

1. Heat oil in a medium pot. Add onion and garlic and sauté until translucent.

2. Add red pepper, raisins, and orange juice. Sauté for 15 minutes.

3. Add lima beans and water. Stir and bring to a boil.

4. Stir in couscous. Remove from heat and let stand for 5 minutes without stirring.

5. Fluff with fork and serve with crispy cucumber or tomato salad.

Couscous is a nutty, aromatic grain. Combined with vegetables, it is an excellent source of energy and a delicious way to lower fat in your diet.

This grain is a staple of Middle Eastern cooking. It is a hard wheat semolina, cracked, ground and rolled in flour.

Among the grains, this is one of the easiest and fastest to prepare. Overcooked couscous will lose its light and fluffy texture.

Asparagus Chicken

MAKES 4 SERVINGS

The appealing and unusual flavors of this dish consistently draw raves from family and friends. Delicate asparagus and mushrooms are dazzled with capers and lemon juice.

1 1/2 tablespoon canola oil
1 onion, finely chopped
2 cups mushrooms, sliced
2 whole skinless chicken breasts, cut into chunks
(1 pound tofu for vegetarian version, drained and cut into chunks)
3 tablespoons all purpose flour
1 cup water
2 pounds fresh asparagus tips or one 15-ounce can (save liquid)
2 tablespoons capers
Juice of 1/2 lemon
1/2 tablespoon sugar
1/2 tablespoon salt
1/2 teaspoon pepper
2 cups Basmati rice
4 cups water
1 tablespoon fresh parsley, chopped

1. Heat oil in a medium pot and sauté onions until translucent. Add mushrooms and sauté until they turn light brown.

2. Add chicken and sauté until it appears white on all sides, about 10 minutes.

3. Sprinkle flour over chicken and stir well. Add water, asparagus and its juice, capers, lemon juice, sugar, salt and pepper. Cover. Cook on low heat for 35 to 40 minutes, stirring occasionally.

4. In the meantime, cook Basmati rice in water; follow directions on package.

5. Serve the asparagus chicken mixture over rice and sprinkle it with parsley.

The festivity of traditional German cooking is captured in this low-fat chicken dish. Capers and asparagus add unmistakable flavor.

Try serving over halved puff pastry shells. Guests love it.

This entrée is easily transformed into a vegetarian meal by substituting tofu for chicken.

Turkey Meatloaf

MAKES 4 SERVINGS

Canyon Ranch has taken the high-fat American standard meatloaf and turned it into a healthful, low-fat meal—not your average, ho-hum meatloaf!

> ¼ cup diced onion
> ¾ pound ground skinless turkey breast
> ¾ cup dry whole-wheat bread crumbs
> 1 egg white
> Pinch salt
> Pinch black pepper
> ½ cup tomato sauce
> 1½ teaspoons Worcestershire sauce

1. Preheat oven to 350°. Lightly spray baking sheet or loaf pan with nonstick vegetable coating and set aside.

2. Combine all ingredients in large bowl and mix well.

3. Form meat into loaf shape on baking sheet or put in loaf pan. Bake about 40 minutes or until loaf is firm to the touch.

This is a perfect meal for you and your family if you are making the transition away from red meat to a more vegetarian-based diet.

◆

Turkey is much lower in fat than red meat. In fact, one serving of this meatloaf has only 4 grams of fat.

Breaded Chicken

MAKES 2 SERVINGS

In Germany, we call this Schnitzel. But instead of pork or veal, traditionally found in most restaurants, this recipe uses chicken. When we are in the mood for a flesh-based meal, this is one of our favorites.

> 2 skinless chicken breast fillets, pounded thin
> Salt and pepper
> 2 tablespoons all purpose flour
> 1 egg white, beaten lightly
> 2 tablespoons bread crumbs
> 3 tablespoons canola oil
> Juice of ½ lemon (optional)

1. Sprinkle chicken with salt and pepper. Dip chicken first, in flour to coat evenly, then dip in egg whites, followed by bread crumbs.

2. Heat oil in a large skillet and fry chicken on both sides on medium heat for about 15 minutes, until golden brown and well done. Shake skillet occasionally to prevent burning.

3. Drain chicken on paper towels to remove excess oil. Squeeze lemon juice over chicken and serve with Potato Salad, noodles and brown gravy.

Poultry, in moderation, can be part of a low-fat, high-energy diet. Many traditional meat dishes can be lightened up by substituting chicken for red meat.

◆

When chicken or other flesh food is a part of your meal, accompany it with lots of vegetables for energy balance. This recipe harmonizes well with Potato Cucumber Salad.

◆

Enjoy this dish hot for dinner, or cold on a sandwich the next day, with some Dijon mustard and sauerkraut. This makes an unusual and delicious sandwich.

Chicken Goulash

MAKES 4 SERVINGS

This was the traditional Sunday meal in my house when I was growing up, but my mother prepared it with pork and beef. I created this healthier version so that I can still enjoy the wonderful fragrance and memories of this meal.

2 tablespoons canola oil
2 medium onions, diced
2 skinless chicken breast fillets, cut into 2-inch chunks
16 ounces of mushrooms (brown if available) cut in half
4 cloves garlic, sliced
1 tablespoon tomato paste
4 cups water
1/2 cup beer (optional)
1 teaspoon sugar
1 teaspoon paprika
Salt and pepper to taste
1 lb. wide noodles

1. Heat oil in a large pot and add onions. Sauté until golden.

2. Add chicken. Stir frequently until chicken is golden brown, being careful not to burn.

3. Add mushrooms and garlic. Stir well. Cook for 10 minutes.

4. Add tomato paste and stir well for about 5 minutes.

5. Turn heat to medium/low. Slowly begin adding water, 1 cup at a time (also add beer). Let each cup cook down a bit before adding more (this creates a nice, strong gravy).

6. Cover and simmer for 45 minutes, stirring occasionally. Add sugar and paprika, then salt and pepper to taste.

7. Serve over wide noodles, with Swabian Cucumber Salad and Swabian Potato Salad for an authentic German dinner.

◆

Traditional goulash is filled with pork and beef—a dish so high in fat it can make your heart race just thinking about it! But this low-fat version replaces red meat with poultry for a hearty and heart-healthy goulash.

◆

Poultry is a good source of protein. To reduce fat from chicken, be sure to remove all skin and any visible fat.

◆

For a strictly vegetarian version, use portobello mushrooms instead of chicken. Portobellos are "meaty" and flavorful, and make a perfect vegetarian goulash.

♦

Halibut on Vegetables

MAKES 2 SERVINGS

Fish and vegetables are a winning high-energy combination. You won't believe how tasty this is.

> 2 halibut steaks
> Salt and pepper to taste
> Juice of 1 lemon
> 1 cup water
> 2 cups carrots, cut in 2-inch slices
> 2 medium potatoes, cut in 2-inch cubes
> 2 cups green peas
> 2 tablespoons Crème Fraîche or low-fat sour cream
> 3/4 tablespoon Dijon mustard
> 1 teaspoon Worcestershire sauce
> 2 tablespoons parsley, chopped

1. Preheat oven to 350°.

2. Clean and wash fish. Sprinkle with salt and lemon juice.

3. In a large pot, pour 1 cup water and add carrots and potatoes. Boil about 10 minutes, until vegetables are crisp tender, but not mushy. Reserve water.

4. While vegetables cook, mix crème fraîche with mustard and Worcestershire sauce until smooth. Add salt and pepper to taste.

5. Add crème fraîche mixture and parsley to pot with water and vegetables and stir well.

6. Transfer vegetable mixture to a 9″ × 9″ casserole dish. Lay halibut on top of vegetables. Cover with foil and bake in the oven on low heat for about 20–30 minutes, until fish is opaque and flaky.

7. Transfer vegetables and fish to plates and serve hot.

Fish has many nutritional and health benefits. We try to eat fish each week.

♦

◆

Fish contains omega-3 fatty acids, the unsaturated fats that may help lower cholesterol levels in the blood. Fish also provides niacin, riboflavin, vitamins B_6 and B_{12}, and at least a dozen important minerals, including calcium, magnesium, and potassium.

◆

Halibut is very lean and nutritious. If halibut is unavailable, select any other fresh, light fish, such as sea bass. This recipe also works with swordfish, shrimp or scallops. Also experiment with other seasonal vegetables, such as cauliflower and red pepper.

Turkey Burgers

MAKES 4 SERVINGS

These patties are delicious as an entrée, served with red cabbage, potatoes and gravy, or served between a whole-wheat bun or sour-dough bread with mustard, ketchup, and thinly sliced pickles.

> 2 *slices bread*
> 1 *medium onion, minced*
> 2 *tablespoons canola oil*
> 24 *ounces ground turkey, extra lean*
> 1 *tablespoon parsley, minced*
> 1 *egg*
> 1 *teaspoon salt*
> *Pepper to taste*
> 1 *tablespoon Maggi seasoning*

1. Soak bread in water for 5 minutes, then squeeze out all water, completely.

2. In a large skillet, sauté onion in 1 teaspoon oil until browned, stirring frequently.

3. In a large bowl mix sautéed onion with turkey and bread, parsley, egg, salt, pepper, and Maggi. Add a little water if too dry.

4. Form palm-sized patties and fry in remaining tablespoon oil until golden brown on each side until well done. Use a nonstick pan if possible. Drain on paper towel.

Ground turkey makes a much lighter and lower fat burger than ground red meat. Be certain to choose extra lean turkey.

◆

This is a great meal for families making the transition away from red meat toward a more vegetarian-based diet.

◆

The fat content of regular hamburgers gets even higher when cheese and high-fat condiments such as mayonnaise are added. These burgers are so flavorful, they don't need those high-fat extras.

◆

Tin Foil Salmon and Vegetables

MAKES 4 SERVINGS

This is our absolute favorite fish dish. It is easy, fast, and actually fun to prepare, and even more fun to eat. We've experimented with the ingredients from thyme to thyme, but this original recipe is the winning combination.

> 4–6 stalks celery, diced
> 4 spring onions, diced (or regular onions)
> 4 medium carrots, peeled and cut in $1/4$ inch pieces
> $1/2$ tablespoon canola oil
> 2 pounds salmon fillet, cut into 4 pieces
> 2 ripe tomatoes, sliced
> 1 lemon, sliced
> 4 basil leaves
> $1/4$ teaspoon fresh thyme, or a pinch dried
> Salt and fresh-ground pepper to taste
> 4 squares (12 × 12 each) aluminum foil

1. Preheat oven to 450°.

2. In a medium skillet, sauté celery, onions, and carrots in $1/2$ tablespoon canola oil for 5 minutes, or until just tender—don't overcook. Season with salt and pepper to taste.

3. On each foil sheet, layer one-fourth of the ingredients in the following order:
   Sautéed vegetables
   Salmon fillets
   Salt and pepper
   Tomato slices
   Lemon slices
   Bay leaf
   Thyme

4. Fold the packets securely, tucking edges carefully, and place on a baking sheet.

5. Bake 20 minutes. Slit packets before serving and transfer to plates, or allow guests to open their own (be careful of the escaping steam).

6. Serve with basmati rice.

Salmon is frequently disparaged as a high-fat fish. It is higher in fat than halibut or catfish, but it is still very heart healthy. Salmon has plenty of omega-3 fatty acids, which have been identified as a potential agent in lowering cholesterol levels in the blood.

◆

Often it is the cooking method that adds high amounts of fat to seafood. In this dish, the salmon is oven-baked with just a small amount of added oil for sautéing the vegetables.

Crab Cakes

These are always a favorite at dinner parties. We have to double the recipe to satisfy hungry guests!

⅔ cup drained silken tofu
2 teaspoons canola oil
4 teaspoons freshly squeezed lemon juice
3 tablespoons Worcestershire sauce
Pinch celery salt
Pinch white pepper
Pinch ginger
Pinch paprika
Dash tabasco sauce, or to taste
2 lightly beaten egg whites
1 cup soft whole-wheat bread crumbs
3 cups canned crab meat, flaked and drained well (about 6 ounces)
¼ cup minced onion
2 tablespoons minced celery

1. Using a food processor with a metal blade, blend tofu, oil, lemon juice, Worcestershire sauce, seasonings, and Tabasco sauce until smooth. Transfer mixture to bowl and add all other ingredients. Mix well. Cover tightly and refrigerate until well chilled.

2. Divide chilled mixture into 12 patties. Cook in nonstick skillet over medium heat until brown on both sides.

Traditional crab cakes, fried in lots of oil, are loaded with fat. But it's easy to transform this high-fat favorite into a heart-healthy dish.

◆

Simply use a nonstick skillet and leave out the egg yolks, and you will have a delicious crab cake with half the fat of the traditional recipe (just 5 grams) and a healthy 27 grams of protein.

◆

We use canned crab in this recipe. Be sure to pick crab canned in water, not oil. To lower the sodium content, the Canyon Ranch chefs who created this recipe recommend soaking the crab meat in skim milk for 30 minutes in the refrigerator and draining with a colander before using.

Salmon Tomato Rigatoni

MAKES 2 SERVINGS

This quintessential Italian dish was inspired by a meal we had in northern Italy, where the lakes in the region bring fresh fish to the restaurant tables every night.

> 1 tablespoon olive oil
> 1 medium onion, finely diced
> 2 cloves garlic, mashed
> $\frac{1}{2}$ pound fresh salmon fillet, cut in 2-inch pieces
> $\frac{1}{2}$ tablespoon Italian herbs (i.e. basil, parsley, oregano)
> 2 tablespoons tomato paste
> 1 cup water
> $\frac{1}{2}$ cup walnuts, chopped
> Juice of 1 small lemon
> 1 teaspoon sugar
> Sugar, salt and pepper to taste
> $\frac{1}{2}$ pound rigatoni

1. Heat oil in a large frying pan. Add onion and garlic and sauté until translucent.

2. Add salmon pieces, herbs, and tomato paste to the pan and stir very well for 5 minutes.

3. Add water, walnuts, lemon juice, sugar, and season with salt and pepper to taste. Sir well and cover.

4. Simmer on low heat for 20 minutes. Meanwhile, boil pasta, and cook to al dente.

5. Be sure to check the taste of the sauce while it cooks. Remember—add salt and pepper slowly. You can always add more, but you can't take it out.

6. Serve sauce over plates of rigatoni. *Mangia bene!*

Variation: if salmon is not available, you can use canned tuna. Be sure to use tuna packed in water, not oil. If you use canned tuna, do not cook the fish, just mix it in once all the other ingredients are thoroughly cooked.

For heightened flavor and pizzazz, add a handful of capers.

Tips for cooking pasta: boiling water is easy, but the perfect pasta requires a few tricks. Use a large pot filled with water; too little water doesn't give pasta enough room to expand and results in sticky pasta.

Don't add oil to the water. It's not necessary and will make pasta so slippery your sauce won't mix well.

Catfish with Tomatoes

MAKES 2 SERVINGS

Catfish is one of the healthiest types of seafood available. We eat it regularly.

Juice of ½ lemon
2 catfish fillets, cleaned
1 teaspoon canola oil
1 medium onion, finely diced
1 green bell pepper, cut in thin rings
10 medium fresh tomatoes, sliced, or one 28-ounce can whole peeled tomatoes, mashed
Salt and pepper to taste
2 tablespoons parsley, chopped fine

1. Preheat oven to 350°.

2. Squeeze lemon juice over catfish fillets and sprinkle with salt and pepper.

3. Heat oil in medium-size pot. Add onion; sauté until translucent. Add bell peppers and tomatoes. Season to taste with salt and pepper. Cook on low for 10 minutes.

4. Spread half of the bell pepper and tomato-mixture across the bottom of a small ovenproof cassserole dish. Lay catfish fillets on top and cover with remaining mixture.

5. Cover with foil and bake in a preheated 350° oven until fish is opaque in the center, approximately 30 minutes.

6. Remove foil. Sprinkle with parsley and serve hot from the oven with mashed potatoes or rice.

Catfish is our preferred seafood because it is farm-raised, which guarantees that fish are raised in a quality controlled environment. They are raised in water from underground wells and are fed a high protein mixture of soybean, wheat, corn, vitamins, and minerals.

Salmon Croquettes

MAKES 2 SERVINGS

This recipe always pleased the hungry Taub boys when they were growing up. These croquettes are light and taste so good.

2 6-ounce cans salmon, skinned and boneless
Juice of ½ medium-size lemon
1 tablespoon parsley, finely chopped
1 egg white
¾ cup matzoh meal or plain bread crumbs
1½ tablespoons canola oil for frying

1. Mix salmon in a medium bowl with the lemon juice, parsley, egg white, and matzoh meal (or bread crumbs). If mixture is too wet, add more bread crumbs. Season to taste with salt and pepper.

2. Form flat patties, the size of your palm.

3. Heat oil in a frying pan and fry patties until medium golden brown on each side.

4. Serve with a light cucumber salad, or between two slices of crusty sourdough bread.

Salmon is one of the best sources of omega-3 fatty acids, which have recently been shown to be very beneficial to your health.

♦

This recipe is a wonderful substitute for hamburgers, and makes great leftovers for sandwiches the next day.

◆

Sue's Jambalaya

MAKES 4 SERVINGS

Our good friend Sue Myers served this flavorful dish to us and brought good old Southern hospitality to a New York city high-rise apartment! The meal inspired the same celebratory spirit characteristic of Mardi Gras in New Orleans . . . We nearly forgot we were in the Big Apple!

> 4 skinless chicken breasts, cut into strips
> 1 tablespoon canola oil
> 1 medium onion, diced
> 2 ribs celery, diced
> 1/2 green bell pepper, diced
> 2 cloves garlic, minced
> 2 teaspoons paprika
> 1 cup tomato juice
> 1/2 cup vegetable broth
> 1 teaspoon Creole seasoning
> 3/4 cup long grain rice
> 1/4 cup scallions, sliced
> Salt and fresh ground pepper to taste

1. Season chicken with salt and pepper. Heat oil in large skillet or stock pot and fry chicken on high heat until brown on both sides. Remove chicken from pot and set aside.

2. Reduce heat to medium and add vegetables, garlic, and 1 teaspoon paprika. Sauté for 3 to 5 minutes, or until just tender. Return chicken to pot and add tomato juice, vegetable broth, 1 teaspoon paprika, and creole seasoning.

3. Bring mixture to a boil and add rice. Stir thoroughly to distribute rice evenly. Return to a boil, cover, reduce heat and simmer for 10 minutes.

4. Remove cover and stir well to turn the rice from top to bottom. Cover and continue cooking for another 15 minutes.

5. Uncover, stir well, add scallions, and serve.

Traditional Southern food is typically high fat and heavy on meat. But with a little imagination, the spicy, smoky flavors of the South can be captured in variations that reduce the meat and fat.

This healthful, light variation on a Creole classic highlights fresh vegetables and authentic Southern seasonings.

For a strictly vegetarian and absolutely delicious variation, simply omit the chicken.

Stuffed Bell Peppers

MAKES 4 SERVINGS

These peppers take little time to prepare but will impress your taste buds and your family.

> 1 cup vegetable bouillon or vegetable broth (see recipe page 237)
> 2 red or green bell peppers, cut in half lengthwise and seeded
> 1 medium onion, finely diced
> 1 teaspoon butter
> 5 medium potatoes, cooked, peeled, and mashed
> 1 tablespoon parsley, finely chopped
> 2 tablespoons sundried tomatoes, chopped
> 1 pinch marjoram
> 1 cup green peas, fresh or frozen, defrosted
> Salt, pepper and nutmeg to taste
> 1 cup low-fat plain yogurt
> 4 tablespoons chives, finely chopped (or spring onion greens)

1. Pour vegetable bouillon into a casserole dish and place pepper halves in dish.

2. Sauté onions in butter until golden brown.

3. Mix with mashed potatoes, then add parsley sundried tomatoes, marjoram, green peas, nutmeg, salt and pepper, and mix well. If filling is too dry or stiff, add a bit of hot water.

4. Spoon filling into peppers and cover with tin foil.

5. Bake on lowest oven rack for 40 minutes at 350°.

6. While peppers bake, mix yogurt and chives and season with salt and pepper.

7. Top baked peppers with yogurt mixture and serve hot.

◆

A savory stuffing transforms these bell peppers into a satisfying and tasty main dish.

◆

Look for plump, fresh red peppers. Red peppers are sweeter than green varieties, and easier to digest. They are also loaded with vitamin C.

◆

Give this unusual medley of tastes a try. Even the most "confirmed" meat-eaters will be in for a nice surprise!

◆

For a variation lower in fat and dairy free, omit the yogurt and accompany peppers with brown rice on the side.

Turkish Black-eyed Peas Over Rice

MAKES 5 SERVINGS

This delicious recipe uses black-eyed peas creatively.

2 *cups brown rice*
8 *cups water*
2 *large onions, peeled and finely chopped*
1 *tablespoon olive oil*
2 *10-ounce boxes of frozen black-eyed peas*
1 *cup lemon juice*
6 *ripe tomatoes, chopped*
Salt and pepper to taste

1. Cook rice in 5 cups water in a large pot until done. Meanwhile, stir-fry onions in oil for 2 minutes in a large pot.

2. Add black-eyed peas, 3 cups water and lemon juice.

3. Cover pot and simmer for 30 minutes, stirring occasionally.

4. Add tomatoes and seasonings and simmer 10 minutes longer, stirring occasionally.

5. Serve hot over cooked rice.

Many thanks to Deborah Wasserman for this high-energy dish.

It is also a wonderful source of dietary fiber, with 12 grams per serving.

Fast Cuban Beans

MAKES 4 SERVINGS

This dish is so healthy and bursting with the flavors of Cuba.

> 1 tablespoon canola oil
> 1 medium onion, diced
> 4 cloves garlic, mashed
> 2 green bell peppers, cubed
> 2 tomatoes, ripe and quartered
> ½ teaspoon cumin
> 2 15-ounce cans black beans, drained
> ½ cup of water
> 1 tablespoon Cilantro, chopped
> Juice of 1 small lime
> Salt and pepper to taste
> 1 teaspoon sugar

1. Heat oil in large pot. Add onion, garlic, and bell pepper. Sauté on medium heat until onion is translucent, stirring often.

2. Add tomatoes, beans, cumin, and water. Stir well. Simmer on low 20 minutes. While cooking, add cilantro, lime juice, salt and pepper to taste, and sugar.

3. Serve with Basmati or simple white rice.

This dish will delight your taste buds and ignite your energy.

◆

Black beans are a rich source of protein. Combined with lots of fresh vegetables, this is a healthy, high-fiber meal.

◆

Tomato and Lima Bean Stew

MAKES 4 SERVINGS

An autumn afternoon in the French countryside, surrounded by vineyards . . . that's what this delightful stew, created by my French sister-in-law, always brings to mind.

I cup lima beans, dried. Soaked for 6 hours or overnight
5 cups water
I tablespoon olive oil
6 garlic cloves, mashed
1/2 teaspoon Rosemary
Salt and pepper to taste

The sauce:
I 28-ounce can whole peeled tomatoes, stems removed
1/2 tablespoon sugar
Juice of I medium orange
Salt and pepper to taste

1. Rinse beans after soaking. In 3 cups fresh water bring beans to boiling point. Remove beans from heat, drain, and rinse. Pour beans into medium casserole dish. Add 2 cups water, olive oil, garlic, rosemary, salt, and pepper to taste. Stir together well. Cover tightly with aluminum foil and bake at 175° for 2½ hours.

2. While the beans bake, prepare the tomato sauce. In a medium pot add tomatoes, orange juice, salt, pepper, and sugar. Mash together and cook for 10 minutes.

3. When the beans are done, add them to the tomato sauce.

4. Serve with crusty French bread . . . et voila! Bon appetit!

One bowl of this hearty stew contains tremendous amounts of soluble fiber. Even small servings of cooked beans appear to have have a cholesterol-lowering effect.

◆

Soaking beans and rinsing them with plenty of fresh water decreases the gas-producing elements and makes them easier to digest.

◆

If you don't have time to cook dried beans, frozen or canned beans are a fine alternative but bake only for one hour. Choose a brand with no salt added and rinse them well.

Vegetable Chili

MAKES 6 SERVINGS

This chili has great character! I like to make it in abundance so there will be leftovers. After the spices and vegetables mingle overnight, the chili is even more tasty.

1 tablespoon olive oil
1 large onion, finely diced
5 carrots, peeled and sliced
2 red bell peppers, cored, seeded, and diced
3 stalks celery, diced
3 cloves garlic, finely minced
1 teaspoon cumin
1 ½ tablespoons chili powder
1 small jalapeño pepper, minced (optional)
Salt and pepper to taste
1 cup water
1 28-ounce can chopped tomatoes
2 tablespoons sherry, or ¼ cup beer (optional)
1 15-ounce can black beans
1 15-ounce can red kidney beans
Nonfat plain yogurt, chopped scallions, shredded cheddar
    cheese (optional) for garnish

1. Coat the inside bottom of a large, heavy saucepan with olive oil and heat over medium-high heat. Add onion, carrots, red bell pepper, celery, and garlic. Cook, stirring frequently, for 10 minutes, or until the onion is transluscent.

2. Stir in cumin, chili powder, jalapeño pepper, water, tomatoes, and sherry or beer. Season to taste with salt and pepper. Bring to a boil.

3. Lower heat and cover. Simmer for 15 minutes.

4. Add beans, cover, and cook for 5 minutes. Uncover the pan and continue cooking until the liquid has thickened slightly.

5. Top each serving with a spoonful of yogurt, chopped scallions, and shredded cheese.

A good, hearty vegetable chili provides a high-energy, healthful meal. This chili contains only healthy monounsaturated fat and is loaded with fiber, protein, and vitamins.

◆

Chili is a versatile dish. Served over brown rice, you'll get even more fiber. Alternatively, this is delicious over couscous or noodles. Kids love to eat this chili wrapped up in a tortilla.

◆

However you serve it, vegetable chili is spicy and satisfying.

DESSERTS

Apple Pie Nany

MAKES 6 SERVINGS

This pie is easy to prepare and tastes heavenly. It proves you can indulge in dessert without loading up on fat and calories.

> *One half of a 17¼-ounce package frozen puff pastry*
>   *(Pepperidge Farm is excellent; use 1 sheet)*
> *3 large apples, peeled and shredded*
> *2 tablespoons honey*
> *2 tablespoons raisins, rinsed with water*
> *3 tablespoons walnuts or pecans, chopped and toasted*

1. Preheat oven to 400°.

2. Thaw puff pastry sheet until it unfolds easily without breaking. Lay it in a round 9- or 10-inch glass pie plate.

3. Combine apples, honey, raisins, and nuts. Spread evenly over pastry sheet.

4. Bake pie on lower oven rack for 20 minutes or until sides are just turning brown.

5. Let cool and serve.

Apple pie is an American classic, but most traditional recipes are heavy with butter and sugar.

♦

Instead of a high-fat, buttery crust, this recipe uses a light puff pastry. A bit of honey enhances the natural sweetness of apples without adding lots of sugar.

◆

Enjoy this treat especially in fall, when apple orchards are overflowing with fresh fruit.

◆

For a tart variation, use raspberries instead of apples. In summertime, use fresh strawberries.

◆

This low-fat apple pie will satisfy even the sweetest tooth!

◆

Orange Raisin Muffins

MAKES 1 DOZEN MUFFINS

These muffins are fast and simple to prepare. Serve them fresh out of the oven for a delightful, healthy breakfast.

   1 1/2 cups all-purpose flour
   1 teaspoon baking powder
   1 teaspoon baking soda
   1/8 teaspoon salt
   2 egg whites
   1/2 cup low-fat buttermilk
   2 tablespoons canola oil
   3 tablespoons honey
   2 tablespoons apple sauce, unsweetened
   1 large orange, juice and zest
   1/2 cup raisins

1. Preheat oven to 350°. Lightly coat a 12 cup muffin tin with vegetable spray, or fill with paper liners.

2. Sit flour, baking powder, baking soda, and salt into a medium bowl and set aside.

3. In another bowl, using a whisk, beat egg whites until very foamy. Add buttermilk, canola oil, honey and applesauce and beat well.

4. Add dry ingredients and raisins to wet ingredients and stir *just* until flour is combined. *Do not* overmix.

5. Fill muffin cups about 3/4 full.

6. Bake approximately 12–15 minutes or until muffins are golden brown.

7. Remove muffins and cool on wire rack.

Most muffins in cafes and bakeries are really just breakfast cakes—high in fat and sugar.

◆

"Healthy" muffins tend to be so dry and flavorless they are no fun to eat.

◆

Here is a healthy muffin that is moist and tasty, and very good for you. The applesauce and orange juice give this muffin moisture, adding fat and a natural sweetness without adding sugar.

◆

Variation: Soy milk can be substituted for buttermilk to reduce fat even more.

Baked Apples with Dried Plums

MAKES 4 SERVINGS

The aroma of baked apples always reminds me of autumn and winter weekends in Germany, when the fragrance of apples, honey, and brown sugar seemed to linger in the kitchen all day long.

4 large apples
3 tablespoons rolled oats
2 tablespoons corn flakes
2 tablespoons raisins
3 tablespoons honey
1 teaspoon cardamom (optional
6 dried plums, finely chopped
1 tablespoon brown sugar

1. Preheat oven to 350°.

2. Core apples. Make a large opening at the top and leave a bit of core at the bottom of each apple to hold in filling. Place apples in casserole dish.

3. Combine oats, corn flakes, raisins, honey, cardamom, and dried plums. Spoon filling into apples and top with a sprinkle of brown sugar.

4. Bake apples at 350° for approximately 35 minutes until they are soft. Check for softness with tip of a knife. Remove from oven and spoon some baking juice over apples before serving.

This delicious, homey dish is perfect for breakfast or for dessert. It is especially good in the fall when apples are at their best.

♦

Choose a tart, flavorful baking apple. Braeburn or Granny Smith are good because as they bake they become tender but not mushy.

♦

Apples are a superb source of nutritional fiber.

♦

As a dessert variation, top with a spoonful of low-fat whipped cream or low-fat vanilla ice cream.

Toasted English Muffins with Fruit Topping

MAKES 4 SERVINGS

This is a nourishing high-energy breakfast. Fresh fruit is delicious spread on toast. For an especially wholesome breakfast, use whole-wheat English muffins.

> 4 *English muffins*
> 1 *banana, mashed with 2 teaspoons lemon juice*
> 1 *tablespoon honey or maple syrup*
> 1 *small inner tender celery stalk, finely minced*
> 1 *apple, peeled and minced or shredded*

1. Split and toast English muffins.

2. While muffins toast, mix mashed banana with honey or maple syrup.

3. Add celery and apple bits and mix well.

4. Spread evenly on each muffin and serve warm.

Mom was right—breakfast *is* the most important meal of the day. Especially if you are trying to lose weight. People who skip breakfast tend to eat more later on in the day.

◆

You need energy in the morning. A cup of coffee is not enough. If you think skipping breakfast will help cut down your daily calorie intake, think again. When you skip breakfast, you rob your body of the energy it needs to gear up for the day ahead. You will be more likely to crave high-fat junk foods later, when your energy in running on empty.

◆

This simple breakfast is fast to prepare and loaded with nutritional goodness. Parents and kids alike will enjoy it!

◆

For a variation, substitute pears, strawberries, or walnuts.

Fresh Fruit Freeze

MAKES 4 SERVINGS

Children and adults alike will devour this dessert. This is especially refreshing on a hot summer night.

> 6 *frozen bananas (Peel bananas and wrap in plastic wrap*
>   *before freezing), cut into chunks*
> *or*
> 2 *cups any frozen fruit, cut into chunks*
> 1 *tablespoon honey (optional)*
> ½ *cup vanilla soy milk (optional)*

1. Place frozen fruit in a food processor or blender. Add honey and soy milk (if desired) and process or blend until creamy but some small chunks of fruit remain.

2. Transfer to bowls and serve immediately.

There are many wonderful, low-fat as well as non-dairy alternatives to ice cream. Our favorite is this pure fruit dessert. It is so simple and it's sweetened by nature.

◆

Frozen bananas make an especially creamy fruit freeze, but you can try this recipe with all of your favorite fruits—strawberries, peaches, raspberries . . . Use your imagination!

◆

Honey and soy milk make a creamier dessert but are optional.

Part Eight

EXERCISE–WISE

I have mulled over the best way to approach the subject of exercise now for days. Should I list all the health benefits derived from exercise? Should I shock you with the damaging side effects of not exercising at all? Or should I simply encourage nonexercisers to get up on their feet and out the door?

The longer I debated how to begin, the more aware I became of the ache spreading across my back. After three days of sitting in my desk chair with little more than a few fifteen-minute breaks to answer phone calls, my lower back was so sore I could barely sit still.

That back pain made me aware that, in trying to think and write about exercise, I had neglected my own regular exercise. Each time my wife invited me out for beach walks and wellness yoga stretching, I insisted I could not interrupt my work then, and that she should enjoy the walk and stretching in the sunshine on her own.

Now the pain in my lower back forced me to remember that, even at the busiest moments in life, it is crucial to get up out of your chair, put on your walking shoes or sneakers, and get in motion. After thirty minutes of walking on the beach, my back pain subsided—and I knew exactly how to open this part of the book!

Most of us probably *think* about exercise more often than we *do* exercise. Indeed, we spend lots of time thinking our way *out* of exercising. Do any of these statements sound familiar to you?

- It's too cold.
- It's too hot.
- I'm too busy.
- I'm running late.

- I'm too tired and really need a nap.
- It can wait until tomorrow.

How easy it is to fall into these traps. Even as I was thinking about how to persuade readers to start exercising regularly, I let my own daily exercise fall to the wayside. It took intense back pain for me to become aware of this irony. I put the computer to sleep, pushed back my chair, grabbed my walking shoes, and headed for the beach. Even the smallest dose of exercise is powerful medicine!

I called my brother on the phone to tell him about my experience. "Guess what cured my writer's block on the exercise chapter? *Exercise!*" My brother, who has been a physician almost as long as I have, said, "Ed, if exercise can cure your writer's block, it can probably cure *anything!*"

Although my brother was innocently exaggerating, there is some truth to his statement. Even small amounts of regular exercise encourage a healthy body and mind as well as help protect against and treat many chronic illnesses and diseases. You have almost certainly heard news reports or seen headlines about the health benefits of exercise. Perhaps you paid attention, perhaps you didn't pay attention. Either way, after learning about your body's energy system and the cycles of your life, you can now truly appreciate the information and use it to your best health advantage.

To be exercise-wise, you need to understand the exercise *whys*. Why is exercise so important to your health? Why is it absolutely essential that you begin exercising now? Consider these facts:

- Exercise is effective prevention and treatment for coronary heart disease. Brisk walking and other aerobic exercises strengthen and reduce strain on the heart muscles. People who exercise regularly have an amazingly lower risk of heart attack compared to people who lead sedentary lives. A study of forty male runners between the ages of fifty and eighty showed that most of them had hearts as healthy as athletes half their age. In fact, research at the National Institutes of Health has shown that the heart of an older person, when free of disease, functions comparably to that of a much younger person. Exercise helps protect against coronary heart disease while inactivity ranks fourth as a major risk factor for heart disease just behind overweight, hypertension, and smoking, as determined by the American Heart Association.

- The *New England Journal of Medicine* has reported that regular exercise is an essential factor in the treatment of high cholesterol. Researchers at Stanford tracked the cholesterol levels of 197 men and 180 postmenopausal women for one year. At the beginning of the study, all the men had moderately high blood levels of LDL cholesterol (the cholesterol that damages the heart) and were considered at high risk for coronary heart disease. Participants were divided into four groups: one group followed a low-fat, low-cholesterol diet and did weekly aerobic exercise; the second group followed the low-fat diet but did not exercise; the third group did regular exercise but ate as they normally did; the last group made no changes, continuing with their regular lifestyle. After a year, the study found that there were no significant reductions in LDL cholesterol levels for those who followed a low-fat diet alone. In fact, the only group that showed any improvement was the group that combined a low-fat diet with exercise.

- Studies have shown a link between exercise and a lower risk of colon cancer. At Harvard Medical School, a study of Harvard alumni found that those who took brisk thirty-minute walks five times a week had half the incidence of colon cancer than a group of less-active alumni.

- Studies have also shown that women who exercised one to three hours per week had 20 percent to 30 percent fewer cases of breast cancer. *Women who exercised at least four hours a week demonstrated a 37 percent decrease in the incidence of breast cancer!*

- Exercise helps create and maintain healthy bones and is essential for preventing bone mass loss as we advance in the cycle of life. Small doses of regular exercise are the best medicine for preventing osteoporosis, or slowing down its progress if it has already set in. Research has shown that just thirty minutes of exercise three times a week slows bone mass loss among women. While calcium consumption is essential to preventing and treating osteoporosis, exercise combined with calcium strengthens bones and makes them more dense. Weight-bearing activities (such as walking), in which you use your bones and muscles against gravity, increase bone density. Resistance activities, such as light weight lifting, strengthen the bones. In fact, research has shown that postmenopausal women who did forty minutes of resistance activity twice a week gained 1 percent in bone density after one year, compared to a group of sedentary women, who lost between 2 and 2½ percent during that same period. Studies have found that people who do light weight-lifting activities have as much as 10 percent greater bone density compared to people who do not exercise.

- As we advance in the cycle of life, not only our bones but also our muscles become more frail. Frailty contributes to a number of health problems among older adults, such as falls and hip fractures. A frail body has a harder time recovering from even minor spills or stumbles. But even in the mature stages of the life cycle, physical frailty can be reversed with small doses of exercise. Regular physical activity strengthens muscles and improves mobility. A physically active ninety-year-old may be less frail than a sedentary sixty-year-old. In a study of men and women between the ages of eighty-six and ninety conducted by the National Institutes of Health, those who exercised with light weights increased the strength of their leg muscles three-fold! With greater leg strength and knee and hip flexibility, this group was proactive in preventing weakness-related injuries that commonly occur among older adults.

- As the process of entropy unfolds in the later years of the human lifecycle, it is not uncommon for the body to lose its ability to utilize glucose efficiently and normally. This results in what we call non-insulin dependent, or adult-onset, diabetes. Active people are less likely to develop this form of diabetes than sedentary people. Even after the onset of this disease, however, regular physical activity helps in treatment by improving the body's insulin sensitivity and blood glucose level.

- It's no secret that physical activity is necessary for achieving and maintaining your optimal weight; not only by burning excess calories, but by increasing your energy and bringing it back into balance. Exercise is a magic key!
- Perhaps the most important benefit of exercise is the effect it has on your psychological and spiritual outlook. Exercise makes your feelings of self-value and self-esteem soar. When you feel better about yourself, when you feel empowered and energetic, you make healthier choices in your eating and lifestyle habits.

Those are some of the most important exercise *whys*. Generally speaking, exercise is a naturally powerful medicine. Exercise empowers people to *prevent disease before it occurs because exercise helps to prevent energy imbalance*. Especially as individuals advance in the cycle of life (as the force of entropy gains momentum), exercise becomes a key to slowing down this process. The American College of Sports Medicine and the Centers for Disease Control and Prevention recently sent out a call to action: For optimal health, every adult should do moderate physical activity for thirty minutes most, if not all, days of the week.

As a physician, one of the most important prescriptions I can give my patients is an "Exercise Rx."* The combination of a healthful diet and regular physical activity stimulates your own internal pharmacy to help prevent the majority of illnesses and diseases related to being overweight. You see, this is not just another "diet book"—there are plenty of those already available. Perhaps losing weight is your goal. But as I have emphasized throughout, if you do not address the actual factors that are *causing* you to be overweight, you will never lose weight healthily and permanently. If you are overweight, your energy is out of balance. My goal is to help you increase and balance your energy—so you will lose weight naturally and permanently. *This is Total Health Rejuvenation.*

---

*The "Exercise Rx" has been expanded in this revised edition to include "Simple Strength Training." Please see Part Nine.

Exercise is one of the most powerful tools for creating more energy in your life. It is just as important as eating well. Starting to exercise is just as important, from an energy wellness perspective, as quitting smoking. With more energy, through a combination of exercising and eating wisely, you will extend your life, slow the process of entropy, and live a more fulfilling, productive life, even at the most advanced stages of the lifecycle.

We cannot defy age—aging is natural, healthy, and necessary. In many cultures, age is associated with strength, beauty, wisdom, and esteem. But in our culture, advertising-driven standards of beauty and strength emphasize youth and encourage us to fight aging tooth and nail, as if age itself was a disease! The approach I advocate is much different. Aging is not a disease, but a natural process. It's how we live and the choices we make that are catalysts for either the premature onset and speedy progress of entropy, or for extending and enhancing nature's cycles of life.

Especially as we reach the later stages of our lifecycle, what we don't use we are more prone to lose. For example, as older adults become less active, and as bone and muscle mass naturally decrease, the hip muscles and joints become more fragile. Hip fractures are among the most common injuries for seventy- to ninety-year-olds. Adults in this age group however, who use their hip muscles and joints through gentle stretching, light weight lifting, walking, and swimming, greatly improve their bone density and strengthen their muscles.

Entropy and its effects on the body are natural. But exercise is the best tool for countering the negative effects of entropy. I recently received a letter from a seventy-four-year-old woman who is so convinced of the benefits of regular walking that she formed a wellness walking club in the retirement community where she lives.

Dear Dr. Taub,

I thought you would be proud to know what a positive impact you have had on my life and health, as well as on my community. I never thought exercise was possible because of nagging arthritis in my knees and hips that developed about five years ago. Since that time, I'd spent most of my days sitting in a chair, enjoying the sunshine and company of dear friends. But now I know that all of that sitting around just made the stiffness and pain worse! After reading one of

*your books, I adopted your "use it or lose it" attitude and now I walk
twenty minutes every day. The pain in my hips and knees comes back
only when I skip my walks.*

*All it took was one step, then another; it was as easy as that. Six
months later, I'm leading a group of ladies in daily walks around our
community, and all of us feel younger and more energetic than ever
before! Tell your patients that we found the secret fountain of
youth—in our feet!*

Thanks from all of us,
Greta M.

Greta discovered what so many people are learning: Regular exercise, especially walking and simple stretching, is the best tool for achieving optimal health, no matter your cycle of life, and *especially* if you are upwards of fifty. Remember that chronological age influences but *does not determine* your health and energy. Greta, as an active seventy-four-year-old, is chronologically older than a fifty-year-old inactive woman, but she is more physiologically fit than her younger counterpart.

Indeed, there is a difference between your body's age in actual years and your body's age in terms of energy and fitness. Greta's body is much younger than her seventy-four years. Regular exercise has slowed the process of entropy and elevated her energy and fitness. Science still hasn't found a way to turn back the clocks, but exercise is, as Greta says, the closest thing to a fountain of youth. Regular physical activity is a fountain of energy. The more you drink from it, the younger you will feel in body and mind. And, the more you drink from it, the thirstier you will be for more exercise and the energy it imparts.

Is your physical age in or out of sync with your chronological age? Do you think your body is older or younger than your chronological years? Flexibility, strength, and energy are the keys to building a fit body. A fit body is one that is at least as young as, if not younger than, your chronological age. Here are some simple questions to help you determine your fitness level:

1. Most days, I feel _____ flexible.
   (a) very
   (b) somewhat
   (c) not very

2. Standing up, I can bend from the waist and touch _____.
   (a) the floor
   (b) my toes
   (c) my knees
   (d) I can hardly bend from the waist

3. Most days, I feel _____ energetic.
   (a) extremely
   (b) very
   (c) moderately
   (d) not very

4. Walking up a flight of stairs makes me feel _____.
   (a) energized
   (b) a little huffy and puffy, but I could make one more flight
   (c) exhausted

5. Most days, I feel _____ strong.
   (a) very
   (b) pretty
   (c) not very

6. I can carry a few bags of groceries into the house without feeling exhausted.
   Yes   No

7. I can rake the leaves in the yard without feeling like I need to sit down.
   Yes   No

8. I can play with my kids or grandkids without getting too tired.
   Yes   No

What is most important is that you have the energy and vitality to accomplish your daily tasks productively and with enthusiasm. If you can run 10 kilometers, that's wonderful. But what matters more is that you are getting the most out of your daily activities so they don't get the best of you.

People commonly give up on exercise for one or all of these reasons:

- They choose an exercise they don't like.
- They set unrealistic goals.
- They don't stick with it long enough to experience the benefits.

For many people, beginning to exercise is so difficult and quitting is so simple. If, however, you choose an exercise that you enjoy, one you can stick with and that produces visible benefits, you will not be discouraged and give up.

Of all the exercises and sports activities commonly practiced, brisk walking is the simplest and has the lowest drop-out rate. I advocate walking because it is so easy to do and so easy to stick with. Other activities may burn more calories faster, and may produce more muscle mass or lower body fat more quickly. But if it is difficult to stick with over time, its benefits will be limited. People start and stop exercise programs every day. Walking has the staying power to produce long-term health benefits, especially permanent weight loss!

Walking is the oldest form of exercise. Unlike other activities, such as running, swimming, skiing, and tennis, participation does not decline among people in their mid and later years. Almost everyone can walk. The only lessons you need in walking are those you received when you were a toddler. It doesn't cost an arm and a leg to participate, and the only gear you really need is a good pair of walking shoes. Walking is easy to do almost anytime and anywhere; you don't have to rely on a team, and even inclement weather doesn't have to stop you. You can walk alone or in a group like Greta's.

Because walking is so easy to do, it is much easier to stick with over time than other forms of exercise. Think about it this way: You are already walking; now it's just a matter of increasing the amount of time and the pace of your walk. It's easy to turn a stroll into a workout. Just pick up the pace and sustain it.

Unlike many kinds of exercise, there are virtually no health risks associated with walking. Walking does not strain your muscles or bones the way jogging and high-impact aerobics do. It's easy on your arms, legs, and back. In fact, it's so easy to do, you may be wondering, *how can it be a serious form of exercise*? Just because walking is easy does not mean it is ineffective. Walking briskly and regularly promotes all the health benefits associated with exercise, but without the injuries commonly suffered. Walking regularly strengthens the heart and lungs while improving the body's ability to consume oxygen, and it reduces blood pressure. By lowering blood pressure and burning excess calories through walking, you are taking preventive measures against heart attack and stroke.

If your goal is to lose weight, there is nothing to lose with walking except pounds. When you walk, you burn just about the same number of calories per mile as if you were jogging. Since walking is a weight-bearing activity, a person who weighs more will burn more calories than a lighter person walking the same distance at the same pace. The dropout rate for new joggers is much higher than the rate for brisk walkers, which makes it more effective for your health over the long haul.

The fact that walking is easy is the very reason why walking works. Walking completely satisfies the body's need for movement and energy. Walking is a simple but surprisingly effective way to lift us out of the sedentary lifestyle into which so many of us have settled. It's no wonder that, in 1996, the Surgeon General of the United States declared such sedentary habits the cause of a rising public epidemic. Most people know that physical activity will improve their health, but many still struggle against that truth or are not motivated to put it into action in their own lives. That is partly because the first steps seem so hard.

Actually, walking makes the first steps quite easy. Many of us have been misled to believe in the "no pain, no gain" slogan of the 1980s. Exercise does not, indeed *should not*, hurt your body. Even the most moderate physical activity will have a tremendous positive impact on those who have led a lifetime of inactivity. Walking just twenty to thirty minutes, at a steady clip, five times a week will reduce your risk of falling prey to obesity, heart disease, hypertension, breast cancer, colon cancer, osteoporosis, diabetes, and many other illnesses.

In her letter to me, Greta also indicated another health benefit of walking: Regular walking helped relieve the chronic pain associated with arthritis in her joints. I've heard from many readers who find that even after a few days of walking, the pain associated with all kinds of illnesses subsided. Walking has helped many of my own patients reduce the number of medications they depended on for years. My own mother has made a remarkable recovery from triple bypass heart surgery with the help of daily walks in the sunshine. Walking lifted her spirits and increased her energy while strengthening her body and attitude. Her doctors were amazed by her will to get well. She literally walked herself to wellness! Although they cautioned her that too much activity might sap her energy, she demonstrated to them how sensible walking was, and it made her energy soar!

The Surgeon General emphasizes the important health benefits of exercise in preventing risk of many major diseases. Just as important, however, are the benefits of walking for your mood and outlook. In fact, one way that walking benefits your health is by its capacity to reduce stress. Many people walk to lose weight but discover they're shedding stress as well as pounds. Remember that stress is the leading cause of illness. When you are stressed, your energy is out of balance, and that's when illness strikes.

One of my patients, Jerry, invited me to share his story with readers. Jerry is a business executive whose physiological age was much older than his chronological age of forty-five.

Dr. Taub,

A year ago, I dragged myself into your office overweight, stressed out, chain-smoking—literally hopeless. The best advice you gave me was to leave my car at home and start walking to work. Eager to rid myself of the stress of rush-hour traffic, I complied. You assured me it would be worth leaving an hour early in the morning. Doc, that change actually saved me time. It turned out that walking was faster than sitting in rush-hour traffic! But it saved me more than just time—it truly saved my life.

I was on a collision course with a heart attack; my blood pressure was already through the roof. As I began walking, everything fell into balance. I began to lose weight, not just because of the exercise, but because as I started to feel better about myself, I made smarter, healthier choices about what I ate, what I did. Even quitting smoking was much easier than I thought it would be. It was keeping me from enjoying my walks, so it naturally felt good to stop.

I smoked and overate because I was so stressed. The level of stress in my life did not change (except for eliminating the stress of rush hour), but my ability to deal with it changed. Walking proved to be incredibly effective for releasing stress. Even if I began my walk with a wrinkled brow, tight shoulders, and a scowl, after only a few blocks I couldn't resist feeling better. I began to appreciate my surroundings, the trees, people who smiled as they passed. I stopped worrying about the pile of work waiting for me on my desk, the phone calls that had to be made and the e-mail that needed a response. When I

*arrive at work, I can now tackle those things more productively, and
without all of the stress and anxiety. Walking truly did wonders!*

*Oh, and how can I forget? I lost twenty pounds. I have so much
more energy, strength and stamina. Little things that exhausted me
before are no big deal now. I am forty-five but feel physically better
and more optimistic than I did when I was twenty.*

Jerry's letter goes on to describe how he met the love of his life
on one of his morning walks to work! Walking helped eliminate the
stress in his life, and when that happened, a world of opportunities
was just a few steps away. Jerry gained a partner in walking, and in
life.

Why does walking help eliminate stress? Walking, like other exercise, triggers the release of substances known as endorphins.
These substances are what produce the "runner's high." The good
news is, you don't have to be a runner to experience the beneficial
rush of endorphins from the brain. When you walk, your brain releases endorphins that naturally flow to the parts of your body in
need of repair or rejuvenation. Endorphins are the brain's natural
healers that not only stimulate physical healing but mental outlook
as well. A walk in the sunshine (with sunscreen) is even better, because the light of the sun boosts the level of serotonin in the brain.
Nothing cures a sad heart or brooding mood like a walk outdoors
(except, perhaps, a walk outdoors with a companion!).

Endorphins soothe your stress and let your positive side shine
through. This is why walking has proven so beneficial to relationships at work and at home. Groups of co-workers who walk together at lunch or before or after work interact better with each
other during the day. Walking together positively influences the
way coworkers relate to each other. The same is true with couples.
My wife and I walk together daily and both feel our communication
with each other reaches exceptional clarity during and after our
walks. Walking, and the release of endorphins, makes us feel so
good about ourselves and each other.

Walking also soothes stress on another level. When you walk outside, in nature, you can see the issues and events that trigger your
stress anew. Spending time in nature reminds you that you are part
of something much bigger, that life has greater meaning than, you

are able to see while you work. When you feel connected with nature, you make choices that are more in tune with nature, including what you eat. New walkers always tell me that they feel better about their bodies, about themselves, and have a more positive mental outlook. Such feelings inspire your will to be well, and continue to be well in every aspect of your life.

Remember that you are only as well as you feel. In other words, your feelings and attitude have a profound effect on your health, energy, and weight. Physical and mental health are deeply intertwined. When your mental energy is out of balance, for example, because of negative feelings or stress, your physical energy will be shaken out of balance. Therefore, you need an exercise program that inspires total wellness, in body and mind.

The best workout for body and mind combines walking with stretching and strength training. Both walking and stretching generate greater energy and help restore energy balance. Combined, walking, stretching and strength training play a tremendous role in slowing down the process of entropy and reducing the negative effects of premature aging. While walking provides the weight-bearing activity so important to strengthening bones and muscles, stretching and weight lifting contributes to bone strength and density.

Stretching is a gentle form of resistance exercise for everyone, but weight lifting is especially important as you age. Instead of using free weights or barbells, however, stretching uses the weight of your own body. Regular stretching complements walking. The increased flexibility and relaxation that stretching provides protects you against straining muscles during walking. Furthermore, serious walkers sometimes become inflexible as the muscles in the back and legs become tighter and stronger. Stretching helps prevent stiffness and inflexibility, and keeps your stride long and smooth. So, ideally, it is preferable to do some stretching before you do your walking. I am personally an advocate of what I call "wellness yoga stretching." We will address that shortly.

Early in life, from the time you are an infant through about age thirty, your body builds its bones. Your bone mass is at its peak between ages twenty and thirty. Exercise is essential for children to achieve their optimal growth and to establish good bone health early on. Yet today, young people are more inactive than ever before. Inactivity among children already contributes to poor bone health in later life, putting them at risk for osteoporosis and other degenerative bone diseases.

As we progress through the cycle of life, our bone mass begins to diminish. By the time we are thirty or forty, bone mass loss begins to occur, sometimes at the rate of 1 percent each year. The rate of bone mass loss depends largely on how active we were as children, current physical activity, and calcium consumption. At this age, a minimum of thirty minutes of weight-bearing activity, such as walking, stretching, and strength training at least every other day is essential.

For women, loss of bone density speeds up during menopause. Some women eventually lose as much as 20 percent of their bone mass. The best steps to slow down bone mass loss are those you take with your own two feet. Plenty of brisk walking, combined with stretching and strength training, will slow down bone mass loss and strengthen your bones significantly. Arm yourself against osteoporosis: *Use your legs!*

At the age of sixty and beyond, both men and women continue to lose bone mass. At this age, it is especially important to combine walking, stretching and strength training. In addition to these bone strengthening exercises, men and women at this age should increase their intake of calcium and vitamin D. Exercise and supplements are your best tools for preventing the loss of height, or "dowager's hump," that results from bone mass loss. It is never too late to begin exercising. Even in the later stages of your lifecycle, exercise imparts major health benefits.

Now that you are wise to the exercise *whys*, and have a clear understanding of the benefits exercise imparts to body, mind, and spirit, your motivation to begin exercising is hopefully at a peak. You're ready to begin; you just need a sensible, enjoyable, and effective program to help you attain your health and weight goals. In the remainder of this part of the book, you will learn a simple but powerful combination of walking, stretching and strength training—my "Exercise Rx": a prescription for energy that will make entropy smooth sailing through *Total Health Rejuvenation*. So, before you lace up your walking shoes, read on!

As long as you have no serious health conditions that prevent you from walking, there are only a few basics to cover before you begin. (If you have any concerns, check with your primary care physician before you start.) First, when you walk or do any other form of exercise, keeping yourself hydrated with water is essential. Even if it's cold outside, as your body heats up inside, it requires water to move efficiently. Drink water before, during and after your walk. If you are walking outdoors in sunlight, be sure to wear a cap and/or protective sunscreen. If you are walking in cold weather, wear layers of clothing instead of a heavy coat so that you are warm but can remove layers and tie them around your waist as your body heats up. A warm wool cap will keep your head warm and protect you from the cold.

Your common sense may tell you to avoid walking outdoors in cold weather, but regular walking has been shown to actually help reduce the risk of catching the common cold. In my experience, people who walk at least twenty minutes a day, five days a week, have cold symptoms half as frequently as non-walkers. Walking also boosts immune cell activity and empowers the body to protect itself from bacteria and viruses.

Shoes that fit right are essential. If your shoes are too tight, your feet will ache. When purchasing walking shoes, remember that your feet are smaller at the beginning of the day and larger at the end of the day. Just as your car runs best when it has good tires, your body walks best when there are good, comfortable shoes on your feet.

Remember, it is preferable to do some stretching before you begin walking. When you set out on your walk, spend the first few minutes walking at a leisurely pace to warm up and loosen your muscles. After you've walked for a few minutes, stop at a curb or beside a tree to do a brief stretch. Use the tree for support and stretch one leg back and press your heel toward the ground, feeling the stretch in your calf. Stretch the other leg and then continue with your walk.

You learned everything you needed to know about walking when you were a child. A few reminders will help you get the most out of your walk and help minimize the risk of straining muscles. The basic things to remember are:

1. Begin with good posture. Walk with a straight spine. Lift your chest; relax your shoulders and pull them back slightly. Gently contract your abdominal muscles to support the muscles of your lower back. Keep your chin parallel to the ground and look straight ahead. If you stare at the ground as you walk, you may end up with a stiff neck.

2. Loosen up your arms and relax your shoulders. Let your arms swing loosely by your side at first. Shake out your hands and wrists, wiggle your fingers, and release any tension in your arms and hands. To increase the flow of energy, bend your arms at the elbow and let them pump at your side as you walk. Relax your hands in loose fists. Boost your heart rate and speed by swinging your arms, bent at the elbow, in an arc from waist to chest.

3. Relax your knees and keep them slightly flexed. If you walk with locked knees, you are more likely to develop soreness. Walk with short, fast, gliding steps, heel to toe. Let your heel naturally touch the ground first, then roll along your foot and lift off your toes. People who walk on their toes tend to experience shin splints, or pain in their lower front legs. Glide from heel to toe and avoid a choppy step.

4. Remember to breathe. As you walk with good posture, your chest and rib cage are open and expanding, allowing you to take full, deep breaths.

5. When walking and stretching, always wear comfortable clothing that is loose but not too baggy. Anything that restricts your movement limits the benefits of your workout.

6. Smile and have fun! Exercise is most beneficial when you are enjoying yourself.

Now, just when you think you're finally ready to start, you may find yourself up against the "walker's wall." The walker's wall refers to the million and one reasons your mind will erect to block your walk. Especially if you have been leading an inactive life for a while, your mind and body have settled comfortably into inertia and may resist attempts to break out and work out. Pay attention to the messages your mind is sending your body. Recognize your mind's resistance, and then determine that your will to be well is infinitely stronger than your mind's stubborn resolve to stay at rest. Maggie Spilner, the walking editor of *Prevention* Magazine's Healthy Ideas website (www.healthyideas.com), suggests the following exercise: Repeat a word or phrase that is meaningful to you and has the power to propel you out the door. Some examples she gives are: "I love how I feel when I'm walking"; "I am strong and healthy"; "walking works wonders." My favorite is, "I am walking to wellness." Such affirmations have the power to raise your energy and lift your spirits. The hardest part is getting out the door—once you are walking, the good feelings the activity generates take care of the rest.

Wellness Walking Week-by-Week

WEEK ONE

For the first week, walk at least four times. If you are new to fitness, begin with just three times a week. During the first week, walk as long and as briskly as you can while still feeling good about it. Try at least ten minutes each walk but just do whatever you can. No excuses! The aim this week is to gradually begin integrating exercise into your daily life. The key is to build walking into a habit, as integral to your day as brushing your teeth. If you start gradually, walking will become a highlight of your day, not a drag. Getting started may be hard at first, but as it becomes a habit, your exercise will seem as essential to you as the air you breathe.

It is especially important during this first week that walking be enjoyable. Remind yourself that each walk is a time out you are taking for your health and happiness. If you enjoy and value the time spent walking, you will stick with it.

WEEK TWO

Gradually increase the frequency and duration of your walks. Add five minutes to each walk you take, and be sure to take at least four walks this week. So, for Week Two, walk a minimum of fifteen minutes on four days, and spread the days out if you can.

As you walk, be aware of your posture and pace. If you find that your eyes are fixed on the sidewalk, lift your chin. Put a smile on your face and enjoy the scenery. Correct shrugged shoulders. Focus on walking heel to toe. How is your pace? Increase your speed by taking short, fast steps, rather than big, gaping steps.

WEEK THREE

You've been walking almost every day for two weeks. Congratulations! You should be feeling great, enjoying more energy throughout the day, and sleeping more soundly through the night. This week, increase your walking time to at least twenty minutes a day for at least four days.

If you find it hard to set aside twenty straight minutes each day, it is fine to occasionally split your walking time in half, walking ten minutes in the morning and the remaining ten in the afternoon or evening. Twenty consecutive minutes is optimal, because it takes about ten minutes to get your heart rate up to the point that you are a little huffy and puffy. Even if you don't have twenty consecutive minutes, however, ten minutes here and ten minutes there is much, much better than not walking at all.

And remember, the goal is to find ways of integrating physical activity into your daily life. As walking becomes a habit, you will find it increasingly easy to set aside your exercise time. In time, it will become the activity around which you schedule other things.

WEEK FOUR

You are steps away from a full month of regular walking. Congratulations on our resolve and dedication! By now you are probably finding that walking has become its own reward. You look and feel great, your skin glows, your attitude is improved, and stress affects you less and less. Even those who have never exercised until now have begun to experience the benefits of physical activity.

For this week, increase the duration of your walk by another five minutes and boost the frequency of your walks one more day. Your goal this week is to walk a minimum of twenty-five minutes on at least five days. In any case, just do the best that you can.

Have you hit the walker's wall? If excuses spring to mind before you set out on a walk, take a long, hard look at them. Is it a legitimate excuse? In other words, should it really stand between you and your walk? Unless you are truly sick or injured, overcome the excuse by repeating an affirmation such as, "I am walking to wellness." Repeat it over and over until your walking shoes are on, your laces are tied, and you are out the door, arms pumping, feet gliding, energy soaring!

If at any point the prescribed pace begins to feel uncomfortable and you are feeling exhausted, reduce the duration of your walk by five minutes. While you are establishing the exercise habit, the frequency of your walks is much more important than the length of time you walk. Frequency is also more important than pace. If you are getting huffy and puffy in the first five minutes of your walk, feeling breathless and unable to speak comfortably, you are walking too fast. Make your pace as brisk as feels comfortable given your current state of fitness. If you are moving so fast that you are uncomfortable, you will not enjoy your walk and will be missing out on one of the greatest benefits of exercise. Use the "talk test" to determine the right speed. If you are too huffy and puffy to be able to speak, you are walking too fast. Walking almost every day is essential, especially in the beginning. It's the habit of actually getting motivated, putting your walking shoes on and getting yourself out the door, that is most important to ingrain in your mind and body right now.

If at any point you are feeling more ambitious than the program prescribes, there are many enjoyable ways to increase the intensity of your walk. Find a path that includes hills. Slight grades will work muscles harder, burn calories faster, and get your heart pumping more vigorously. If you live near the beach, walk barefoot in the sand. Walking in sand adds a level of resistance that works your calf muscles especially well. At one time, fitness experts encouraged the use of small hand or ankle weights to increase workout intensity, but now most agree that even the lightest weights invite injury to the joints and muscles.

The most common reason people get waylaid on their walk to wellness is lack of time. I cannot count the number of times people have told me, "I'm too busy to exercise." In fact, I cannot count the number of times I've said this to myself! There are some creative ways around that particular walker's wall, as I know from firsthand experience. The exercise program can easily be integrated into even the busiest schedule with just a little bit of imagination and flexibility.

Remember Jerry's story, told earlier? Jerry found room for walking in his hectic life by leaving the car in the garage and trading tires for a pair of walking shoes with good treads. He walked thirty minutes to and from work each day. At first, when he was just starting out, he woke up an hour early to give himself enough time to walk to work. He was very out of shape and needed extra time to walk at a very moderate pace. Within two weeks, however, walking at a comfortable pace, the walk to work took only twenty minutes.

If you live too far from work to walk the entire way, continue to drive but park three or four blocks from your workplace. Alternately, spend half of your lunch hour walking. Just bring a pair of walking shoes to work with you. You will be amazed at how much energy you have after lunch, and how much more focused and productive you are in those afternoon hours.

There are other excellent ways to integrate a workout into your work day. Skip the elevator and take the stairs. Climbing stairs, like walking, is a weight-bearing activity that builds stronger muscles and bones. This is true of both walking up and down the stairs. This healthy habit will probably save you time as you no longer wait for the elevator to arrive.

Throughout the day, be aware of your posture. Both sitting and standing, your spine should be elongated, your chest open, and your shoulders relaxed. So many shoulder, neck, and backaches are the result of poor posture at work. Slouching in your chair puts tremendous pressure on your lower back, and hunching over your desk strains the muscles of the back, neck, and shoulders. Poor posture is usually a manifestation of stress. When stress makes you feel tired and sluggish, it shows in your shoulders. When stress makes you feel constrained and under pressure, your chest tends to collapse inward and literally does constrain your breathing capacity. Remember, you are learning to prevent stress and all of the manifestations of stress, especially overweight and illness.

Small corrections in your posture at work can help relieve tension and discomfort and help you have more productive workdays. My patients often tell me that as they became aware of correct posture, they felt less tense and pressured. By learning to sit straight and lift up out of your hips, elongating your spine, you will breathe deeper, feel taller and lighter, have more energy, and experience pain and discomfort much less frequently.

Simple Wellness Yoga Stretching Is Simply Essential

As I mentioned previously, walking is most beneficial when combined with simple stretching. The combination of walking and stretching has a powerful impact on your health, weight, and energy. Like walking, stretching is an activity suitable for all fitness types, no matter how flexible you are right now.

Before introducing you to nine easy wellness yoga stretches that you can easily and joyfully incorporate into your daily activities, it is important that you understand how stretching fits into the overall health and weight goals you are ready to achieve. The stretches included in this program are especially beneficial because they are based on yoga, an ancient art and science that has become so popular in the West because it balances body, mind, and spirit.

Let's stick with stress for a moment. Remember, stress is the trigger that sets off energy imbalance. Being overweight is one of the most common effects of energy imbalance. Stretching is an ideal strategy for relieving stress. Freeing yourself of harmful stress is the first and most important step to freeing yourself of excess weight.

♦

Physical and psychological health are deeply intertwined. Only an exercise program that works out your body and mind will be effective. Physical energy imbalance affects your mood and attitude. When your energy is low, self-esteem and body image tend to plummet. Similarly, when your self-esteem is waning and you feel bad about yourself, you tend to make less than optimal choices about what you eat and what you do. The health of the body and mind go hand in hand.

The regular practice of stretching helps strengthen and tone muscles, increases flexibility, and relaxes both body and mind. Stretching makes the joints more loose and supple, and it relaxes the large muscle groups in your legs and back. Slow, gentle stretching relieves stress in the body and in the mind, improving your mental focus and clarity, reducing worry and anxiety, strengthening your overall well-being. Remember: Mental well-being is necessary for a **well being**.

Stretching also incorporates methods of breathing that help increase the capacity of the lungs. Not only does this strengthen your respiratory system, but improving the flow of oxygen throughout your body also helps bring essential nutrients to the muscles. After stretching, most people experience a surge of energy and feel refreshed. That feeling results because stretching enhances the circulation of blood throughout your entire body.

For adults in the later stages of the cycle of life, wellness yoga stretching has another major benefit: The regular practice of stretching improves your balance and equilibrium. As we age and entropy speeds up, balance begins to decline. In 1997, the *Journal of the American Geriatrics Society* published a study showing that for adults over age sixty, poor balance contributed to a more than 50 percent increase in their risk of a fall-related injury.

Just as exercise strengthens bones and slows bone mass loss, regular physical activity can improve balance. Stretches that build balance are especially important for women forty and over, who experience the most rapid loss of balance. In her book, *Strong Women Stay Young*, Miriam Nelson writes that most women in this age group can hold their balance on one leg for less than fifteen seconds. Men, she says, because of their tendency to have more physical strength, don't begin to lose balance until about age fifty.

Remember that chronological age is usually different from physiological age. Very active older adults have greater balance than inactive younger people. The more physical activity you get, the more balance you will have.

Test your own balance now: Stand firmly on both feet, eyes focused straight ahead on a point that is not moving. Slowly shift your weight onto what you consider to be your strongest leg. Slowly lift your other foot off the floor. Count the number of seconds you remain balanced. Dr. James Rippe, a cardiologist at Tufts University School of Medicine in Boston, gives the following formula to assess your equilibrium: If you can stand on one leg for twenty-two seconds or more, you have the equilibrium of a twenty-year-old; fifteen seconds compares to a thirty-year-old; 7.2 seconds to a forty-year-old; 3.7 seconds to a fifty-year-old; and 2.5 seconds to a sixty-year-old.

No matter what age you are, you can develop the equilibrium of a twenty- or thirty-year-old. Exercises such as walking and stretching strengthen and tone the muscles in your legs and back which give you balance. Greater balance reduces your risk of falls and fall-related injuries.

Stretching has all the wonderful attributes of walking. It's enjoyable, you move at your own pace, and it encourages physical well-being as well as peace of mind. Like walking, stretching stimulates the flow of energy throughout your body. This energy is vital for weight loss. Many patients tell me that after struggling to lose weight for years, the breakthrough came, surprisingly, with stretching. Gentle stretching calms and balances your energy, and when energy is balanced, weight loss occurs naturally.

Like walking, stretching is meant to be enjoyed. Never strain, pull, or bounce while you stretch. Everybody, depending on their level of flexibility, has a different comfort zone. Whether your body is limber or stiff, all you have to do is find your point of comfort and stay there. Stretching is a challenging but noncompetitive activity. As long as you enjoy it, you will continue to practice it.

Let's cover some basics before introducing you to wellness yoga stretches.

1. Stretching will be easier and more comfortable if you do not eat a meal just before you begin. If you stretch in the morning,

a piece of fruit beforehand is fine. But consuming a large meal will make you sluggish, and much of the energy you generate will be diverted to the process of digestion.

2. Try to pick a regular time to stretch. If possible, stretch just before your wellness walk. Stretching at a regular time will help create the habit of stretching in your daily life.

3. Wear loose and comfortable clothing, but nothing too baggy that will interfere with your range of movement. Use an exercise mat or blanket if the floor is hard or cold. Preferably, stretch with bare feet or socks only.

4. Find a quiet place with fresh air to practice your stretching. If weather permits, outdoor stretching is ideal—you get the benefits of stretching, sunlight, and fresh air. Indoors is fine, as long as it is mostly free of distracting noises and smells. If possible, stretch near an open window.

5. Honor your body. The purpose of stretching is to relax. Many people have a tremendously difficult time succumbing to relaxation. The more you relax in your stretches, the greater the health benefits. Remember that the goal is to relieve stress in the body, so don't push yourself too hard. Be comfortable and enjoy.

6. Breathe. Many people tend to hold their breath during stretching, which adds tension and strain to the activity. As you stretch, breathe freely and smoothly. The point is to unwind, not get yourself all wound up. How can you decompress if you are holding in all of that stale air?

Breathing is so important to your health and energy. Because we breathe naturally, you may think a breathing practice is unnecessary. Most of us, however, do not breathe to our full capacity because stress and tension get in the way. Try this simple breathing exercise, which will help you breathe more fully and deeply:

Lie down on your back with your legs outstretched and your feet relaxed. Place your hands on each side of your rib cage. Now, inhale slowly and deeply, and feel your breath rise up through your abdomen, then your lower lungs, then your upper lungs and entire chest. Exhale slowly and feel your chest, ribs, and abdomen relax as the breath goes out. You can also do this while sitting up comfortably with good posture while gently relaxing your shoulders.

This may be the opposite of how you presently breathe. To get into the habit of breathing this way, place your hands on your abdomen and feel it expand when you inhale and constrict when you exhale. If it helps, you can also imagine your lungs and abdomen as a balloon that fills with air as you inhale and releases air as you exhale. Repeat this breathing practice three more times, each time following the breath as it expands up through the body as you inhale, relaxing the body as you exhale.

Practice this basic full breath during and between each stretch. Breathing deeply and slowly will help you relax into each stretching position. In between stretches, deep, full breathing will heighten your awareness of the wonderful feeling of energy flowing through your body.

This breath is also excellent to practice in situations or moments when you feel inundated by stress. No one even has to know you are doing anything out of the ordinary. Just focus on your breath, breathe deeply, and feel the breath rise and fall in your chest and torso. This breathing exercise will loosen up a tight chest, relax pinched shoulders, calm nerves, and cool body temperature.

Now you are ready to learn the wellness yoga stretches. Many may feel familiar to you. Just keep in mind that the goal here is to relax and restore your energy. Practice the stretches in the order described below, as the sequence takes the body through a deliberate range of motions and movements. This series of stretches will give your body a thorough and balanced workout. Like walking, stretching is easily adaptable to all body types and fitness levels. People at all ages and fitness levels can benefit from these stretches. To increase the intensity of a stretch, hold it longer. Each stretch can be modified for those with less flexibility. Listen to your own body's limits and keep the stretches comfortable. This entire cycle of wellness yoga stretches requires a minimum of fifteen minutes to complete. As your flexibility and strength improve, as well as your ability to relax, you will find yourself taking more time, holding stretches longer, relaxing more deeply. You can spend fifteen minutes or an hour with this cycle. Its up to you. But take at least the necessary fifteen minutes, at least five times a week, to get the full benefits of stretching.

Leg Stretches

As walking builds and strengthens your leg muscles, it is important to do stretching that keeps these muscles limber and loose. These stretches promote flexibility, which balances the strength-building effects of walking. Strong and flexible legs improve your balance and provide protection for your lower back.

1. Lie on your back and let the muscles of your back relax against the floor. Bend your knees so that both feet rest on the floor beneath your knees. Let your arms relax by your sides with palms upturned. Wiggle your fingers to relax them. Breathe deeply and relax.

2. Begin drawing your knees toward your chest. Wrap your arms around your knees and slowly hug your legs to your chest while taking full, deep breaths. Each time you exhale, allow your legs to relax further toward your chest. As you relax into this stretch, let your lower back raise slightly off the floor.

3. Continue breathing deeply and lower your left foot to the floor with your knee bent. Now gently stretch the right leg by raising your foot toward the sky. Use your hands to support your leg if necessary, and if your legs are stiff, keep the knee slightly bent. Hold this stretch for a while, remembering to breath deeply. Lower the leg and repeat with your left leg.

4. After stretching your right and left legs, bend your knees and pull both legs to your chest once more. Feel the stretch in the lower back while breathing and relaxing After several deep breaths, lower your feet to the floor and stretch out your legs fully. Let your legs and back relax.

The Cobra

With this position, you stretch the chest and strengthen the muscles of the lower back. The Cobra improves flexibility in your spine, which is essential for balance. It also unties the knots of tension that tend to build up in your back, allowing you to move more freely and comfortably in all your daily activities. The Cobra is excellent therapy if you suffer from low back pain.

1. Roll over on your belly, legs outstretched. Place the palms of your hands on the floor just beneath your shoulders. Keep your elbows tucked in close to your sides. Lift your head gently so your chin rests lightly on the floor. (For a gentler stretch, turn your fingers toward each other with your elbows turned out.)

2. While slowly inhaling, begin raising your chin and upper chest off the floor. Focus on using your back muscles, not your arms, to lift yourself. Your palms should be resting lightly against the floor, not pressing against it. Take a deep, full breath and, as you exhale, relax your shoulders and pull them away from your ears. Hold this stretch, while taking several breaths, only for as long as it is comfortable.

3. Gently lower your chest back to the floor. Turn your head and rest your cheek against the floor, and let your arms relax loosely at your sides. Continue breathing, nice and deep.

4. Return your palms to the floor beneath your shoulders. Lengthen your legs out behind you. Lift your head and rest your chin on the floor. This time, as you inhale, press your palms against the floor as if you are doing a push-up (unless you are doing the gentler stretch). Now tighten your buttocks, lift up your torso, and extend the arch in your back, keeping your stomach and hips on the floor. You should feel a gentle stretching of the muscles in your middle and lower back. Arch your back only as far as it is comfortable and without straining. Remember to take slow, deep breaths.

5. As you exhale, begin slowly lowering your body to the floor. Rest your cheek on the floor, breathe deeply, and relax your entire body.

The Cat

After the Cobra stretch, it is important to continue to fully stretch and relax your spine and back. The Cat stretch flexes and stretches your back all along the length of your spine, building greater flexibility and encouraging healthy alignment. This stretch is also especially good for people with tight or sore lower backs. If you wake up in the morning with a stiff back, this is a wonderful stretch to do first thing, even before stepping into the shower.

1. Kneel on the floor with your knees just under your hips and your hands lined up with your shoulders. If your knees are stiff or tender, place a folded blanket under them. Turn the palms so your fingertips point directly ahead. Straighten your spine and neck so that your eyes are directed at the floor beneath you.

2. Take a deep breath, and as you exhale, curl your back, just like a stretching cat. Tuck your chin to your chest to round your neck and upper back, and gently tuck your pelvis under your hips. Press your palms against the floor so your arms are straight but not locked at the elbows. Take several slow, deep breaths.

3. Now, while inhaling, slowly flatten your back, raise your chin to look straight ahead, and gently arch your spine to create a small dip in the middle back. Stretch the front of your neck without hyperextending it and allow your shoulders to pull away from your ears to create more length in your neck. Hold the stretch for several seconds while breathing deeply and feeling the stretch down the length of your spine. Keep your elbows straight and your head relaxed.

4. Take a full, deep breath and, as you exhale, slowly move into the rounded stretch again, curling your back toward the sky. Repeat the rounding and arching sequence three times slowly.

Seated Shoulder Stretch

Now that you have stretched your legs and spine, the shoulders and upper body need attention. Many people carry a good deal of tension in their shoulders and upper back. Tension in the upper spine can throw your whole back out of balance.

1. Sit comfortably on the floor with your legs crossed. First concentrate on good posture, lifting up out of your hips and elongating the spine. Rest your palms in your lap, fingers intertwined. Inhale deeply and raise your arms above your head, turning the palms towards the sky. As you slowly exhale, pull your shoulders down away from your ears.

2. Continue to breathe deeply and gently press your arms back behind your head, feeling the stretch down the inside of the arms and in the shoulders. While exhaling, slowly lower your arms and return your palms back to your lap.

3. Shake your arms out by your side, wiggling the fingers, shaking out the wrists. Rest your palms back in your lap and feel the energy in your shoulders.

4. Intertwine your fingers again. This time, as you inhale, stretch your arms out in front of you and lift your hands to chest level. Turn your palms away from you and press them outwards, and round your upper back gently, creating a stretch down the upper back and shoulders, down the length of your arms. To create a deeper stretch, pull your shoulders down away from your ears. Hold the stretch for several breaths, exhale, and release.

5. Shake your arms out by your side again, releasing any tension in your upper back and shoulders. Finally, wrap your arms around your shoulders as if you are giving yourself a hug. Sit up with good posture and gently tuck your chin into your chest. Pull your shoulders away from your ears and feel the stretch in your neck and shoulders. Take several deep breaths, then relax.

♦

The Rag Doll

A great way to relieve tension in the back is to let gravity do its magic. The Rag Doll works with the flow of gravity to stretch and relax your entire spine, neck, and shoulders. The stretch is also wonderful for flexibility in the legs. If you have a history of dizziness or high blood pressure, be cautious and hold this stretch only briefly.

1. Stand upright, feet together and firmly planted on the floor. Lift your chest, pull your shoulders down and back, tuck in your pelvis, and keep your knees fairly firm but relaxed bent about 2–4 inches. Your chin should be level with the floor, your eyes focused straight ahead. Let your arms dangle loosely by your sides.

2. Begin with a slow deep breath. As you exhale, tuck your chin gently into your chest and begin to slowly round your upper body from the waist, while curling your chest over your legs. Let your arms swing loosely in front of you, without tension.

3. As you breathe, bend over as far as is comfortable for you. If your legs are stiff or if you feel strain in your hamstrings or shins, bend your knees a little bit more. Continue breathing fully and deeply, relaxing further with each exhalation.

4. While inhaling, very slowly come back up to a standing and upright position. Make sure to keep your knees soft, while tucking in your pelvis and keeping your chin pressed toward your chest until you are standing upright in order to avoid dizziness.

5. Stand still and with good posture for a while. As you breathe, release any lingering tension or tightness in your back and legs.

The Warrior

This standing stretch strengthens the legs while improving flexibility in your back. While stretching the upper back, this stretch opens up your chest area, improving your breathing capacity. The Warrior also improves your balance.

1. Stand upright with good posture, feet firmly pressing against the floor. Bring your palms together at your chest, in a prayer position, and relax your shoulders. Inhale deeply, expanding your ribcage and filling your lungs with air. As you exhale, take a step forward with your left foot, creating between one and two feet of space between your feet. Keep your hips squared forward and your knees firm but not locked.

2. Continue breathing deeply and fully while bending your left knee until it is just over your ankle (not your toes). Bend your knee only to the point you are comfortable—do not strain your leg or knee. Stretch your right leg firmly behind you, heel pressing into the floor.

3. With palms together, lift your arms above your head and gently back, creating a slight arch in the upper back. Keep your eyes focused forward and hold the stretch for as long as it is comfortable for you.

4. Breath deeply again, and as you exhale, lower your hands back to your chest, step your right foot forward to your left, and slowly come to an upright, standing position. Breathe deeply and relax your arms to your sides.

5. Let the muscles in your legs and back relax. When you are ready, repeat the stretch with your right leg coming forward and your left leg stretched behind you.

The Half Moon

It is important during stretching to use your back's full range of motion to promote maximum flexibility. Arching and bending stretches need to be balanced with sideways bending stretches. The Half Moon stretches the sides of your back and promotes suppleness in the spine. This stretch is also wonderful for increasing circulation and strengthening your breath. Moreover, it tones the muscles of the waist and abdomen.

1. Stand upright with good posture, feet firmly together with your knees relaxed. Inhale deeply and raise your arms above your head until your palms meet lightly.

2. Exhale slowly and bend your upper body to the right. Bend from the waist and keep your hips squared straight ahead. Hold your head relaxed and centered in between your arms and be sure you are not hunching your shoulders to your ears.

3. Hold the stretch for as long as it is comfortable—hopefully for at least three complete breaths. Now inhale as you come back to the center, rising up onto your toes and stretching the soles of your feet with your arms reaching toward the sky. Exhale as you lower yourself back down onto your feet while relaxing your arms by your side. Relax.

4. Repeat the stretch again, this time bending to the left. Focus on your lower back, making sure it is not swaying and that it is gently tucked forward. As you hold the sideways stretch, roll your shoulders gently backward so that your rib cage expands.

Gentle Spinal Stretch

Having stretched the spine forward and back and side to side, now it is important to gently twist the spine. Twisting stretches restore suppleness to the disks between each vertebrae and help keep your spine in proper alignment. A limber spine is truly the backbone of health and fitness. If your spine is inflexible, it effects all of the muscles in your back and hips. Twisting stretches also stimulate energy in the digestive area and help promote healthy digestion.

1. Stretch out on your back on your floor. Stretch your legs out in front of you with your arms at your side. Inhale deeply and use your abdominal muscles to pull both knees up to your chest. Hug them gently there for a moment and then, keeping your legs bent and your knees together, lower your legs to the right side. Let your legs rest against the floor, or, if they don't reach the floor, rest them on a pillow beside you.

2. Outstretch your arms at shoulder height and flatten your upper back and shoulders against the floor. With your legs resting to the right, turn your head gently to the left to increase the twist. Continue breathing deeply and fully, relaxing more into the twist each time you exhale.

3. Take a deep breath and use your abdominal muscles to help draw your knees back to your chest. Now slowly lower your feet to the ground and stretch out your legs. Relax your arms by your side and consciously let go of any tension you are holding in your back or legs.

4. Repeat this stretch, twisting your legs to the left and gently turning your head to the right.

Relaxation Stretch

In stretching it is important to combine rigor with relaxation. The benefits of stretching are deepened and more fully felt when you take a few moments after stretching to consciously relax the entire body. As you relax, you can feel all the energy generated from your stretching coursing through every muscle of your body. This is also a wonderful time to reaffirm your commitment to wellness to yourself. Relaxed and refreshed, your body and mind are receptive to such positive input.

1. Lie on your back, legs stretched out before you. Let your legs and feet relax, toes pointing comfortably outward. Rest your arms easily by your sides, palms upward, fingers free of tension. Gently close your eyes so that you are not distracted by anything in your environment. If you are cold, cover yourself with a warm blanket.

2. If your back is sore in this position, modify the stretch by placing a chair in front of you and resting your lower legs on the seat of the chair. The chair will help support your lower back.

3. Lie still in this position, being aware of how your body feels. Find any tension lingering in the body and imagine that as you exhale, you release the tension. Breathe slowly and deeply, letting the slow smooth rhythm of your breath relax you further.

4. Remain in the Relaxation stretch for at least five minutes, giving your body a chance to experience all of the effects of stretching. Slowly open your eyes and come to a seated position, and feel how refreshed and energetic you are.

Summing Up Exercise

Whether you practice your walking, stretching and strength training together, or do them at separate times of the day, the combination of activities is a powerful prescription for health, energy, and weight loss. As you notice your progress, you will be motivated to continue and make exercise an essential part of your daily life, as natural as getting dressed in the morning.

To help make your progress visible, take the time each day to note a few things about your exercise and how you are feeling in the journal you are keeping about your eating patterns. These notes are important reminders to yourself of how much you are learning, growing, achieving, and gaining (or, in most cases, losing!). If you skip a day of exercise, write down how you feel then, too. Do you notice a change in your energy level? How about your sleep? Take note of all your changes. After a month of walking, or other exercise, stretching and strength training, turn back the pages and read your notes in those early days and weeks. See how far you have come!

If you are ill, physically disabled, or for any reason unable to walk, stretch or lift weights as much as I have suggested, then just do as much as you can. Just do it and please remember that there should be no excuses.

Before going on to Simple Strength Training (Part Nine of this revised book), I want to alert you to a new scientific report: a study of 72,000 nurses published in the August 26, 1999 issue of *The New England Journal of Medicine*, indicated that the women who walked briskly for just three hours a week reduced their risk of heart disease by more than a third!

Part Nine

SIMPLE STRENGTH
TRAINING

In 1999, since the first edition of *Balance Your Body, Balance Your Life* was published, the American College of Sports Medicine issued an official recommendation urging people over 50 to do strength training two to three days a week.

Now that I've reached 60 and I can feel and see the positive results of strength training, I sure wish I had started at 50. But like many people my age, I didn't because I thought it would be too tedious, complicated, and frankly not necessary for better health. I was wrong! Strength training is easy, enjoyable and beneficial—*especially because the results occur so simply.*

Moreover, strength training is the only type of exercise that substantially slows down and even reverses the loss of muscle, bone density and overall strength that used to be considered inevitable in the second half of our personal human life cycle. A study in the prestigious *New England Journal of Medicine* reported that in just 10 weeks of a strength training program, 50 frail men and women were able to increase their weight-lifting ability by more than 100 percent! *There's no way to stop time—but you can help to make entropy smooth sailing.*

Don't worry if you're not athletic. Don't worry if you have never done anything like this before. You should be comforted by the fact that this is an ideal form of exercise because it doesn't require athletic prowess—*just a willingness to concentrate on what you are doing and a commitment to stick with it.* Strength training reshapes your body, makes you feel younger, and helps you lose weight naturally and permanently. It's ideal for women, not only to help prevent and reverse osteoporosis, but also to help decrease symptoms of **PMS** and menopause. After strength training for just six months, women as well as men are extremely likely to stay with it forever!

The eight exercises featured in this chapter are perfect for beginners and non-beginners. Motivation is the biggest challenge until you establish a routine, so designate a specific time of the day—preferably before breakfast or before lunch.

You may wish to start your strength training at a gym or, if you can afford it, hire a personal trainer to help get you into a routine and keep you motivated. You may also decide to work out with a friend. But all you really need to get started, working out in the comfort and convenience of your own home, is three sets of weights!

Purchase Three Sets of Two Weights
SMALL FRAME: Fair Strength (most women)
3 pounds • 5 pounds • 8 pounds
LARGER FRAME: More Strength (most men)
5 pounds • 8 pounds • 10 pounds

The goal is to condition your major muscles by lifting weights heavy enough to achieve two to three sets of 10–15 repetitions before the muscles become fatigued. Two or three days a week for 20 to 30 minutes a session is ideal. Take a day or two off between strength training sessions to give your muscles a rest. *Just enjoy your increased energy!*

It's very important to do at least a few stretches to get limber before strength training, so try doing your wellness yoga stretches. Also, it's best to get your heart beating faster and work up a little bit of a sweat, so try some brisk "wellness walking" before starting.

Whether you are a beginner or not, you should start slowly and progress gradually. Women especially should choose lighter weights and go easy on themselves, rather than experience too much exertion.

- Start with what really feels like a light weight for you.
- Breathe properly by exhaling . . . *slowly* . . . while lifting weights, and inhaling while returning weights to the starting position.
- Do the exercise slowly, 15 times in a perfect form, by concentrating on the involved muscles.
- If it was no challenge at all, then move up to the next heavier weight for the next set.
- If it was too heavy for you to be comfortable, then move down to the lower weight.
- If it was challenging but something you were able to accomplish, then that is your weight!
- From now on, do three sets of 10–15 repetitions with this weight until it becomes way too easy. You may wish to purchase two heavier weight in a month or two.

STRENGTH TRAINING AT HOME

- Lunges—for your buttocks, thighs and legs
- One Arm Row—for your back
- Pectoral Fly—for your chest
- Lateral Raise—for your upper arms
- Upright Row—for your shoulders
- Biceps Concentration Curl—for front of your upper arms
- Triceps Extension—for back of your upper arms
- Abdominal Crunches—for your abdomen

Lunges: Stand up straight with your feet slightly apart and your abdominal muscles tightened. Take a large step forward with your right foot, while bending both of your knees. Keep your right foot flat while your left knee is pointing towards the floor. It's very important that the knee of your forward leg is over your foot, not in front of it. Pause for a moment and then push back with your right leg, raising yourself upright again. Do this 10–15 times and then repeat the exercise with your left leg in front of you. If you have difficulty balancing, you can always hold onto a chair by your side with one hand for support.

One Arm Row (Use medium weights.): Start with your right foot on the floor and your left knee on a bench or a chair seat. Keep your back parallel to the floor rather than hunching up, and let your right hand hang down while holding the weight. Tighten your abdominal muscles, bend your right elbow and pull your upper arm as far back as it will comfortably go. Keep your palm facing your body and don't swing your elbow out to the side. Pause and slowly lower the weight. Except for the arm raising the weight, keep the rest of your body still. After you do this 10–15 times with one arm, repeat with your other arm. Do two or three sets with each arm, pausing briefly between sets.

Pectoral Fly (Use medium weights.): Keep your feet flat and your hips and shoulders on the bench. Tighten your abdominal muscles and push your arms up until your elbows are almost straight with your palms facing each other. Pause and slowly lower your arms. Move your arms up and then back in a smooth arc as if you were wrapping and then unwrapping your arms around someone. Don't lower your arms much below the level of the bench. Make sure to visualize your pectoral muscles doing all the work. Do 10–15 repetitions of this exercise. Do two or three sets.

Lateral Raise (Use light or medium weights.): Start with your feet at hip-width apart, your knees slightly bent, your abdominal muscles tightened and both hands hanging down at your sides while holding the weights. Now straighten (but don't lock) your elbows and lift both arms simultaneously away from your sides until they reach shoulder level. Pause and slowly lower your arms back to your sides. Don't lean forward during this exercise and make sure to keep your palms turned downwards as your lift. Do 10–15 repetitions of this exercise. Do two or three sets.

Upright Row (Use light or medium weights.): Start with your feet hip-width apart, your knees slightly bent and your abdominal muscles tightened. Both hands should be holding the weights and let them hang down in front of your thighs with your palms facing in. Now slowly lift your arms up until the weights are slightly higher than your shoulders. Pause and slowly lower the weights back down. Don't lean back or forward as you lift and don't swing the weights around. Do 10–15 repetitions of this exercise. Do two or three sets.

Biceps Concentration Curl (Use medium to heavy weights.): Sit on a bench or a chair with your feet more than shoulder-width apart. Holding a weight in your right hand, lean forward and place your right elbow against the inside of your right knee. Tighten your abdominal muscles and slowly curl the weight toward your shoulder as if you were cracking a walnut between your elbow. Focus on squeezing your biceps at the top of the curl and lower the weight at the same speed that you lifted it. Do this exercise 10–15 times before switching sides. Do two or three sets with each arm.

Triceps Extension (Use medium weights.): Sit comfortably with your feet flat on the floor. Tighten your abdominal muscles. Push the weights up until your arms are straight and your palms are facing each other. Pause and slowly bend your elbows while keeping your upper arm straight. Lower the weights until you feel a stretch in your triceps (or the weights are close to touching your shoulders). Pause and straighten your elbows, keeping your upper arms still while slowly lifting the weights back up in an arc so you don't hit your head. Keep your elbows pointed up so they don't flare out to your sides during the movement. Do 10–15 repetitions of this exercise. Do two to three sets.

Abdominal Crunches: Keep your knees bent and feet flat on the floor. Imagine that you are pushing the small of your back into the floor. Place your hands behind your head with your elbows comfortably out to your sides. Use your hands only to keep your neck supported, not to lift it or push your chin up or forward. Tighten your abdominal muscles and raise your head, shoulders and upper back just a few inches off the floor. Come up about 30 degrees, hold for a moment while squeezing your abdominal muscles, and then slowly lower your shoulders all the way back down. Keep going until you do three sets of 10–15 crunches, pausing very briefly in between sets.

Part Ten

NUTRITIONAL SUPPLEMENTS . . . BEYOND DEFICIENCY

Descartes Was Wrong!

Scientific progress took a wrong turn during the seventeenth century, when philosopher Rene Descartes claimed that good science consisted only of those things that could be measured objectively. The impact of Descartes's pronouncement has been profound. Based on this paradigm, medical students are trained to see the body as a collection of cells and organs constantly in need of repair. From the paradigm of wellness, I view the body as an energy system always seeking balance and remembering wellness. The treatments I prescribe for patients assist their body's own efforts to restore balance and remember wellness. I prescribe treatments that assist the body's natural internal pharmacy—the healing force known as homeostasis. Homeostasis is the key to *Total Health Rejuvenation* and permanent weight loss.

Homeostasis baffles the traditional scientific paradigm because it is difficult to observe and measure. Keep in mind, however, that just because something cannot be measured or observed under a microscope does not disprove its existence.

Homeostasis is always at work in your body, even as youth eventually gives way to entropy. Constant changes encoded in your DNA began in your body from the moment your father's sperm united with your mother's egg. Every minute, hour, day, month, and season of your life has reflected this incredible journey. Even as you approach the last stage of your lifecycle, you'll be powered by the very same energy that first breathed life into you. When used properly, vitamins and minerals stimulate homeostasis and permanent weight loss. It may sometimes be difficult to measure such factors, but they do exist. *Descartes was wrong.*

Vitamins and minerals are some of nature's best catalysts for energy balance. Your body uses the chemicals in these substances to build, maintain, and repair your tissues and organs. Unfortunately, the medically recommended uses of vitamins and minerals established years ago no longer address our modern understanding of energy and total wellness.

There is an entirely new and evolving science of nutritional supplementation—much of it beyond the scope of this book—that addresses many everyday but significant problems: "Social drinkers" require more vitamins C, B_6, B_{12}, and zinc; smokers require extra vitamin C and folic acid; sexually active men need more zinc; people regularly using antacids need more thiamin and calcium; antibiotics may deplete the body of vitamin C, riboflavin, and zinc; cholesterol-lowering medicine may lower blood levels of vitamins A, B_{12}, D, K, and folic acid; even regular laxative use can deplete the body of vitamins A, C, D, E, and K.

Medical doctors have been trained to recommend supplemental vitamins and minerals only for infants, children, pregnant women, chronic alcoholics, and very ill adults. Additionally, physicians have been trained to diagnose and treat the diseases caused by vitamin deficiency, such as beriberi (thiamin deficiency), scurvy (vitamin C deficiency), and pellegra (vitamin B_6 deficiency). In the meantime, hundreds of studies have emerged documenting that nutritional supplements can help prevent congenital abnormalities of the spine, cataracts, heart disease, stroke, and cancer. *It's obviously gone way beyond deficiency!*

How many vitamins and minerals should you take? Which kinds? Why? How do you compensate for special circumstances? Here, I hope to make you aware of the importance of vitamins and minerals and to motivate you to take them every day. You rely on manuals for the proper operation of your car, computer, VCR, microwave oven, and much more. Why not refer to one for the most important pieces of equipment you'll ever operate—your body?

What follows is a road map for the sensible use of vitamins and minerals to keep your energy in balance. I believe the best way for me to guide you is to share what I personally take, and what I recommend to my family and patients. First, however, I'll tell you about vitamins and minerals.

The "Vital Amines"

The term *vitamins* originated in the beginning of the twentieth century, when medical scientists discovered that the body couldn't manufacture proteins from amino acids that were necessary to life without the presence of certain substances. These substances, which were found only in foods, were called "vital amines." Eventually the term was shortened to *vitamins*.

Vitamins are organic substances that nature supplies to support human life. They carry out their specific functions by supplying certain life-giving codes that regulate the metabolism within our cells. They are responsible for efficiently converting food into energy and are necessary for good vision, healthy blood, and strong bones and teeth. They ensure the proper functioning of the heart, the nervous system, and the reproductive system. These vital amines indeed contribute to our vitality!

Minerals are also essential to life and vitality. These are single-chemical elements found concentrated in all parts of the body. Some are present in abundance, like calcium and magnesium; others are found in mere traces, such as zinc and copper. Most are essential to life, and because our bodies are unable to manufacture them, we must obtain them through the foods or supplements we ingest.

Free Radicals and Antioxidants

Free radicals are highly reactive, unstable oxygen molecules. They possess an unpaired electron that causes them to search out more balanced molecules, snatch their electrons, and leave them unstable in return. This is the chemical process called *oxidation*. Oxidation is the scientific term for *rust*.

Every cell in the human body is constantly exposed to the oxidation process from free radicals normally generated by our daily metabolism and natural aging process. Problems only occur when there are too many of these renegade electron-thieves. You can't see them or feel them, but modern life tends to cause an explosion of free radicals because of inner influences such as stress, anxiety, and depression, and outside influences such as cigarette smoke, air pollution, pesticides, contaminants, and unhealthy food. In these times, it's estimated that each of our cells experience many thousands of free radical "hits" a day!

Antioxidants are chemicals that protect our bodies against the harmful effects of free radical damage. They inhibit free radicals and impede the damage they cause. Naturally occurring antioxidants help prevent or repair oxidative damage, but once the amount of rust we accumulate exceeds our body's ability to repair it, degeneration and disease occur—free radicals accelerate aging, weaken immunity, and cause cancer. Your body makes many of its own antioxidants to combat free radical damage, but it also depends on you to ingest sufficient amounts of antioxidants such as vitamin C, vitamin E, vitamin A, beta-carotene, and selenium.

Vitamin C: Cancer, Cataracts, and Colds

Vitamin C possesses a remarkable ability to reduce the havoc caused by free radicals. It plays a vital role in building healthy bones and teeth, promotes wound healing and tissue repair, and appears to be particularly effective in cleaning up some of the damage from cigarette smoke. Moreover, vitamin C helps to maintain a healthy heart by working in synergy with vitamin E and other antioxidants to prevent atherosclerotic plaque in the coronary arteries.

More than thirty scientific studies have demonstrated that vitamin C has a protective effect against cancer. People with low vitamin C intakes have significantly more cancer of the mouth, larynx, esophagus, breast, lung, stomach, colon, rectum, and cervix than people with higher vitamin C intakes. One large study of people ingesting more than 200 mg. per day showed a 60 percent decreased risk of salivary gland cancer.

There is also very strong evidence that vitamin C, along with vitamin E and beta-carotene, protects against cataracts. Vitamin C is normally sixty times more concentrated in the lens of the eyes than in the blood. It has been estimated that the number of cataract operations in the United States would decrease by at least 50 percent if people took adequate amounts of antioxidant vitamins. The Harvard Nurses' Study of over eighty-thousand women demonstrated an 83 percent decrease in the incidence of cataracts among those consuming at least 250 mg. of vitamin C for ten years as compared to those who were not taking supplements.

What about the common cold? The body's natural response, when it senses a cold coming on, is to crave foods rich in vitamin C, such as fresh orange juice. An entire book could be written on the controversy over whether vitamin C protects against the common cold, but that is not my purpose here. However, my strong belief, after practicing pediatrics and family medicine for over three decades, is simply: Yes, vitamin C protects against colds. I take 750 to 1,000 mg. vitamin C every day, and I usually double or even triple my daily vitamin C intake when I feel I am "coming down with something"—*and it helps*.

Vitamin E: The Miracle Antioxidant

Vitamin E is required for the formation of DNA and blood cells. It also prevents premature aging by reducing oxidation. Vitamin E is found naturally in green leafy vegetables, as well as nuts and vegetable oils. Strong evidence also suggests that vitamin E supplementation helps prevent heart disease, cataracts, strokes, and cancer. In a major study involving over four hundred colon cancer patients and a similar number of healthy individuals, it was found that the use of multivitamins containing 200 IU of vitamin E for ten years was associated with a 57 percent reduction in the risk of colon cancer. Finally, vitamin E also appears to improve immunity, especially in the elderly. In a study of over eleven thousand elderly people conducted by the National Institute on Aging, it was found that users of both vitamin E and vitamin C supplements had a 53 percent decreased risk of mortality from heart disease and a 42 percent decreased risk of mortality from all causes, compared to those who did not take supplements. No wonder vitamin E is called the miracle antioxidant!

The Harvard Nurses' Study demonstrates a 41 percent reduction in heart disease for women ingesting at least 200 IU of vitamin E for more than two years. The Cambridge Heart Antioxidant Study of men with heart disease showed that those who ingested 400 to 800 IU of vitamin E every day for eighteen months reduced their risk of heart attack by 75 percent compared to those men who didn't take a vitamin E supplement. Almost all studies show that people with high intakes of vitamin E, taken as a nutritional supplement, have lower risks of heart disease. Supplements are an extremely important means of increasing vitamin E consumption because most foods provide just small amounts of vitamin E. A cup of almonds contains about 20 IU of vitamin E; a cup of hazelnuts has about 30 IU. We would need to ingest more than four quarts of olive oil a day to provide 400 IU of vitamin E!

Beta-carotene and Vitamin A

Vitamin A and beta-carotene, called carotenoids, are required for healthy mucous membranes, skin, bones, and teeth. Beta-carotene is converted into vitamin A in the body. Carotenoids are also essential for general and night vision. Vitamin A deficiency is one of the five major malnutrition problems in the world, most commonly found in children who consequently develop infections, pneumonia, and diarrhea, and who tend to die prematurely. Deficiency in adults can cause general and night blindness, rough, scaly skin, and increased susceptibility to infections. Beta-carotene is found naturally in yellow and green vegetables and fruits: carrots, pumpkins, spinach, corn, turnips, apricots, cantaloupe, mangoes, papaya, and sweet potatoes. Vitamin A is found mostly in dairy products, eggs, and fish liver oil. These potent and effective antioxidants help our body to defend itself against free radical activity and, while doing so, help protect us against cataracts, stroke, heart disease, and many types of cancer.

Carotenoids are also essential for the prevention of age-related macular degeneration (AMD), which is the most common cause of visual impairment and legal blindness in the United States. AMD occurs in about 20 percent of the population above the age of sixty-five. No treatment is available for most people, and their ability to read, drive a car, or even recognize familiar faces may be lost. The effect on the quality of life is so severe that we should be doing everything we can to prevent this condition. Since our body does not synthesize carotenoids, we are dependent on food sources and nutritional supplements. For this reason, beta-carotene and vitamin A supplementation is highly recommended. While beta-carotene can be used in larger doses, the dose of vitamin A should be limited to 5,000 IU a day.

Selenium: Team Player and Cancer Knockout

Selenium is a mineral and a highly effective antioxidant found naturally in seafood, as well as in grains and seeds grown in soil containing selenium. A deficiency of selenium weakens the effect of some of the antioxidants that the body itself produces to counter free radical damage. Selenium actually helps protect other antioxidants, such as vitamin C, vitamin E, and beta-carotene, while working right alongside them to combat free radicals.

A stunning thing happened in scientific research on selenium recently. While studying the effects of selenium, researchers halted the study prematurely when they discovered the results were so important that they had to be announced to the public without delay. The research found a dramatic lowering of rates of cancer in people who were taking 200 mcg of selenium for up to ten years, compared to those who were not taking selenium. In the group taking selenium, rates of prostate cancer were 69 percent lower, rates of colorectal cancer were 64 percent lower, and there was a 30 percent lower incidence of lung cancer.

Calcium, Vitamin D, and Osteoporosis

Calcium and vitamin D work in remarkable synergy. The mineral calcium is necessary for healthy bone growth and essential for the heart and proper nerve and muscle function. We obtain vitamin D, which our body requires to absorb calcium, from our intestines, primarily from our being exposed to sunlight.

Increased intakes of calcium and vitamin D help to build healthy bones during childhood and adolescence and slow the bone loss that comes with aging and entropy. The combined effects of calcium and vitamin D are crucial for helping to prevent osteoporosis and the bone fractures associated with this condition. Research indicates that adequate calcium and vitamin D supplementation in premenopausal women can prevent the loss of more than 1 percent of bone mass per year. That can amount to a substantial decrease of bone loss by the onset of menopause. The right combination of calcium and vitamin D dramatically reduces the risk of nonvertebral fractures among men as well as women. The incidence of hip fractures can be reduced by as much as 50 percent.

In light of abundant new evidence linking calcium and vitamin D intakes to bone health, the prestigious Institute of Medicine recently increased its calcium and vitamin D recommendations for adults. The recommendations for vitamin D were doubled to 400 IU daily for people aged fifty-one to seventy and tripled to 800 IU daily for people over the age of seventy. It is now recommended that people over the age of fifty consume 1,200 mg. of calcium daily, compared to the previous recommendation of 800 mg. daily for this age group.

Most people don't ingest anywhere near these amounts of calcium. And while most people identify cow's milk and dairy products as sources of calcium, these foods, as we've learned, are not ideal. Green leafy vegetables, peas, beans, nuts, whole grain bread, and fish are much healthier sources of calcium. At the same time, most people do not get enough vitamin D because they are sunlight deprived. Although some vitamin D is present in oily fish (sardines, salmon), fortified cereals, and milk, our body depends primarily on sunlight to manufacture this vitamin. The destruction of the ozone, which necessitates avoiding direct sunlight, and all the daylight hours spent indoors, is an evolutionary surprise that our bodies are ill-equipped to handle.

Our skin contains a chemical that changes to vitamin D when exposed to the ultraviolet rays of sunlight. That's why our bone mass actually decreases during winter and spring and rises in summer and fall. Vitamin D supplementation is especially helpful to people who always wear sunscreen or sit in the shade while outside, because they don't synthesize adequate amounts of vitamin D. Finally, with age and entropy, the amount of vitamin D the stomach can absorb decreases while simultaneously people tend to be outdoors even less. Studies demonstrate that approximately 50 percent of Americans and Europeans over the age of sixty are vitamin D deficient.

Here's the bottom line: The key to preventing one of the worst problems occurring during the later stages of the human lifecycle is to *begin the process of prevention earlier*. Osteoporosis, characterized by a serious loss of bone material, predisposes us to softened, easily breakable bones. Osteoporosis is so common that about 50 percent of women over age fifty experience broken bones because of it, including fractured vertebrae. About 30 percent of men also experience broken bones from osteoporosis. Thus, it is crucial for you to know that the proper use of calcium, vitamin D, and magnesium supplements can potentially decrease the rate of osteoporotic fractures almost by half.

Magnesium: A Very Essential Mineral

Magnesium, found in green leafy vegetables, nuts, soybeans, whole grain cereals, bananas, and fish, helps ensure the strength of our bones and the proper functioning of our heart, muscles, and nerves. It is necessary for strengthening our immunity and is also a crucial catalyst for the body's entire energy production system. Diuretic medications used for high blood pressure may cause the body to lose magnesium through the urine. Diets that are deficient in magnesium may lead to osteoporosis, diabetes, kidney and heart disease, as well as cause feelings of low energy and a general lack of vitality. Several excellent clinical studies demonstrate that magnesium supplementation may be useful for the treatment and prevention of cardiac arrhythmia, asthma, chronic obstructive pulmonary disease, and migraine headaches.

The science of nutritional supplementation requires an understanding of the underlying nutrient interrelationships within the body. Proper *balance* is necessary. The balance between magnesium and calcium is especially crucial. Magnesium is instrumental in keeping calcium in solution within our bloodstream, as well as converting vitamin D into a form the body can utilize. Thus, calcium and vitamin D increase our daily magnesium requirements. Studies demonstrate a steady rise in the rate of cardiovascular disease in countries where people ingest small amounts of magnesium in relation to their amounts of calcium intake. As your calcium intake increases, your magnesium intake should also increase. The optimum calcium/magnesium ratio appears to be between 2 and 2½ to 1. Thus, a 1,000 mg. calcium supplement should be balanced with 400 to 500 mg. of magnesium.

Iron: A Double-Edged Sword

The mineral iron plays an essential role in building healthy blood, enhancing our immunity, and supporting the complicated metabolism of virtually all our cells. Besides red meat, excellent food sources for iron include green leafy vegetables (such as spinach), peas, nuts, soybeans, and whole grain cereals. Well-balanced, mostly vegetarian diets are perfectly compatible with adequate iron intake. Moreover, it is important to be aware of the fact that milk and dairy products may seriously interfere with the ability of our intestines to absorb iron from foods.

Iron deficiency is a prevalent nutritional condition in the United States in women of child-bearing age. Recent national surveys indicate that about 10 percent of adolescent girls and menstruating women in the United States are iron deficient. This translates to about 10 million adolescent girls and women of child-bearing age who would benefit from more green vegetables as well as iron supplementation! On the other hand, too much iron in the body may increase the risk of liver and heart disease and cancer. Thus, men and postmenopausal women should generally avoid nutritional supplements containing iron.

Zinc: Just a Little Bit Does a Lot

Zinc is an indispensable mineral. It is required for the synthesis of DNA, protein, and insulin, and it is vital for the proper functioning of our eyes, liver, kidneys, muscles, and testicles. Yet only 2 to 3 grams of zinc are present in the entire body, where it concentrates mostly in the bones, eyes, and prostate gland. Zinc deficiency leads to infertility, impaired immunity, abnormal night vision, and delayed healing of wounds. Men require more zinc than women.

It is important also to be aware that an excess of zinc may lead to serious problems, including nausea, vomiting, diarrhea, lethargy, and fatigue. It may also lead to a deficiency of copper in the body. Thus, it's important to be careful about the amount of zinc contained in nutritional supplements. Besides red meat, zinc is found naturally in nuts (Brazil nuts, cashews, pecans, and peanuts), whole grains, sesame seeds, black-eyed peas, garbanzo beans, poultry, and seafood. Oysters contain an incredibly high amount of zinc.

As a result of a study at the prestigious Cleveland Clinic, zinc has been enjoying wide popularity in the form of a throat lozenge to lessen the severity and shorten the duration of colds. Unfortunately, the study was conducted with an unusually small amount of people, the beneficial results were not very dramatic, and other researchers have not been able to consistently replicate the findings. So, in my opinion, it's doubtful—for now. It reminds me of the old adage I tell my patients: *I can treat your cold with medicine and it will go away in a week—or we can do nothing and it will take seven days.*

Vitamin B₁₂: The Great Masquerade

Vitamin B_{12} is necessary for our body to release energy from the food we eat. It is required for cell growth, healthy blood, a well-functioning nervous system, and reproduction. Remarkable as it seems, about 50 percent of people over the age of sixty in North America and Europe may be deficient in vitamin B_{12}. We used to think the major reason was that older people lose the ability to secrete gastric acid in their stomachs. Now we know that is not so.

Vitamin B_{12} deficiency causes damage to the sheath that surrounds nerves so that electrical impulses cannot travel along them. When the nerve sheath falls into disrepair, it can cause mental confusion, memory loss, dementia, and various psychiatric problems. Older people with significant memory loss should have their vitamin B_{12} blood levels checked. Vitamin B_{12} deficiency can also cause neurological deficits that lead to a lack of balance, a stumbling walk, and numbness in the body and limbs. In general, vitamin B_{12} deficiency can result in severe, health-destroying pernicious anemia.

The signs and symptoms of vitamin B_{12} deficiency are seldom correctly diagnosed because they mimic the findings of so many other mental and physical illnesses. To further complicate the diagnosis of vitamin B_{12} deficiency, the common blood tests that medical doctors perform to establish this diagnosis are usually not helpful. (The proper test to perform is a specific serum B_{12} level or a test of a certain B_{12} derivative.)

It's important to know that folic acid supplementation, now common in breads and cereals, tends to mask the symptoms of pernicious anemia. Consequently, the National Academy of Sciences has recommended that people over the age of fifty should be taking vitamin B_{12} supplements—orally! American and Western European physicians traditionally have been taught that B_{12} could only be given by injection. Now it is common knowledge that, in appropriate dosages, *oral B_{12} works just fine*.

Vitamin B_{12} is truly an all-purpose vitamin, and it requires only a microscopic amount to do the job. I strongly urge all adolescents and adults to take this remarkable substance as a nutritional supplement each day.

Preventing Congenital Birth Defects and Living Healthfully with Folic Acid

The human body requires folic acid to regulate cell division and maintain a healthy immune system. Folic acid is a B vitamin found in green leafy vegetables, nuts, peas, and beans. One of the most surprising breakthroughs in nutritional science in the last fifty years has been the discovery that folic acid supplementation helps prevent several types of serious birth defects. Women who ingest nutritional supplements containing 400 mcg. of folic acid within one to three months of becoming pregnant and during the first trimester of their pregnancy will dramatically lower their risk of having babies with neural tube birth defects such as spina bifida (an opening in the spine, which leads to paralysis or a severe handicap) or anencephaly (partial or complete absence of the brain). The degree of protection against these catastrophic defects is remarkable—up to an 80 percent reduction!

The neural tube of the fetus is the earliest phase of the spinal cord and brain. It develops within the first month of pregnancy, when many women are not even aware they are pregnant. The scientific evidence is strong—all women who are capable of becoming pregnant should consume 400 mcg. of folic acid throughout their child-bearing years to reduce the risk of having a baby with spina bifida or anencephaly.

It's important to note that in all the scientific studies, the risk reduction has been seen when a supplement of 400 mcg. of folic acid was consumed *in addition to* the usual diet. Thus, the effective level of folic acid is not a total of 400 mcg. but *an increase of 400 mcg.* over the amount of folic acid consumed naturally.

There is also evidence that women who take folic acid as part of a comprehensive multivitamin formula help protect their infants against other birth defects, including cleft lip, cleft palate, urinary tract defects and defects, involving the arms and legs. Additionally, it has been demonstrated that women ingesting multivitamins with minerals during pregnancy are less likely to deliver premature or low birth weight infants.

Important new scientific data indicates that multivitamins containing folic acid may not only protect against birth defects, but may also substantially reduce your risk of cancer, heart disease and stroke. This groundbreaking information is discussed in the following pages.

Understanding Homocysteine

It is important that you read this again, even though we've touched upon it in Part Four. You have the opportunity to launch a preemptive strike against a major enemy: atherosclerosis. Atherosclerosis refers to the buildup of fatty deposits in your blood vessels that could trigger heart attacks and strokes. The current scientific understanding of atherosclerosis is based upon the very simplistic notion that the cholesterol we ingest is somehow deposited on the walls of our heart and brain arteries, eventually causing an obstruction and subsequent heart attack or stroke. I do not believe this simple explanation. It is much more likely that injury to the inner linings of our blood vessels allows the fatty deposits to build up that then lead to heart attacks and strokes. The health of our heart and brain vessels has to be compromised before plaque builds up and obstructs them.

But there is something much larger to consider: The human body isn't so poorly constructed that it would just deposit excess fat on the inner linings of the very blood vessels that support life by nourishing its brain and heart. Indeed, mounting scientific evidence supports the notion that the fatal buildup of atherosclerosis occurs *after* the inner linings of our arteries have become thickened and damaged. Moreover, I believe that the deposition of fatty material upon these injured cells represents our body's ill-fated attempt to protect the injury and halt the damage—an inadequate Band-Aid for the ravages of civilization.

Stress, hypertension, smoking, and elevated homocysteine, a toxic amino acid, appear to be the major causes of injury to the inner linings of our blood vessels. Recent findings indicate that stress and stress-related high blood pressure promote injury to the endothelium of the arteries feeding blood to our brain and heart. It has been demonstrated that "type A" individuals who have blood pressure rises in response to mental stress also have the most atherosclerosis and thickening of the inner lining of their carotid arteries.

Homocysteine has a direct toxic effect on the inner lining of human blood vessels. It appears to cause coronary artery disease and strokes by injuring the lining of the arteries *regardless* of the level of cholesterol in the blood. Actually, the *majority* of people with significant coronary artery disease have been found to have normal cholesterol levels.

Widespread interest in the United States regarding homocysteine began with the 1992 publication of a Harvard study of nearly fourteen thousand male physicians. A striking three-fold increase in the rate of heart attack was found in the men with elevated homocysteine levels. More recently, the 1998 publication of the Harvard study of female nurses found that those consuming 400 mcg. of folic acid and 3 mg. of vitamin B_6 a day lowered their incidence of coronary artery disease and heart attack almost by half!

Homocysteine seems to interfere with the ways that endothelial cells use oxygen and results in an excess of damaging free radicals in the lining of the arteries. It also promotes deposition of collagen between the cells, which causes a thickening and hardening of the arterial walls. Additionally, it seems to increase the potential for platelets to aggregate together, which can lead to clot formation.

What causes homocysteine levels to build up? The most important factor causing elevated blood homocysteine levels appears to be the inadequate intake of B vitamins, including folic acid, B_6, and B_{12}, which are required to break down homocysteine in the body.

It is important to be aware of the fact that homocysteine is mostly a by-product of the body's metabolism of red meat, cheese, and other dairy products. Other factors proven to increase homocysteine are cigarette smoking, lack of exercise, and coffee consumption. Extensive research carried out in Holland indicates that merely the combination of smoking, coffee consumption, and low folic acid intake can increase the rate of cardiovascular disease by 40 percent!

Age and hormones also matter. Premenopausal women have homocysteine levels about 20 percent lower than men of the same age. After menopause, the levels approach that of men of the same age. Homocysteine levels then continue to increase with age in both sexes. Moreover, deficiency of the thyroid hormone also causes a rise in homocysteine levels.

How can you best prevent the buildup of homocysteine in your blood? Take a daily nutritional supplement with 400 mcg. of folic acid. I also recommend a *minimum* of 6 mg. a day of B_6 for all adults, a *minimum* of 40 mcg. a day of B_{12} for adults under the age of fifty, and a *minimum* of 400 mcg. a day of B_{12} for those over fifty years old.

Also, as you read earlier in this book, regular exercise is extremely important. Of course, quitting smoking is crucial. It makes sense to limit coffee to no more than two cups a day. Finally, limiting your red meat and dairy intake should have a significant impact on keeping your homocysteine level within a normal range.

European scientists have never been as convinced about the importance of dietary cholesterol in heart disease and stroke as American scientists. Now there is ample evidence that first our most important blood vessels are injured, and then our body responds by coating the injury with fat. *Isn't that enough reason to take your vitamins and minerals every single day?*

Recipe for Wellness

Many studies show the wonderful benefits of vitamins and minerals for the efficient functioning of our bodies throughout our human lifecycle. One consistent finding stands out in all the research: Taking a daily comprehensive nutritional supplement, proper daily exercise, and eating foods that are filled with life-energy are the keys to maintaining optimal health and wellness.

The following formula is what I take every day and recommend to my family and patients, both adolescents and adults:

- **vitamin A (as beta-carotene)**   **10,000 IU**
- **vitamin B$_1$**   **20 mg.**
- **vitamin B$_2$**   **20 mg.**
- **vitamin B$_6$**   **20 mg.**
- **vitamin B$_{12}$**   **100–1,000 mcg.** *(increase with age)*
- **niacin**   **20 mg.**
- **biotin**   **30 mg.**
- **pantothenic acid**   **30 mg.**
- **folic acid**   **400 mcg.**
- **vitamin C**   **750 mg.**
- **vitamin D**   **400–600 IU** *(increase with age)*
- **vitamin E**   **400 IU**
- **vitamin K**   **25–80 mcg.**
- **calcium**   **500–1,200 mg.** *(men/women, increase with age)*
- **selenium**   **200 mcg.**
- **magnesium**   **250–500 mg.** *(men/women)*
- **iron**   **18 mg.** *(only menstruating women)*

- copper   2 mg.
- zinc   15–40 mg. *(women/men)*
- manganese   5 mg.
- chromium   100 mcg.
- molybdenum   75 mcg.
- iodine   75 mcg.
- boron   3 mg.

A Vitamin and Mineral Update

Since the first edition of this book was published, there has been a major explosion of new scientific data that validates the information as well as the underlying concept in Part Ten: *A scientifically-based formula of vitamins and minerals can help your body prevent cataracts, osteoporosis, heart disease, stroke, and cancer!*

So it is now more important than ever for you to keep in mind that your body doesn't manufacture vitamins and minerals (except for tiny amounts such as vitamin B-12). Therefore, the only way for you to get the vitamins and minerals your body requires is through the food you ingest, nutritional supplements, and sunshine (vitamin D). However, even if you eat properly, it is *highly unlikely* that you will get the amounts of vitamins and minerals that your body requires to maintain it's energy balance—*The key to total health rejuvenation and permanent weight loss.*

Data in an important Finnish study recently published in the *Journal of the National Cancer Institute* strongly suggests that vitamin E supplementation greatly reduced the risk of prostate cancer: Finnish men taking vitamin E supplements demonstrated a 36 percent lower incidence of prostate cancer than men who took a placebo!

Moreover, data in a study of women nurses recently published in the *Annals of Internal Medicine* has provided the strongest evidence yet that folic acid might help prevent colon cancer—our nation's second largest cancer killer. *Only lung cancer kills more Americans.* The study of more than 80,000 nurses being followed by researchers from Harvard Medical School suggests that the women who took multivitamins containing folic acid for at least 15 years had a 75 percent decrease in their risk of colon cancer!

Dr. Edward Giovannucci, the head researcher, commented that, although only women were studied, other research suggests that folic acid has similar effects in men. He also pointed out that supplements aren't a panacea. Exercise and a diet rich with fruits and vegetables remain essential to colon cancer prevention. *I wholeheartedly agree!*

It is also noteworthy that the decrease in colon cancer was considerably less in women who were taking multivitamins for only a short time. This supports a previous finding in the same nurses' study showing an 83 percent decrease in cataracts among the women who were taking Vitamin C supplements for *over ten years.* So it's important for you to realize that there are no "quick fixes." In other words, it's crucial to take a comprehensive formula that contains sensible amounts of high quality ingredients in the proper balance, over an extended period of time, to build up your immunity to disease. *This plea for your good health cannot be overemphasized.*

Part Eleven

PREVENTIVE
THEOLOGY

"BEHIND EVERY BLADE OF GRASS IS ITS VERY OWN
ANGEL THAT FOREVER WHISPERS . . . 'GROW, GROW' "
(The Talmud)

I believe there is only one religion: *the religion of love.*
The point was made clearer to me this morning when my wife Anneli, who is Christian, came into my office wearing a Jewish "Star
of David" around her neck. I thought to myself, *"What an honor for
Judaism!"* It clarified what Dr. Robert H. Schuller, minister of the
Crystal Cathedral, meant when he said to me during an interview
on his "Hour Of Power" television show: "Dr. Taub, like Jesus, you
are a Jew, and I believe you and He are on the same wavelength."
Afterwards, he took me aside and said, beaming, "You are developing 'Preventive Theology' . . . *what an honor for Christianity!"*
   Preventive Theology constitutes the beginning of what I hope will
be a true "Healing Testament" for this new millennium. It's for
everyone seeking health and well-being as well as permanent
weight loss. It's generally based on the principles of Judaism and
Christianity because both faiths would be so much better served by
living with each other's wisdom. Christians might well consider the

special covenant between the Jews and God, which after more than 5000 years remains very much alive and is still mentioned daily in prayers throughout the world! Jewish contributions in science, medicine, philosophy, psychology, literature, music, and charity have been enormous as a result of this special covenant, which requires Jews to live ethical lives, be charitable, seek justice, and walk humbly before God. On the other hand, Jewish people might well consider the magnificence of the Sermon on the Mount preached by Jesus. It is the essence of Christianity, yet the beauty and wisdom radiating from it can inspire all of us to seek new vistas of personal health and healing.

In the Twenty-Third Psalm, perhaps the most beloved part of the Jewish Torah (first five books of the Old Testament), King David shares an epiphany: God is *accessible* to us:

> "The Lord is my shepherd: I shall not want.
> He makes me lie down in green pastures.
> He leads me beside the still waters. He restores my soul.
> He guides me in straight paths for His name's sake.
> Yea, though I walk through the valley of the shadow of death,
> I will fear no evil, for *Thou art with me* . . .

To this, the New Testament adds the essence of the greatest story that has ever been told: *Love one another.* The Bible is indeed a *good* book!

Now that I have become a physician with Jewish roots and Christian wings (and a Buddhist and Hindu outlook), I can see that healing miracles are occurring every moment! No wonder Saint Augustine wrote 1,700 years ago: *"Miracles never contradict nature. Miracles only contradict what we know about nature."* And no wonder, more recently, the French scientist and Christian theologian Teilhard De Chardin was inspired to write:

> "Some day, after we have mastered the winds, the waves, the tides and gravity, we shall harness the energies of love. Then for the second time in the history of the world, Man will have discovered fire."

I believe I learned everything I needed to know about God before I went to kindergarten. I recall asking my mother, as she was giving me a bath one evening when I was about three years old, "Where is

God?" I vividly remember her reply: "God is everywhere." I also remember asking: "Do you mean God is right here?" and her reply: "*Sure . . .* just put your toes up against the water where it's running into the bathtub and feel how good it feels . . . *God is in that water.*" I still recall how delighted I was with this *terrific* bit of information—*as well as how wonderful my toes felt just wriggling around in that water!* Then I remember asking my mother, "Is it ever possible to see God?" "Absolutely," she said, "You can see God wherever you see love, because God is love."

By the time I did get to kindergarten, I knew I wanted to be either a fireman, a policeman, or a doctor, so I could help take care of people. I felt God would appreciate that, since after all, as my mother had said, God was love. Then, while preparing for my Bar Mitzvah at 13 years-old, I began feeling that God would also appreciate my being a good Jew . . . especially the way that Rabbi Maimodenes, a major theologian as well as the greatest Jewish physician of all time, described being Jewish. Referring to Micah in the Old Testament, he said: "To be a good Jew is to do charity, seek justice, love goodness and walk humbly before God." Then the great rabbi and physician went on to say: "Everything else is mere commentary." *That sparked my decision to go to medical school.*

I also went to medical school because I felt driven to serve as an educator and a healer. I wanted to help keep my patients well in the first place and, if they became ill, to help get them well as quickly as possible. It was 1960, when iron lungs for polio victims were fortunately being wheeled into storage and penicillin was rapidly evolving into a whole new group of antibiotics. We students, as well as our teachers, were enthralled with developing more vaccines and more antibiotics for preventing and treating disease. Indeed, we anticipated making special "magic bullets" for every major illness. Who could have imagined then that the major epidemic we'd have to confront in the new millennium would be obesity and its related diseases? Being overweight certainly causes more illness and death than smallpox or polio ever did! Thus, while we were searching for magic bullets, modern physicians steadily lost sight of the importance of stimulating in our patients an abiding will to be well.

I am reminded of Sandra, a young woman who was diagnosed with cancer at the age of 27. She described her initial experiences with doctors at a teaching hospital in New York City as being "poked, stabbed and poisoned . . . *and they just referred to me as 'the neck mass.'* " "The treatment was so horrible and I felt so unloved by the doctors that I wanted to die," she said. After a relapse one year later, she moved to California where she found a new group of doctors, and a new attitude. She told me she knew she was going to be OK when her oncologist said to her, "Medical science can only do so much. *You have to help, too.* I want you to beat this cancer. You have to want to beat it, too." He prescribed surgery and radiation therapy along with good nutrition, less stress, happiness and prayer. *Sandra has been healthy ever since.*

By now you know what is in my heart. So I will share something I have discovered after 35 years of being a physician, without softening it or pulling any punches: *It's absolutely ridiculous for physicians to ignore the fact that their patients' spiritual outlook and behavior can profoundly affect their capacity for health and healing!* People who love God and who live ethical lives are happier, less fearful, and far less likely to become sick from stress. And when they are ill, they also get better more quickly. Finally, people who believe in a completely loving supreme being are able to conquer their addictions more successfully—*including urges to eat and cravings for junk food.*

As a matter of fact, miracles of healing occur thousands of times everyday in America. We physicians call this phenomenon an *"idiopathic spontaneous remission,"* which means that we haven't got the slightest idea what happened! But I have asked hundreds of patients with idiopathic spontaneous remissions, especially involving serious diseases (lupus erythematosis, periarteritis nodosa, rheumatoid arthritis, leukemia, cancer), to tell me what happened. Virtually every patient says the same thing, *"I just prayed and put myself totally in God's hands."*

> *LOVE THE LORD THY GOD WITH ALL THY HEART, AND*
> *WITH ALL THY SOUL, AND WITH ALL THY MIND"*
> (The New Testament)

Preventive Theology entails loving God with a totally trusting heart, which requires us to be loving, kind, charitable and ethical human beings . . . *for Jews, this means listening to Jehovah; for Christians, it means following the teachings of Jesus. For Jews and Christians alike . . . it means following the Ten Commandments.*

Preventive Theology is also based on the notion that your health is primarily determined by our own personal responsibility, self-value and reverence for life. This means it is necessary to do whatever *you* can do to help make your body a healthier environment for your soul to flourish in. You see, Preventive Theology is a verb as well as a noun; its goal is to make you feel completely *worthy* of saying *"I Love You God."*

When you begin naturally changing the silent refrain in the meditation introduced in Part One of this book from *"I Have Strength"* and *"God loves me,"* to *"I Love You God,"* with a sense of total surrender, then you will truly know in your heart how much you can really determine your own health destiny . . . *and by doing so, you release God's Healing Force in you.*

You see, God *already* loves you, since God is love. What it all boils down to is that *you* need to feel completely worthy to love God. There is no question about it, your spiritual outlook and behavior is a very significant factor in determining whether you will stay healthy or become ill, and certainly whether you'll lose weight permanently. Furthermore, most people are seriously questioning the deeper purpose of their existence. A *USA Today* article during 1999 reported that when Americans were polled about what they would ask God if they were allowed just one question, the majority answered, *"What is my purpose here on earth."* So please, would you, *just for a moment*, imagine God's presence everywhere and in every living thing? Would you also, *just for a moment*, imagine that all life emanates from God's heart? *Good*, now please take some time to reflect upon your purpose in life.

All human beings are on a spiritual pilgrimage back to the source of infinite energy—*God's heart.* Our purpose is to love one another, and strive always towards goodness. Human beings are most reminded of their purpose when they are extolling the divinity of life through charity, meditation, prayer, and ingesting life-energy food from the top steps of the Food Energy Ladder in Part Six of this book.

Your spiritual pilgrimage back to the heart of God can be a glorious experience if you assist nature by nourishing your mind while also supporting your body with regular exercise and good food. Or you can subject yourself to the effects of stress by lacking love in your heart and neglecting your body. Remember, I.L.L. is often equivalent to *I Lack Love*. To love one another while striving always towards goodness . . . this is the ultimate spiritual effect. *Can you imagine how wonderful the world would be if each person lived by this ideal?* Ethics and integrity emanate from the whispers of your heart—the voice of truth propelling you toward goodness. When you listen to the whispers through meditation and prayer, you are making a major spiritual effort. We truly reap what we sow and our life is a consequence of our actions. Remember, beliefs are not spiritual unless they are manifested by spiritual conduct. Actions speak louder than words and virtue moves our soul towards God. Therefore, our health and well-being flowers only when it is watered by personal responsibility, self-value and reverence for life. **This is Preventive Theology.**

If you are ill or obese it means *your energy is out of balance.* Therefore, any efforts to preserve or restore your health, or to lose weight permanently, should logically be efforts to bring that energy back into balance. Since your body and your mind are a complete and total ensemble, what is in your heart and on your mind can help keep you well or make you sick. Toxic emotions such as fear, loneliness, or anger hurt your body, while love, hope and forgiveness are transformed into natural medicines that *balance your body and balance your life.*

I'm sure you would agree with me that the basis of health care should be as *spiritual* as it is *scientific.* Therefore, if you will allow me the privilege of being your Wellness Medical Doctor, I want to remind you about the spiritual essence of *Total Health Rejuvenation*: If you are willing to take one genuine, heartfelt step towards God, then God will take a thousand steps toward you. *With this in mind, I wish to respectfully ask you to consider signing the following contract, as your genuine and heartfelt step . . . To-Life.*

> I PROMISE ON MY INTEGRITY AND MY WORD OF
> HONOR, THAT I WILL FOLLOW, TO THE BEST OF
> MY ABILITY, THE 28-DAY PLAN FOR TOTAL HEALTH
> REJUVENATION AND PERMANENT WEIGHT LOSS,
> BEGINNING WITH MY ONE DAY PERSONAL
> WELLNESS RETREAT.
>
> Signed: _____
>
> Dated: _____

*"START THE DAY WITH LOVE, FILL THE DAY WITH
LOVE, END THE DAY WITH LOVE . . . THIS IS THE WAY
TO GOD."*
(Sathya Sai Baba)

There is only one religion and that is the religion of love . . . love for ourselves, others, and God. *This inspiration is the basis of all our major faiths: Judaism, Christianity, Buddhism, Hinduism, and Islam.* Do you have to be religious to experience health, well-being and permanent weight loss? Perhaps not, but in my experience there are very few atheists in emergency rooms or coronary care units! This was very recently brought home to me. It began with a phone call I received at 4 A.M.

I almost lost my mother.

"I'm sorry to wake you up son, but I've got chest pain and I'm really scared."

"Mother, I want you to call 911 and then take a baby aspirin. I'll see you at the hospital."

By the time I arrived at the emergency room, she was already hooked up to a heart monitor, breathing oxygen, and receiving intravenous nitroglycerine and morphine. *But she was still having severe pain.*

The ER physician said to me, "It sure looks like a coronary, or at least unstable angina, even though the EKGs and vital signs are normal. We've got an IV morphine drip going now so we'll see what happens with the pain."

He asked my mother, "On a scale of 1–10, with 10 being the worst pain you've ever experienced, including childbirth, what is the level of pain you're having now?"

"It's the worst pain I've ever had. Ten plus!"

Finally, with more morphine, her pain diminished. The ER doctor reviewed the situation with me: "Her EKG looks perfectly normal, which is amazing considering her pain. Plus her X-rays and blood tests are normal. But I still can't believe it's not a coronary artery problem. Sometimes a dissecting aorta could do this, but her aorta looks normal on the chest film. I suppose we should consider esophageal spasm because it can wake people up with this type of crushing chest pain too—it's called "The Great Imitator" because everyone thinks it's a coronary. *But no, I don't think it's that.* Until we have evidence to the contrary, it's a myocardial infarct or a threatened myocardial infarct. The cardiologist has been called and is on the way."

Later, the cardiologist explained to my mother, "You have three major coronary arteries and I believe one or more of them is significantly blocked even though your EKG is normal. This means your heart muscle is struggling for oxygen to keep itself alive. Fortunately, I don't think you've damaged any heart muscle yet."

"Can I just go home then?" my mother said, "on nitroglycerin or maybe some beta-blocker pills like some of my friends take for their angina?"

"Oh no!" the cardiologist replied. "We need to monitor you constantly because you are not at all out of the woods. I also propose doing a cardiac catheterization—threating a tube up your femoral artery in your groin, and then injecting dye into your coronaries. If they are OK, then we'll put you on the proper medications and send you home. If there's a blockage, then we'll inflate the artery with a balloon or a plastic device. The procedure has very few complications and it's very safe."

Twenty-four hours later, I stood in front of a video screen reviewing the cardiac catheterization results with the cardiologist. My own heart raced as he explained, "There's at least a 70 percent blockage in each of your mom's three main coronary arteries, and I'm afraid I might dislodge a calcium deposit if I go in there with a balloon—it could cause a catastrophic event such as a myocardial infarction, an embolism, or even a stroke—who knows."

Already knowing, yet dreading the answer, I asked, *"What's the bottom line?"* "Open heart surgery," he replied, "probably at least a triple bypass. Your mother's heart muscle is still perfectly healthy, so we could decide to wait . . . but if we do it now, then we avoid the possibility of having to do it later when it's an emergency and her heart has already been damaged by an infarct."

What would you do if this was your mother? Well, what I did was call two other cardiologists who were old friends of mine. I needed reassurance because my mother had been perfectly healthy just yesterday! I posed the same question to each of them: "What would you do if this was your mother?" *"Operate now,"* each of them said.

Our family prayed together the night before open heart surgery. My brother and son, who are also medical doctors, my daughter, who has a Ph.D. and with whom I have a very close relationship, and my wonderful father joined hands with my wife and I as we formed a circle around my mother in her bed, each of us asking for God's help, and each of us remembering what she had written to all of us, for what seemed almost forever, on all our birthday cards—*"Love is all there is."* That was all there was in her hospital room that night. I knew more than ever that there was only one true religion . . . the religion of Love, so I prayed in the simplest, purest, most meaningful way I have ever experienced: *I Love You, God . . . I Love You God . . . I Love You God.*

After a seven hour surgical procedure the next day, my heart sank when I saw the heart surgeon's exhausted expression as he came into the family waiting room. After all, a decision had been made to take my mother through an unforeseen and dangerous journey, when just two days ago she was perfectly fine. *Should we have just done nothing? Did we make the wrong choice?*

"She's fine," the doctor said. Simply. Exquisitely. *"She's fine."*

I Love You, God.

WHAT READERS ARE SAYING ABOUT

BALANCE YOUR BODY
BALANCE YOUR LIFE

"A textbook for nutrition and health for the 21st Century, **Balance Your Body, Balance Your Life** is a must read for all who struggle with weight control. Thank you, Dr. Taub, for providing such a sensible and scientifically sound book that I can enthusiastically recommend."

—Dr. John H. Sklare, author of *The Inner Diet*

"This book is the very best presentation of a scientifically valid, humanly balanced approach to nutrition and physical activity. It brings the reader an ideal prescription for good health for the new millennium."

—Stanley E. Green, M.D., Professor Emeritus of Psychiatry, University of Toronto

"**Balance Your Body, Balance Your Life** is one of the most amazing books I've ever read. It has really changed my life. I will never think of food in the same way again. Thank you for such wonderful insight. This book is a must read for everyone.

—Sheila, Nashville, Tennessee

"**Balance Your Body, Balance Your Life** is simply the most honest and best researched book on permanent weight loss that has ever been written! I believe that just reading it will inspire people to lose weight forever . . . and it could change their lives."

—Joan, Registered Physical Therapist, Laguna Beach, CA

"I am so happy I got your book, **Balance Your Body, Balance Your Life.** I declared it my health bible. I've read it, I think, three times. I cannot tell you how thankful I am to have found you!"

—Gertrude, Texas

"A true healer . . . where were you when I was 20 and foolish? **Balance Your Body, Balance Your Life** is well grounded and very much an idea that can be implemented as a way of life for me. Dr. Taub's book is more like me and the way I am naturally.

—Susan, Chicago

"I just finished reading your book, **Balance Your Body, Balance Your Life.** I have dramatically increased my intake of fresh fruits and vegetables. Eating fruits and whole grains before noon is perfect, and does leave me with more energy during the day."

—Maria, New Hampshire

"I have your book, **Balance Your Body, Balance Your Life,** and I think it's wonderful."

—Rosemary, South Dakota

"I have read your book, **Balance Your Body, Balance Your Life,** and learned *so* much. Thank you for taking the time to cut through all the misinformation we are bombarded with, and teaching us how we can take responsibility for our health, by following your guidelines."

—Lisa, California

"I love your book, diary—and especially the Wellness Retreat Plan."

—Lynn, Pennsylvania

"I am writing to tell you of the wonderful change in my life, and it all started with your book **Balance Your Body, Balance Your Life.**

I have lost 12 pounds in all, one pound each week, which I know is the safest way to lose. After reading your book fresh fruits and vegetables actually started tasting much better to me than they ever had. I'm eagerly searching for vegan recipes everywhere and have enjoyed many of the recipes you included in the book. We also take your vitamins and wish to thank you for caring enough to give us the true secret to losing weight . . . thank you, thank you, Dr. Taub!"

—Marcia, Colorado

MEET DR. TAUB

◆

Edward A. Taub, M.D., is an accomplished author and esteemed physician. After graduating from the State University of New York Medical School in Syracuse in 1963, Dr. Taub completed his internship at the University of California Medical School at Irvine and then served two years with the United States Public Health Service and the United States Coast Guard, achieving the rank of lieutenant commander. His pediatrics residency was served at the University of Southern California—Los Angeles County General Hospital, and he completed National Institutes of Health fellowships in Community Psychiatry and Adolescent Medicine. He is a Fellow of the Academy of Pediatrics. Dr. Taub has been a family doctor and pediatrician for over thirty-five years, served as a member of the clinical faculty of the University of California Medical School at Irvine for two decades, and is a member of the American Medical Association.

From 1968 to 1983, Dr. Taub was the President and Medical Director of the Tustin-Irvine Pediatric Medical Group, Inc., in California, caring for over a hundred thousand children. He also served as Director for the Chapman University Health Center, and has been studying and developing weight loss programs for his patients since 1979. In addition, he founded a clinic for troubled adolescents and received a Disneyland Distinguished Community Service Award.

Currently, Dr. Taub directs the Wellness Medicine Institute. He was the first physician ever to hold the position of wellness medicine director at a major hospital in the United States. In this capacity, Dr. Taub teaches physicians, as well as patients, about *Integrative Medicine*. In the United States, he is pioneer in this field.

In May 1997, Dr. Taub became the Wellness Medical Doctor for QVC, Inc., America's largest home shopping channel, which reaches over 65 million homes—live, seven days a week, twenty-four hours a day. As chairman of a joint venture company with QVC called Health Ventures Partners, Dr. Taub develops wellness products, programs, and books for QVC viewers. Dr. Taub's *Nature's Code* **Multivitamin Nutritional System** received QVC's treasured Q Star Award for "Most Innovative Product of the Year" in 1998.

In addition, Dr. Taub has been a leader in the battle against cigarette addiction. He was the national spokesperson, team leader, and stress management consultant for **HOW TO QUIT**, the National Wellness Stop Smoking Campaign. For achieving a remarkably high success rate of 95.6 percent, Dr. Taub's is the only smoking cessation program to date ever to be reviewed, approved, and supported by the prestigious American Medical Association.

Dr. Taub has broadcast his teachings widely among diverse audiences. He became organized labor's first Wellness Director for the AFL-CIO and Teamsters unions (1981–85). He has addressed the American Medical Association, the President's Association of the American Management Association, the California Medical Association, the American Academy of Pediatrics, and the National Education Association. Dr. Taub has been featured on "Good Morning America," "CBS This Morning," CNN, and numerous television and radio shows across the nation. He has delivered many keynote speeches and currently conducts Integrative Medicine seminars for physicians, nurses, businesses, and educational organizations. He also has provided consulting services for NBC-TV; James River, Inc.; Fit For Life, Inc.; and the General Nutrition Company. Additionally, he has directed more than fifty "Voyage to Wellness" programs for Cunard, Carnival, and Windstar cruise lines.

Among Dr. Taub's literary accomplishments are four other books: *Voyage to Wellness, Prescription for Life, The Wellness Rx*, and the *Seven Steps to Self-Healing* Pack (recent winner of Golden Book Award from *Body, Mind, Spirit* Magazine).

Dr. Taub has also authored the path-breaking foreword to *Fit For Life*, the best-selling nutritional book of all time.

RESOURCES

◆

INTRODUCTION

Skinner, J.D., et al. Fruit juice intake is not related to children's growth. *Pediatrics* 1999; 103: 58–63.

Smythe J.M., et al. Effects of writing about stressful experiences on symptom reduction in patients with asthma and rheumatoid arthritis. *Journal of the American Medical Association* 1999; 281:1304–1309.

Wolk A., et al. Long-term intake of dietary fiber and decreased risk of coronary heart disease among women. *Journal of the American Medical Association* 1999; 281:1998–2004.

Wootan, M. "USDA's food guide pyramid for children should promote healthful food choices, not heart disease." *Center For Science in the Public Interest Press Release*: March 25, 1999.

PART ONE

The American Dietetic Association, 1997 Nutrition Trends Survey.

Fraser, Laura. *Losing It: America's Obsession With Weight and the Industry That Feeds On It*. NY: Dutton, 1997.

"Heavy Losses: New study shows that you can keep weight off." *Washington Post*, Monday, September 8, 1997.

Iggers, Jeremy. *The Garden of Eating: Food, Sex, and the Hunger for Meaning*. NY: Basic Books, 1996.

1996 Surgeon General's Report on Physical Activity and Health, www.cdc.gov/nccdphp/sgr

"Number of overweight children doubles." *USA Today*, February 2, 1998.

PART THREE

Chronic Care In America, A 21st Century Challenge. The Robert Wood Johnson Foundation, Princeton, NJ; November 1996.

Eisenberg, D. M., et al. Unconventional medicine in the United States; prevalence, costs, and patterns of use. *New England Journal of Medicine* 1993; 328; 246–52.

For Our Patients, Not for Profits: A Call to Action. The Ad Hoc Committee to Defend Health Care. *Journal of the American Medical Association* 1997; 278:1733–34.

Herrick, J.B., Clinical features of sudden obstruction of the coronary arteries. *Journal of the American Medical Association* 1912; 59:2015–2020.

Hill, J. O., et al. Environmental Contributions to the Obesity Epidemic. *Science* 1998; 280:1371–74.

Landmark Report on Public Health Perceptions of Alternative Care. Landmark Healthcare Company. Sacramento, CA; November 1997.

Munoz, K. A., Food intakes of U.S. children and adolescents compared with recommendations. *Pediatrics*, 1997; 100:323–29.

Troiano, R. P., et al. Overweight prevalence and trends for children and adolescents: the National Health and Nutrition Examination Surveys, 1963 to 1991. *Archives of Pediatrics & Adolescent Medicine* 1995; 149:1085–91.

PART FOUR

Bahna, S. Common Manifestations of Cow's Milk Allergy in Children, *Lancet* 1978; 1:304–22.

Beeson, W. L., et al. Chronic disease among Seventh-day Adventists, a low-risk group. *Cancer*, 1989; 64:57–81.

Cheskin, L. J., et al. Gastrointestinal symptoms following consumption of Olestra or regular triglyceride potato chips; a controlled comparison. *Journal of the American Medical Association* 1998; 279:150–52.

Cryan, J., Johnson, R. K., Should the current recommendations for energy intake in infants and young children be lowered? *Nutrition Today* 1997; 17:69–72.

Cumming, R. G., et al. Breastfeeding and other reproductive factors and the risk of hip fractures in elderly women. *International Journal of Epidemiology* 1993; 22:684–91.

Cunningham, A. S. Morbidity in breast-fed and artificially fed infants. *Journal of Pediatrics* 1977; 90 (5):726–29.

Davis, M. K., et al. Infant feeding and childhood cancer. *Lancet* 1988; 2:365–68.

Dershowitz, R. A. *Ambulatory Petiatric Care.* New York: J. B. Lippincott, 1993.

Dewey, K. G., et al. Differences in morbidity between breast-fed and formula-fed infants. *Journal of Pediatrics* 1995; 126:696–702.

Duncan, B., et al. Exclusive breast-feeding for at least four months protects against otitis media. *Pediatrics* 1993; 91:867–72.

Feskanich, D., et al. Milk, dietary calcium, and bone fractures in women: a 12-year prospective study. *American Journal of Public Health* 1997; 87:992–97.

Ford, R. P. K., et al. Breastfeeding and the risk of sudden infant death syndrome. *International Journal of Epidemiology* 1993; 22:885–90.

Frank, A. L., et al. Breast-feeding and respiratory virus infection. *Pediatrics* 1982; 70:239–45

Gerstein, H. C. Cow's milk exposure and type 1 diabetes mellitus. *Diabetes Care* 1994; 17:13–19.

Goran, M. I., et al. Energy requirements across the life span: New findings based on measurement of total energy expenditure with doubly labeled water. *Nutrition Today* 1995; 15:115–50.

Gortmaker, S. I., et al. Television viewing as a cause of increasing obesity among children in the United States, 1986–90. *Archives of Pediatric and Adolescent Medicine* 1996; 150:356–62.

Harvard Report on Cancer Prevention. Volume 2: Prevention of Human Cancer. Published as supplement of *Journal of Cancer Causes & Control* 1998.

Howie, P. W., et al. Protective effect of breast feeding against infection. *British Medical Journal* 1990; 300:11–16.

Kassirer, J. P., Angell, M. Losing Weight—An Ill-fated New Year's Resolution. *New England Journal of Medicine* 1998; 338: 52–54.

Kovar, M. G., et al. Review of the epidemiologic evidence for an association between infant feeding and infant health. *Pediatrics* 1984; 74:S615–38.

Melton, L. J., et al. Influence of breastfeeding and other reproductive factors on bone mass later in life. *Osteoporosis International* 1993; 3:76–83.

Meridia advertisement. *Journal of the American Medical Association* 1998 279; 640 AQ–AX.

Meridia advertisement. *New England Journal of Medicine* 1998; 338: 14 (last nine pages).

Morrow-Tlucak, M., et al. Breastfeeding and cognitive development in the first two years of life. *Social Science in Medicine* 1988; 26:635–39.

Newcomb, P. A., et al. Lactation and a reduced risk of pre-menopausal breast cancer. *New England Journal of Medicine* 1994; 330:81–87

Oski, F. A., et al. Don't discount breast-feeding. *New England Journal of Medicine* 1991; 325: 60–61.

———. Don't drink your milk. Teach Services, Inc. 1996.

———. Infant nutrition, physical growth, breast-feeding, and general nutrition. *Current Opinions in Pediatrics* 1994; 361–64.

———. Is bovine milk a health hazard? *Pediatrics* 1985; 75:182–86.

Pisacane, A., et al. Breast-feeding and urinary tract infection. *Journal of Pediatrics* 1992; 120:87–89.

Popkin, B. M., et al. Breast-feeding and diarrheal morbidity. *Pediatrics* 1990; 86:874–82.

Riggs, B. L., et al. Dietary calcium intake and rate of bone loss in women. *Journal of Clinical Investigation* 1987; 80979–82.

Rosenblatt, K. A., et al. WHO Collaborative Study of Neoplasia and Steroid Contraceptives. *International Journal of Epidemiology* 1993; 22:192–97

Saarinen, U. M., et.al. Breastfeeding as prophylaxis against allergic disease: prospective follow-up study until 17 years old. *Lancet* 1995; 346:1065–69.

Sabaté, J., et al. Nuts: a new protective food against coronary heart disease. *Current Opinion in Lipidology*, 1994; 5:11–16.

Sanchez, T. V., et al. Bone mineral in elderly vegetarian and omnivorous females. *Proceedings of the Fourth International Conference on Bone Measurement*. Bethesda, MD: NIAMDD (NIH Publication #80–1938), 1980: 94–98.

Scholl, T. O., et al. Use of multivitamin/mineral prenatal supplements: influence on the outcome of pregnancy. *American Journal of Epidemiology,* 1997; 146(2):134–41.

Spock, Benjamin and Parker, Steven J. Dr. Spock's Baby and Child Care. Pocket Books, 1998.

Thune, I., et al. Physical Activity and the Risk of Breast Cancer. *New England Journal of Medicine* 1997; 336:1269–75.

U.S. Department of Health Education and Welfare. Healthy People: The Surgeon General's Report on Health Promotion and Disease Prevention, 1995.

Wang, Y. S., Wu, S. Y., The effect of exclusive breast feeding on development and incidence of infection in infants. *Journal of Human Lactation* 1996; 12:27–30.

PART FIVE

Camargo, C. A., et al. Prospective study of moderate alcohol consumption and mortality in U.S. male physicians. *Archives of Internal Medicine* 1997; 157:79–85.

Fritz, Robert. *The Path of Least Resistance*. Fawcett, 1984.

Klem, M. L., et al. Patterns of weight loss maintenance. *The American Journal of Clinical Nutrition* 1997; 66:239–46.

Prochaska, James, Norcross, John, and Diclemente, Carlo. *Changing For Good*. Avon, 1994.

Sklare, J. H. *The Inner Diet*. Roswell, GA: Inner Resource, Inc., 1993.

Smith-Warner, S. A., et al. Alcohol and breast cancer in women: a pooled analysis of cohort studies. *Journal of the American Medical Association* 1998; 279:535–40.

PART SIX

Barnard, Neil D. *Food For Life*. NY: Crown Books, 1993.

Heatherton and Renn, Stress and the Disinhibition of Behavior. *Mind/Body Medicine: A Journal of Clinical Behavioral Medicine*, Vol. 1, No. 2, pp. 72–81.

Taub, Edward A. Commentary: Wellness paradigm shift. *Mind/Body Medicine: A Journal of Clinical Behavioral Medicine*, Vol. 1, No. 2, pp. 82–84.

PART EIGHT

Era, P., et al. Postural balance and self-repeated functional ability in 75 year old men and women. *Journal of the American Geriatric Society*, 1997; 45:80–92.

Nelson, Miriam E. Strong Women Stay Slim. Bantam, 1998.

Stefanick M. L., et al. Effects of diet and exercise in men and postmenopausal women with low levels of HDL cholesterol and high levels of LDL cholesterol. *New England Journal of Medicine*, 1998; 339:12–20.

"Recommendations from the Centers for Disease Control and Prevention and the American College of Sports Medicine." *Journal of the American Medical Association*, 273, 402 (1995).

PART TEN

Bales, C. W., Micronutrient deficiencies in nursing homes: should clinical intervention await a research consensus? *Journal of the American College of Nutrition* 1995; 6:563–64.

Block, G. Vitamin C and cancer prevention: the epidemiologic evidence. *American Journal of Clinical Nutrition* 1991 Supplement; 53:270S–82S.

Boucher, B. J. Vitamin D, glucose intolerance and insulinemia in elderly men. *Diabetologia* 1997; 40:344–47.

Chandra, R. K.. Graying of the immune system: can nutrient supplements improve immunity in the elderly? *Journal of the American Medical Association*; 277:1398–99.

Dickinson, V. A., et al. Supplement use, other dietary and demographic variables, and serum vitamin C in NHANES II. *Journal of the American College of Nutrition* 1994; 13:22–32.

Giovannucci, Edward. Multivitamin use, folate and colon cancer in women. *Annals of Internal Medicine* 1998; 129: 517–524.

Graham, I. M., Daly, L. E., et al. Plasma homocysteine as a risk factor for vascular disease: the European concerted action project. *Journal of the American Medical Association* 1997; 277:1775–81.

Hathcock, J. N. Vitamins and minerals: efficacy and safety. *American Journal of Clinical Nutrition* 1997b; 66:427–37.

Looker, A. C., et al. Prevalence of iron deficiency in the United States. *Journal of the American Medical Association* 1997; 277:973–76.

Macknin, M. L. Zinc Gluconate Lozenges for treatment of the common cold: A randomized, double blind, placebo-controlled study. *Annals of Internal Medicine* 1996; 125:81–88.

McCully, Kilmer S. *The Homocysteine Revolution*. CT: Keats Publishing, 1997.

Meydani, S. N., et al. Vitamin E supplementation and in vivo immune response in healthy elderly subjects: a randomized controlled trial. *Journal of the American Medical Association* 1997; 277:1380–86.

Milunsky, A., et al. Multivitamin/folic acid supplementation in early pregnancy reduces the prevalence of neural tube defects. *Journal of the American Medical Association* 1989; 262:2847–52.

Olson, K.B., Pienta, K.J. Further clues for prostate cancer prevention. *Journal of the National Cancer Institute* 1999; 90: 414–415.

Pitkin, R. M. Dietary reference intakes for thiamin, riboflavin, niacin, vitamin B_6, folate, vitamin B_{12}, pantothenic acid, biotin and choline. *National Academy of Sciences; Institute Of Medicine*; April 7, 1998.

Rimm, E. B., Willett, W. C., et al. Folate and vitamin B-6 from diet and supplements in relation to risk of coronary heart disease among women. *Journal of the American Medical Association* 1998; 279:359–64.

———, Stampfer, M. J., et al. Vitamin E consumption and the risk of coronary heart disease in men. *New England Journal of Medicine* 1993; 328:1450–56.

Seddon, J. M., et al. Dietary carotenoids, vitamins A, C, and E and advanced age-related macular degeneration. *Journal of the American Medical Association* 1994; 272:1413–20.

Shaw, G. M., et al. Risks of orofacial clefts in children of women using multivitamins containing folic acid periconceptionally. *Lancet* 1995; 346:393–96.

Snodderly, D. M. Evidence for protection against age-related macular degeneration by carotenoids and antioxidant vitamins. *American Journal of Clinical Nutrition* 1995; 62 (suppl):1448S–61S.

Stampfer, M. J., et al. Vitamin E consumption and the risk of coronary disease in women. *New England Journal Of Medicine* 1993; 328:1444–49.

Stampfer, M. J., Malinow, M. R., Willett, W. C., et al. A prospective study of plasma homocysteine and risk of myocardial infarction in U.S. physicians. *Journal Of The American Medical Association* 1992; 268:877–81.

Stephens, N. G., et al. Randomised controlled trial of vitamin E in patients with coronary disease: Cambridge Heart Antioxidant Study (CHAOS). *Lancet* 1996; 347:781–86.

Thomas, M. K., et al. Hypovitaminosis D in medical inpatients. *New England Journal of Medicine* 1998; 338:777–83.

Welten, D. C., et al. A meta-analysis of the effect of calcium intake on bone mass in young and middle-aged females and males. *Journal of Nutrition* 1995; 125:2802–13.

PART ELEVEN

Eddy, Mary Baker. *Science and Health with Key to the Scriptures*. The First Church of Christ, Scientist, 1994.

Carlson, Paul, R. *O Christian! O Jew!* David C. Cook, 1974.

Gomes, Peter J. *The Good Book*. William Morrow, 1996.

Schneerson, Menachem M. *Toward a Meaningful Life*. William Morrow, 1995.

Teilhard De Chardin, Pierre. Phenomenon of Man. HarperCollins, 1980.

USA Snapshots. Going to a higher authority. *Yankelovitch Partners for Lutheran Brotherhood*. *USA Today* December 30, 1998.

BIBLIOGRAPHY

Atkinson, Brooks (Editor). *Selected Writings of Ralph Waldo Emerson.* Modern Library, 1992.

Benson, Herbert. *Timeless Healing.* Scribner, 1996

Barnard, Neil D. *Food For Life.* Crown Books, 1993.

Bohm, David. *Wholeness and Implicate Order.* Routledge, Kegan and Paul, 1980.

Buber, Martin. *I and Thou.* Scribner, 1958.

Chopra, Deepak. *Ageless Body, Timless Mind.* Harmony, 1993

Cousins, Norman. *Anatomy of an Illness.* Norton, 1979.

Damasio, Antonio R. *Descartes' Error.* Grosset/Putman, 1994

Diamond, Harvey and Marilyn. *Fit For Life.* Warner Books, 1985.

Einstein, Albert. *The World As I See It.* Citadel, 1978

Frankl, Victor E. *Man's Search For Meaning.* Washington Square Press, 1959

Fritz, Robert. *The Path of Least Resistance.* Fawcett, 1984.

Greben, Stanley E. *Love's Labor.* Schocken Books, 1984

Lown, Bernard. *The Lost Art of Healing.* Houghton Mifflin, 1996.

O'Hara, Valerie. *Five Weeks to Healing Stress.* New Harbinger, 1996.

Pellitier, Kenneth R. *Mind As Healer, Mind As Slayer.* Delacorte Press, 1977

Robbins, John. *Diet For a New America.* Stillpoint Publishing, 1987.

Sandweiss, Samuel H. *Sai Baba, the Holy Man and the Psychiatrist.* Birthday Press, 1995

Sarno, John E. *The Mind Body Prescription.* Warner Books, 1998.

Schuller, Robert H. *Self-Esteem: The New Reformation.* Word Books, 1982

Sklare, J. H. *The Inner Diet.* Roswell, GA: Inner Resource, Inc. 1993.

Taub, Edward A. *The Seven Steps To Self-Healing.* DK Publishing, 1996

———. *The Wellness Rx.* Prentice Hall, 1995.

Valliant, George E. *The Wisdom of the Ego.* Harvard, 1993

Wilson, Edward O. *Consilience: The Unity of Knowledge.* Alfred A. Knopf, 1998.

INDEX

◆

RECISE INDEX

◆

DESSERTS